TRANSFORMATIVE RESEARCH AND EVALUATION

© 2009 The Guilford Press
A Division of Guilford Publications, Inc.
72 Spring Street, New York, NY 10012
www.guilford.com

Printed in the United States of America

This book is printed on acid-free paper.

Last digit is print number: 9 8 7 6 5 4 3 2 1

Library of Congress Cataloging-in-Publication Data

Mertens, Donna M.
  Transformative research and evaluation / Donna M. Mertens.
    p. cm.
  Includes bibliographical references and index.
  ISBN 978-1-59385-302-0 (pbk: alk. paper) — ISBN 978-1-59385-985-5
(hardcover: alk. paper)
  1. Evaluation research (Social action programs) 2. Social sciences—
Research—Methodology. 3. Social justice. I. Title.
  H62.M4232 2009
  001.4′2—dc22

                                                          2008037876

Preface

Who Should Use This Text?

This text covers the theory and methods of transformative research and evaluation. In that sense it is complete unto itself. Novice researchers and evaluators, advanced undergraduate students, or beginning graduate students can benefit by using this text to form an understanding of the transformative paradigm, recognizing that other sources are needed to provide full coverage of research and evaluation from other paradigmatic perspectives. More experienced researchers or evaluators or advanced graduate students with knowledge and experience with other paradigms can benefit from this text by gaining understanding of the rationale for the use of the transformative paradigm within the wider context of alternative paradigms. All may benefit from exposure to multiple examples of research and evaluation methods that could be adapted to specific interests.

Organization of This Book

This book is organized as if research and evaluation followed a linear path. In actuality, research and evaluation are dynamic processes that require footwork more akin to salsa dancing. There is a basic set of steps, but there are as many ways to modify those basic steps as there are dancers. Hence, the need for this book to be used in a dynamic way, reading parts, moving on, and then revisiting parts as the research or evaluation study evolves.

The first two chapters provide a framework, rationale, and philosophical bases for the transformative paradigm. Chapter 1, "Resilience, Resistance, and Complexities That Challenge," explores the tensions that coexist in the research and evaluation world in terms of confronting discrimination and oppression, recognizing and supporting resilience and resistance, and taking up the challenge of conducting research that is explicitly centered on issues of social justice. Chapter 2, "The Transformative Paradigm: Basic Beliefs and Commensurate Theories," begins with a general discussion of the meaning of the concept of *paradigm* and illustrates how various paradigms might impact on research and evaluation decisions. It then continues with detailed explanations of the basic philosophical beliefs that underlie the transformative paradigm, along with discussion of specific theories that are commensurate with this paradigm.

Chapter 3, "Self, Partnerships, and Relationships," turns the lens on researchers or evaluators themselves. Knowledge of self is part of the process of recognizing the relation between self and community, which in turn facilitates the building of trusting relationships between study participants and researchers. Establishing this trust is a necessary first step toward working in an ethical and culturally responsive manner throughout the subsequent steps of the research and evaluation process. Relations between the inquirer and the community are a crucial part of establishing the focus of the study. Chapter 4, "Developing the Focus of Research/Evaluation Studies," identifies many sources of support in developing the focus and context of research and evaluation, including funding agency priorities, scholarly literature, web-based resources, fugitive (grey) literature, and group and individual strategies to involve community members.

The philosophical assumptions underlying the transformative paradigm lead to consideration of models for research that reflect the knowledge of self and community as the basis for making methodological decisions. Chapter 5, "A Transformative Research and Evaluation Model," provides a model for transformative research and evaluation that is based on the use of quantitative and/or qualitative methods, with a priority on mixed methods, using short-term or cyclical approaches (with preference given to cyclical studies). The model is rooted in and embraced by community values. More specific methodological choices are presented in Chapter 6, "Quantitative, Qualitative, and Mixed Methods." While the use of mixed methods has intuitive appeal, it necessitates expertise in both quantitative and qualitative approaches. Therefore, the chapter begins with an explanation of quantitative and qualitative approaches and then presents specific mixed methods that allow for the combination of such methods as surveys, experimental designs, ethnography, and focus groups.

The focus of the book then shifts to the participants in the study. Chapter 7, "Participants: Identification, Sampling, Consent, and Reciprocity," discusses the importance of knowing the community well enough to appropriately identify and invite those stakeholders who need to be included, especially if they represent groups that have been excluded historically. In addition, issues of consent and reciprocity are examined in terms of accurate understandings and giving back to the community. The identification of, and invitation to, participants in the study are closely connected to decisions on data collection. Chapter 8, "Data-Collection Methods, Instruments, and Strategies," covers a variety of specific data-collection strategies that can be used in transformative research and evaluation studies. The data that are collected do not speak for themselves. Chapter 9, "Data Analysis and Interpretation," provides strategies for interpreting quantitative and qualitative data with the help of community involvement and within the context of theoretical frameworks that are commensurate with the transformative paradigm. The beliefs of the transformative paradigm lead to serious consideration of what to do with the findings of a study. Chapter 10, "Reporting and Utilization: Pathway to the Future," explores options for reporting and use, with specific emphasis on how research and evaluation findings can be used for social change.

Pedagogical Features

The book includes the following pedagogical features to enhance readers' use of the text:

• Each chapter begins with advance organizers, titled "In This Chapter...."

• First-person narrative style. My experiences in research and evaluation grew from my involvement with the deaf community and the transference of lessons learned from this microcosm of cultural complexity to other community contexts, such as African women and the United Nations Development Fund for Women (UNIFEM), Israeli and Bedouin women, or breast cancer screening in Nova Scotia. The deaf world parallels experiences of other marginalized groups to the extent that children are raised and educated by people who, while well meaning, are usually not part of the child's cultural or linguistic group. Furthermore, historically deaf children have been inappropriately identified as mentally retarded because they do not score high on intelligence or achievement tests that are developed by members of the dominant culture, and because their reading scores, on average, fail to rise above a fourth-grade level for high school graduates.

• Multiple examples of populations and contexts are used throughout the text. These sample studies illustrate the breadth of applicability of a transformative approach to research and evaluation, as well as what makes aspects of such work reflective of a transformative stance.

• Scholarly literature, including sample studies as well as theoretical and methodological pieces, is cited as a major source of insight into transformative research and evaluation.

• Throughout my years at Gallaudet University, I have been privileged to teach very bright and insightful graduate students. As part of my teaching, I use BlackBoard, an electronic, web-based teaching tool that allows for class discussions to occur online. With their permission, I include my students' perspectives when they are applicable to the points being made.

• "Questions for Thought": Because the transformative paradigm is not a cookbook approach to research and evaluation, it functions in many ways to raise questions for the inquirer and community members to consider. In various places in the text, I insert questions to stimulate thinking and discussion.

• Summaries are provided at the end of each chapter.

Acknowledgments

Many people contributed to my ability to complete this book, including my family, my students and colleagues at Gallaudet University (especially Amy Wilson, Heidi Holmes, Raychelle Harris, and Glenda Mobley), and my professional family across the globe (especially Bagele Chilisa, Zenda Ofir, and Barbara Rosenstein). At The Guilford Press, my thanks go to C. Deborah Laughton, Publisher, Research Methods and Statistics, for her support, encouragement, and belief in this project, and Anna Nelson, Senior Production Editor, for her thoroughness and care throughout the production process. I also thank the reviewers of earlier drafts: Katrina Bledsoe, Research Manager, Walter R. McDonald and Associates, Arlington, Virginia; Melvin E. Hall, Educational Psychology, College of Education, Northern Arizona University; Gary W. Harper, Department of Psychology and Master of Public Health Program, DePaul University; and Debra M. Harris, Educational Leadership, California State University, Fresno.

Contents

Introduction

The Intersection of Applied Social Research and Program Evaluation

Research is defined as a systematic method of knowledge construction; evaluation is defined as a systematic method of determining the merit, worth, or value of a program, policy, activity, technology, or similar entity to inform decision making about such entities. Evaluation also includes needs sensing and cost analysis. Despite these straightforward definitions, the exact line between research and evaluation is contested. Trochim (2006) claims that program evaluation is one form of social research that draws its distinctiveness from the organizational and political context in which it is conducted, thus requiring management, group, and political skills not always needed in a more generic research setting. Mathison (2008) argues for a more distinctive line between research and evaluation based on the evolutionary development of evaluation as a discipline that began in the 1960s. Evaluation as a discipline has emphasized the importance of critically examining *valuing* as a component of systematic inquiry, the development of methodological approaches that *prioritize stakeholder involvement*, and use of criteria to *judge quality* that include utility, feasibility, and propriety.

The evolution of program evaluation as a discipline has contributed significantly to our understanding of how to bring people together to address critical social issues. However, parallel developments in applied social research have also been occurring. As a practicing evaluator, I recognize the importance of the development of evaluation as a discipline. However, there is a place at which research and evaluation intersect—when research provides information about the need for, improvement of, or effects of programs or policies. Hence this text encompasses the territory at the intersection of applied social research and program evaluation. Although basic research is essential, it is not the focus of this book.

Approaches that are compatible with social justice—for example, Stufflebeam's (2001) category of social agenda/advocacy in evaluation—are the focus of this book. The terms *research* and *evaluation* are not used interchangeably, as there is uniqueness to each. (Throughout this book I use either *research* or *evaluation* when I cite the text of an author who chooses one term over the other.) Because of the common ground that research and evaluation share, however, this text addresses the shared territory that emerges when research and evaluation are conducted for social justice purposes.

Paradigms

Paradigms became salient in the social research arena with the publication of Thomas Kuhn's *Structure of Scientific Revolutions* (1962), in which he made visible the basic beliefs that guide scientific work and the processes by which these beliefs are challenged and changed to create a paradigm shift. While Kuhn wrote from the world of natural sciences and philosophy, the concept of paradigms and their associated belief systems has provided considerable stimulation in the world of social science research as well. Guba and Lincoln (1989, 1994, 2005) made a major contribution to extending the concept of paradigms in the social sciences in their explanation of (at first) three paradigms: positivism, post-positivism, and constructivism. In their more recent work, they added critical theory, and the participatory paradigm from Heron and Reason (2006). Earlier, I (Mertens, 1998) noted four dominant paradigms in educational and psychological research: post-positivism, constructivism, pragmatism, and emancipatory (building on Guba & Lincoln, 1989, and Lather, 1992). In 2005, I changed the name of the emancipatory paradigm to *transformative* because of a desire to emphasize the agency role for the people involved in the research. Rather than being *emancipated*, we work together for personal and social transformation. For the reader interested in pursuing other paradigms or the philosophy of science further, many texts are available. The purpose of this text is to explore the assumptions of the transformative paradigm and the implications of those assumptions for research and evaluation in the social sciences.

Rationale for the Transformative Paradigm

Many dollars and much effort are put into research and evaluation that are designed to investigate critical issues in society, such as literacy, mental health, addiction, violence, poverty, and sickness and disease. Nevertheless, people who are born into circumstances associated with a greater probability of discrimination and oppression (due to physical, historical, economic, or other factors) continue to experience lower access to resources, as well as a greater likelihood that they will have a lower quality of life (whether due to educational, health, psychological, or social variables). As Kuhn (1962) noted, when anomalies arise that cannot be adequately addressed by the existing paradigm of science, a revolution occurs in such a way as to provide a different avenue of approach to solving those intransigent problems. The transformative paradigm emerged in response to individuals who have been pushed to the societal margins throughout history and who are finding a means to bring their voices into the world of research. Their voices, shared with scholars who work as their partners to support the increase of social justice and human rights, are reflected in the shift to transformative beliefs to guide researchers and evaluators.

In this text, I offer the transformative paradigm as an overarching metaphysical framework to address the anomalies that arise when researchers, evaluators, and community members express frustration that their efforts are falling short of the desired mark in terms of social justice. I put forth this hypothesis:

If we ground research and evaluation in assumptions (covered in Chapter 2) that prioritize the furtherance of social justice and human rights, then we will utilize community involvement and research methodologies that will lead to a greater realization of social change. I argue that the rationale for the transformative paradigm rests in (1) ongoing challenges in the world; (2) the need to acknowledge that addressing issues of power, discrimination, and oppression can play a key role in redressing inequities; and (3) supportive evidence from illustrative studies of the potential for social change when researchers and evaluators operate within the assumptions of the transformative paradigm.

Breadth of Transformative Paradigm Applicability

Some readers may think that because they do not work with African Americans, Latinos, people with disabilities, Africans, Maoris, or deaf people that the transformative paradigm cannot be applied to their work. This reasoning is fallacious for several reasons. The transformative paradigm is applicable to people who experience discrimination and oppression on whatever basis, including (but not limited to) race/ethnicity, disability, immigrant status, political conflicts, sexual orientation, poverty, gender, age, or the multitude of other characteristics that are associated with less access to social justice. In addition, the transformative paradigm is applicable to the study of the power structures that perpetuate social inequities. Finally, indigenous peoples and scholars from marginalized communities have much to teach us about respect for culture and the generation of knowledge for social change. Hence, there is not a single context of social inquiry in which the transformative paradigm would not have the potential to raise issues of social justice and human rights.

To that end, illustrative studies are presented throughout the text that provide specifics as to how assumptions associated with the transformative paradigm lead to methodological choices, involvement of community, and use of results. Many of the examples are derived from my own work with deaf people in regard to sexual abuse (Mertens, 1996), court access (Mertens, 2000), parenting deaf and hard-of-hearing children (Meadow-Orlans, Mertens, & Sass-Lehrer, 2003), and my international work with African, Israeli, and Bedouin women. I also draw on my PhD students' dissertations on experiences of deaf people in international development contexts (Wilson, 2005), the positive aspects of parenting a deaf child (Szarkowski, 2002), resilience in black deaf high school graduates (Williamson, 2007), and discrimination against black deaf students in residential schools (McCaskill, 2005). These studies provide insights into how to conduct research and evaluation within the deaf community, but they also allow for generalization to other communities that are pushed to the margins of society.

I draw on the work of numerous researchers and evaluators who incorporate the transformative spirit across disciplines and methods—and in many marginalized communities—for example:

- Environmental health in Laotian immigrant communities (Silka, 2005)
- HIV/AIDS prevention in Botswana (Chilisa, 2005)
- The Talent Development Model for education of African American students (Thomas, 2004)
- The peace efforts in Northern Ireland (Irwin, 2005)
- Health services for lesbian, gay, bisexual, and transgender youth (Amsden & VanWynsberghe, 2005)

- Mental health services for Native Americans (Duran & Duran, 2000)
- Literacy services in an urban setting for African American and Latino students (Bledsoe, 2005)
- Class-action suit against the State of California on behalf of Latino students (Fine, Weis, Pruitt, & Burns, 2004)
- Algebra classes for low-income and African American students (Moses & Cobb, 2001)
- Appropriate breast cancer screening services for women from multiple ethnic groups (Chiu, 2003)
- Understanding action and inaction with regard to social justice in charter schools (Opfer, 2006)
- Experiences of women in the engineering field (Watts, 2006)
- Cultural conflicts in reactions to the death of a child between the dominant and Maori populations (Clarke & McCreanor, 2006)
- Examination of lesbian, gay, bisexual, transgender, and queer representations in museums and outreach activities to individuals in this community (Mertens, Fraser, & Heimlich, 2008)

Figure I.1 summarizes characteristics of a sample of studies that reflect a transformative paradigmatic stance. These two samples illustrate three common themes in transformative research and evaluation:

- Underlying assumptions that rely on ethical stances of inclusion and challenging oppressive social structures.
- An entry process into the community that is designed to build trust and make goals and strategies transparent.
- Dissemination of findings in ways that encourage use of the results to enhance social justice and human rights.

As I wander through the territory of research and evaluation, I worry that what we do may not make any difference. As I look out in the world, I know that there is such a need to address issues of social inequity, and I believe that research and evaluation do have a place in making visible these inequities and supporting social change to further social justice. Research and evaluation are not the only tools that can be brought to bear to achieve this goal. I have been inspired by many people whose contributions were made outside of the research and evaluation communities, including Nelson

Minority ethnic communities and health care (Chiu, 2003)

- *Underlying assumptions:* Everyone has a fundamental right to access health care, no matter what his or her country of origin, socioeconomic status, or home language.

- *Community entry process:* Chiu contacted the health educators as well as the women the program was intended to serve. She encountered resistance at both levels, but she consciously established trusting relationships with both stakeholder groups.

- *Dissemination techniques:* Chiu used the words of the service providers in focus groups to make visible their (in some cases) unconscious discrimination, based on stereotypical beliefs, against the immigrant women. One outcome was the recognition that the health educators felt they were powerless to exact changes because they needed to convince health care providers of the need to modify their services to be more culturally responsive. As a result, assertiveness training was provided to the educators as a strategy to foster their ability to advocate for the immigrant women.

Sexual abuse (Mertens, 1996)

- *Underlying assumptions:* If sexual abuse were allowed to continue unchallenged at this school, those who would be most damaged would be the deaf students. The evaluation needed to uncover and challenge the beliefs that allowed sexual abuse to proliferate here.

- *Community entry process:* I was asked by a state's Department of Education to evaluate a school setting in which sexual abuse had been well documented in the judicial system. Hence, there was a bit of an adversarial connotation to my appearance at the school to conduct the evaluation. The school administrators attempted to derail the focus of the study. However, I brought the focus back to the need to examine the conditions that allowed sexual abuse to occur by consciously referring to the mandate from the state's Department of Education. My credentials as an American Sign Language user and an expert in program evaluation in programs for the deaf contributed to my efforts to build trust between myself and the stakeholders.

- *Dissemination techniques:* The results of the specific study were provided to the stakeholders at the school and the state's Department of Education. In addition, I made presentations at professional meetings that were attended by educators of the deaf and published in journals read by deaf educators, parents, and members of the deaf community. In the presentations and publications, the name of the school was kept confidential.

FIGURE 1.1. Sample studies reflecting a transformative paradigmatic stance.

Mandela, Martin Luther King, Jr., and Eleanor Roosevelt. These civil rights leaders fought against discrimination and oppression for the furtherance of human rights in the forms of employment, education, housing, health services, and more. It is heartening to see the emergence of scholars whose positioning in the research and evaluation communities is reflective of the values of these great leaders. Much of this book is possible because of the historical legacy of fighters for social justice and the modern-day scholars who are contributing to our understanding of how to use research and evaluation to these ends.

> The hope of a secure and livable world lies with disciplined
> nonconformists who are dedicated to justice, peace and brotherhood.
> —MARTIN LUTHER KING, JR., U.S. black civil rights leader
> and clergyman (1929–1968), *Strength to Love*

> I have walked that long road to freedom. I have tried not to falter; I
> have made missteps along the way. But I have discovered the secret
> that after climbing a great hill, one only finds that there are many
> more hills to climb. I have taken a moment here to rest, to steal a view
> of the glorious vista that surrounds me, to look back on the distance I
> have come. But I can only rest for a moment, for with freedom comes
> responsibilities, and I dare not linger, for my long walk is not ended.
> —NELSON MANDELA, South African statesman (1918–   ),
> *Long Walk to Freedom*

> Do what you feel in your heart to be right—for you'll be criticized
> anyway. You'll be damned if you do, and damned if you don't.
> —ELEANOR ROOSEVELT, U.S. diplomat and reformer (1884–1962)

CHAPTER 1

Resilience, Resistance, and Complexities That Challenge

Can research contribute to social transformation? Gustavsen (2006) cited in Reason and Bradbury (2006a) questions the potential role of research for social transformation: "If we really want to become involved in socially significant practical action with demands for long time horizons, for relating to numerous actors and engaging in highly complex activities, perhaps the notion of linking such involvement to research as traditionally conceived is futile" (p. 25). He calls for a transformation of research to engage in a purer form of democracy that will support the development of social relationships that embody a principle of equality for all participants.

> [For] the radical transformation of social reality and improvement in the lives of the people involved . . . solutions are viewed as processes through which subjects become social actors . . . by means of grassroots mobilizations in actions intended to transform society. (Selener, 1997, as cited in Gaventa & Cornwall, 2006, p. 77)

IN THIS CHAPTER . . .

▼ The transformative paradigm is introduced as a shift in basic beliefs that guide research and evaluation, based on a need to prioritize the role of such inquiries in addressing human rights and social justice.

▼ The need for transformative research and evaluation is supported by examples of inequities in access to culturally appropriate services for people who are pushed to the margins of society.

▼ Deficit perspectives of marginalized communities are challenged by focusing on resilience in such communities and examining sample research studies that are based on transformative principles.

▼ Examples of theoretical frameworks that are commensurate with the transformative approach to research and evaluation are discussed from international development, feminism, queer, disability rights, and critical race theories.

9

▼ Further support for the need for transformative research and evaluation
is provided through the voices of scholars and indigenous peoples, deaf
students, policymakers, and professional association leaders.

▼ Cultural complexities, ethical concerns, and multicultural validity (Kirkhart,
2005) are also explored as a rationale for transformative research and
evaluation.

Social research and program evaluation can be seen as efforts to understand
the reality of social phenomenon as through a prism.[1] Just as a prism bends
the different frequencies of light into an ever-changing pattern of different
colors, dependent upon the light source and the shape and motion of the
prism, so we seek ways to understand social reality as it changes, dependent
upon the diverse qualities and activities inherent in its creation and interpretation. Through the use of transformative, culturally appropriate, and
multiple methods of research and evaluation, we can come to understand
patterns of diverging results and their implications.

The purpose of this book is to examine the basic beliefs and methodological implications of the transformative paradigm as a tool that
directly engages the complexity encountered by researchers and evaluators
in culturally diverse communities when their work is focused on increasing social justice.[2] The transformative paradigm focuses on (1) the tensions
that arise when unequal power relationships surround the investigation of
what seem to be intransigent social problems and (2) the strength found
in communities when their rights are respected and honored. Thus, it does
not support a "blame the victim" mentality, nor does it suggest that communities are powerless to effect change. Rather, the paradigm focuses on
culturally appropriate strategies to facilitate understandings that will create sustainable social change. Understanding the dynamics of power and
privilege and how they can be challenged in the status quo is also a priority.

Recurring tensions coexist somewhat uneasily but, in that way, provide a catalyst for change and hope for a better future. These tensions are
reflected in such facets as the dynamics of discrimination/oppression and
resilience/resistance, as well as exclusion from and inclusion in positions of
power to influence and make decisions. Engagement with participants and
other stakeholders who stand to be affected by the research or evaluation
outcomes evolves from the first encounter to the encounters that become
more complex as the inquiry progresses. Conduct of research and evaluation within the transformative framework is not a linear process; thus,
the writing of a book that is, by definition, a linear artifact is complicated

by the need to lead the reader through a process that allows for emergent understandings and course corrections.

The transformative paradigm recognizes that serious problems exist in communities despite their resilience in the process of throwing off the shackles of oppression, as well as making visible the oppressive structures in society. Researchers and evaluators working in any type of community can learn from those who are engaged in this struggle, just as we learn from each other through a critical examination of the assumptions that have historically guided research and evaluation studies. The transformative paradigm, with its associated philosophical assumptions, provides a means of framing ways to address intransigent societal and individual challenges through the valuing of transcultural and transhistorical stances. Through this reciprocal learning relationship, group processes can be viewed in new ways as venues for research. Challenges arise in the context of research and evaluation concerning such issues as the following:

- Differential privilege accorded to scholarly literature versus lived experience.
- Identification of a research or evaluation problem versus context and focus.
- Doing research or evaluation studies on *subjects* versus with *participants* or *co-researchers/evaluators* from the community.
- The potential role of the researcher or evaluator as an instrument of social change.

It should be noted that the transformative paradigm does not romanticize all that is indigenous and traditional because some traditions, in fact, serve to further oppress the oppressed. One example is the tradition in India associated with widows who were child brides. Consequences associated with the death of a husband include living apart from society, not marrying again, and being forced to help sustain the widow community by whatever means she can, including begging and prostitution. Even though the civil law in India permits widows to marry, the 2,000-year-old sacred scripture prohibits such a marriage, and today over 34 million widows live a life of oppression because of the death of their husbands, in keeping with this tradition. The transformative paradigm supports the integration of the wisdom of indigenous peoples, feminists, people with disabilities, and the poor and invisible toward the creation of a constructed knowledge base that furthers social justice and human rights.

Human Rights Agenda

The transformative paradigm is firmly rooted in a human rights agenda much as it is reflected in the United Nations Universal Declaration of Human Rights (1948). Although the declarations of the United Nations are situated in a multilateral context, they provide guidance in understanding a basis for transformative work domestically as well as internationally. Human rights is a globally relevant issue; "developed" countries are not exempt from violations of human rights.

The U.N. declaration is based on a recognition of the inherent dignity and the equal and inalienable rights of all members of the human family, including the right to life, liberty, security of the person, equal protection under the law, freedom of movement, marriage with the free and full consent of the intending spouses, ownership of property, freedom of thought and religion, freedom of opinion and expression, peaceful assembly, participation in governance, work in just and favorable working conditions, and education. Importantly for this text, article 25 reads:

> Everyone has the right to a standard of living adequate for the health and well-being of himself [sic] and of his [sic] family, including food, clothing, housing and medical care and necessary social services, and the right to security in the event of unemployment, sickness, disability, widowhood, old age or other lack of livelihood in circumstances beyond his [sic] control. (United Nations, 1948)

The U.N. Universal Declaration contains language indicating that everyone is entitled to these rights, without distinction of any kind, such as race, color, sex, language, religion, political or other opinion, national or social origin, property, birth, or other status. However, the United Nations recognized that its declaration has not resulted in enjoyment of the rights contained therein for all people. They noted that specific attention would need to be given to groups who were not being afforded these rights based on race, disability, gender, age, political standing, or status in the work force. Consequently, they approved the following:

- The International Convention on the Elimination of All Forms of Racial Discrimination (1969), which affirms the necessity of eliminating racial discrimination throughout the world in all its forms and manifestations and of securing understanding of, and respect for, the dignity of the human person.
- The Declaration on the Rights of Disabled Persons (1975), which

assures people with disabilities the same fundamental rights as their fellow citizens, no matter what the origin, nature, and seriousness of their handicaps and disabilities. In December 2006, the United Nations strengthened its support for people with disabilities when it ratified the Convention on the Rights of Persons with Disabilities (*www.un.org/esa/socdev/enable/rights/convtexte.htm*).

- The Convention on the Elimination of All Forms of Discrimination against Women (CEDAW; 1979), which provides the basis for realizing equality between women and men through ensuring women's equal access to, and equal opportunities in, political and public life—including the right to vote and to stand for election—as well as education, health, and employment.

These were followed by the Convention on the Rights of the Child (1990a) and the International Convention on the Protection of the Rights of All Migrant Workers and Members of Their Families (1990b). After 20 years of debate, the United Nations finally approved the Declaration of Rights of Indigenous Peoples (United Nations, 2006c). The United Nations International Children's Fund (UNICEF), with the endorsement of the International Organization for Cooperation in Evaluation and the International Development Evaluation Association (IDEAS), prepared a report based on a meeting of 85 evaluation organizations that maps the future priorities for evaluation in that context. This excerpt captures the emphasis on human rights:

> Within a human rights approach, evaluation should focus on the most vulnerable populations to determine whether public policies are designed to ensure that all people enjoy their rights as citizens, whether disparities are eliminated and equity enhanced, and whether democratic approaches have been adopted that include everyone in decision-making processes that affect their interests. (Segone, 2006, p. 12)

The Transformative Paradigm as a Metaphysical Umbrella

The transformative paradigm provides a metaphysical umbrella with which to explore similarities in the basic beliefs that underlie research and evaluation approaches that have been labeled critical theory, feminist theory, critical race theory, participatory, inclusive, human-rights-based, democratic, and culturally responsive. The transformative paradigm extends the thinking of democratic and responsive inquiry strategies by consciously including in research and evaluation work the identification of relevant dimensions of diversity and their accompanying relation to discrimination and oppression in the world. An important aspect of the transformative paradigm is the conscious inclusion of a broad range of people who are generally excluded from mainstream society. Relevant characteristics need to be carefully identified in each context; the wise researcher or evaluator acts with a consciousness of the dimensions of diversity that have been historically associated with discrimination: for example, race/ethnicity, gender, disability, social class, religion, age and sexual orientation.

The transformative paradigm provides a philosophical framework that explicitly addresses these issues and builds on a rich base of scholarly literature from mixed-methods research (Tashakkori & Teddlie, 2003); qualitative research (Denzin & Lincoln, 2005), participatory action research (Reason & Bradbury, 2006a), feminist researchers (Fine et al., 2004; Madison, 2005), critical ethnography (Ramazanoglu & Holland, 2002), culturally responsive research and evaluation (Hood, Hopson, & Frierson, 2005; Tillman, 2006), indigenous researchers (Battiste, 2000a; Chilisa, 2005; Cram, Ormond, & Carter, 2004; McCreanor, Tipene-Leach, & Abel, 2004; McCreanor, Watson, & Denny, 2006; Smith, 1999), disability researchers (Gill, 1999; Mertens & McLaughlin, 2004), and researchers and evaluators in the international development community (Bamberger, Rugh & Mabry, 2006; Mikkelsen, 2005). Framed within a historical perspective, the transformative paradigm is compatible with the teachings of educator Paulo Freire (1970a, 1970b, 1973), who worked to raise the consciousness of the oppressed in Brazil through transformative educational processes that improved their literacy and prepared them to resist their oppressors.[3]

The transformative paradigm also provides methodological guidance for researchers and evaluators who work in culturally complex communities in the interest of challenging the status quo and furthering social justice. It prompts the researcher/evaluator to ask the following questions:

- What is the researcher or evaluator's role in uncovering that which has not been stated explicitly within the context of the current research and evaluation climate?
- What dangers lurk in applying the conceptualization of scientifically based inquiry without consideration of important dimensions of diversity?
- Specifically, what is implicit in the mandate of scientifically based

research and evaluation and in the use of "reliable" and "valid" standardized tests when applied to extremely diverse populations?

- What are the ethical implications of randomly assigning participants to research conditions when other evidence supports a particular course of action as having a higher probability of effectiveness?

- What are the common denominators and unique facets associated with Africans, African Americans, Latinos, feminists, people with disabilities,[4] indigenous peoples, and others who have been pushed to the margins of society when viewed in relation to forces of discrimination and oppression as well as transformation and resilience?

Gilmore and Smith (2005) note that "research not conforming to the prevailing academic genres still risks being either patronized or denigrated as 'not real scholarship'" (p. 78). However, taking the risk to blend academic genre with the conventions of the researched is an indication of community solidarity. Those who take risks in research that detract from the conforming standards imposed by those with academic power in fact teach those in power a thing or two (Lincoln & Denzin, 2005). In fact, researchers have much to learn from the researched. Much work lies ahead for us, to *"rewrite and re-right* existing and often damaging academic research" (Gilmore & Smith, 2005, p. 71, emphasis in original).

Need for Transformative Research and Evaluation

The need for transformative research and evaluation is evidenced by current events, scholarly literature, and the voices of those who live in a world that allocates privileges to some and denies those privileges to others based on inherent characteristics. The inequity and intransigence of social problems glare at us from the headlines of the world's newspapers. The following examples reflect the kinds of salient conditions that could benefit greatly from research and evaluation done from a transformative stance:

- A review of nearly 140,000 mentally ill patients in a national Veteran's Affairs registry revealed that blacks in the United States are more than four times as likely as whites to be diagnosed with schizophrenia (Blow et al., 2004). This disparity in diagnoses is evident even when controlling for differences in income, wealth, educational background, drug addiction, and other variables. Although there is uncertainty about why schizophrenia is diagnosed more in blacks, researchers hypothesized that diagnostic measures developed primarily on a white population do not automatically apply to other groups.

• Two catastrophic natural disasters led to social catastrophes associated with poverty and race. The tsunami that hit South Asia (December 2004) and Hurricane Katrina and the subsequent flooding in the U.S. Gulf Coast (August 2005) resulted in an outpouring of aid, arguments about how that aid should be used, and accusations about who was not yet being served by that aid.

• The U.S. Census Bureau reported that between 2000 and 2004, Hispanics accounted for 49% of the nation's population growth (41.3 million Hispanics out of a national population of 293.7 in 2004; Cohn, 2005). Most of the increase is due to children born to first-generation immigrants. What is the appropriate model of education for Hispanic children who, unlike their parents, arrive at school with some knowledge of English, even if they do not have a full command of the language?

• Following an outbreak of gang-related violence in which six young people were stabbed outside their school and at a local shopping mall, Assistant State's Attorney for Montgomery County, Maryland, Jeffrey T. Wennar, said that the county did not adequately focus on prevention (Raghavan & Paley, 2005). He noted that the county eliminated a full-time staff employee who dealt with gang issues some time ago. Evidence from the Justice Policy Institute, however, shows that cities (such as New York) that use extensive social resources (e.g., job training, mentoring, after-school activities, and recreational programs) make significant dents in gang violence (Greene & Pranis, 2007). In contrast, areas that rely heavily on police enforcement, such as Los Angeles, have far less impact.

• African countries are experiencing ongoing famine that threatens the lives of hundreds of thousands (Devereux, 2006). Despite U.N. efforts to provide food, drought, possible vendor profiteering, loss of productivity due to HIV/AIDS, and ongoing conflicts leave people in Somalia, Ethiopia, Zimbabwe, and Malawi at risk of starvation.

• A federal judge gave state education officials control over a sizable portion of Baltimore, Maryland's troubled special education system (Reddy, 2005). The basis for the decision involves lapses in providing services, such as physical therapy and counseling, which about 10,000 of the city's special education students were supposed to receive during the last school year.

• Aboriginal languages are the basic media for the transmission and survival of Aboriginal consciousness, cultures, literatures, histories, religions, political institutions, and values. These languages provide distinctive perspectives on and understandings of the world. The suppression or extermination of their consciousness in education through the destruction of Aboriginal languages is inconsistent with the modern constitutional rights of Aboriginal peoples (Battiste, 2000b, p. 199).

Deficit Perspectives

Researchers and evaluators are using a deficit perspective when they choose to focus only on the problems in a community and ignore the strengths. Chiu (2003) argues that much research in minority ethnic communities suffers from this destructive theoretical and methodological stance. She contends that the reason many intervention studies yield inconclusive and contradictory results is because they focus on community deficits. Her work in the area of minority ethnic women and health care suggests that researchers tend to focus solely on communication and cultural deficits, without recognizing the social context. She states: "The narrow focus on language and culture as barriers to uptake of services has not only hindered a wider theoretical understanding of the problems, but also has had the effect of perpetuating ineffective health promotion practice" (2003, p. 167). When the deficit perspective is used to frame a group as a "problem" with barriers, then the strengths in that community are not as likely to be recognized. Another picture of deficit-based experiences is provided by the following student perspective:

Student Perspective: Deficit Perspectives and Deafness

Deaf students being held back in school or who were just passed along to the next class because they were just too old to be held back any more . . . "graduating" with special diplomas (and often reading far below grade level) . . . being told in the classroom that their speech was fine, but then finding in the real world that people couldn't understand their speech. Being told [in school] that yes, they can do anything they want to after high school . . . then being limited to menial jobs because they are too far behind in literacy to get better jobs. They cannot even attend community college because they only have a special diploma. Elementary children are being praised for good work in the classroom . . . but being held back because they cannot read on grade level yet. Too much focus on speech instruction and not enough on content instruction. All of this affects adult life, as I have already mentioned— limited to low-paying jobs or dependency on government handouts. Many older deaf adults have given up and will not even consider trying to improve their lives, are bitter toward the world, and fiercely oppose any changes that might reduce or eliminate the monthly checks they get.—Martha Knowles (September 2004)

While this comment is situated in a deaf context, the essential meaning of the statement would still ring true if one substituted many other dimensions of diversity associated with discrimination and oppression.

Combining Social Challenges and Resilience

One of the major principles underlying transformative research and evaluation is the belief in the strength that is often overlooked in communities that are rising to the challenge of addressing seemingly intransigent problems. Battiste's (2000b) justification for giving serious attention to indigenous knowledge is not to prepare Aboriginal children to compete in the non-Aboriginal world. On the contrary:

> It is, rather, that . . . society is sorely in need of what Aboriginal knowledge has to offer. We are witnessing throughout the world the weaknesses in knowledge based on science and technology. It is costing us our air, our water, our earth; our very lives are at stake. No longer are we able to turn to science to rid us of the mistakes of the past or to clean up our planet for the future of our children. Our children's future planet is not secure, and we have contributed to its insecurity by using the knowledge and skills that we received in public schools. Not only have we found that we need to make new decisions about our lifestyles to maintain the planet, but we are also becoming increasingly aware that the limitations of modern knowledge have placed our collective survival in jeopardy. (p. 202)

When theoretical perspectives such as resilience theory, positive psychology, and critical race theory are used to frame a study, then a deliberate and conscious design can reveal the positive aspects, resilience, and acts of resistance needed to promote social change (Mertens, 2005). Ludema, Cooperrider, and Barrett (2006) argue that research has largely failed as an instrument for advancing social-organizational transformation because it maintains a problem-oriented view, rather than focusing on the strengths of a community. Historically, social science research has proceeded from a deficit-based orientation, such that the research problem was derived from the deficits found in the people to be helped by the research. Ludema et al. propose turning away from such a deficit-based view and looking instead at what is positive. Thus, the focus on positive psychology provides one of the bases for developing the appreciative inquiry approach (see Chapter 7 on methods). Thus, social change is seen as emanating from asking unconditionally positive questions that focus on the life-giving and life-sustaining aspects of people and the communities in which they reside.

Challenging the Status Quo

Fals Borda (2006) challenges the traditional scientific requirement of objectivity as follows: "We felt that colleagues who claimed to work with 'neutrality' or 'objectivity' supported willingly or unwillingly the status quo, impairing full understanding of the social transformations in which we were immersed or which we wanted to stimulate" (p. 29).

Maori researchers also articulate a responsibility for those in "minoritized spaces" to challenge the status quo by moving to the foreground issues of inequality and social justice (L. T. Smith, 2004, as cited in Cram et al., 2004). After all, at the heart of the Nuremberg Code[5] is a concern that research ethics, and therefore research, should be an instrument of social justice (L. T. Smith, 2004, as cited in Cram et al., 2004, pp. 156–157). To this end, the Maori call for "decentering whiteness" in their writing about research by, for, and with Maori (Cram et al., 2004):

> People who are pushed to the margins, like Māori and Deaf people, in other words, are "decenterized." The Māori lost their land and family structures, relationships were unsettled, and their languages were repressed, thus pushing Māori people from the center. Cram et al. (2004, p. 167) argue that " . . . Māori researchers are essentially seeking to decentre 'whiteness as ownership of the world forever and ever'" (as discussed by black activist DuBois, 1920, cited in Myers, 2004, p. 8). On a parallel note, research with the Deaf community requires decenterizing "hearingness," so American Sign Language and Deaf culture are given back to Deaf people. Ensuring that research represents the people increases its validity, therefore research in the Deaf community should be by Deaf, for Deaf and with Deaf, like Cram et al. (2004) argue that research involving the Māori has to be done "by Māori, for Māori, with Māori." (Harris, Holmes, & Mertens, 2009)

In addition, the researchers' gaze should be turned to those in "majoritized spaces" who are privileged by the status quo (McCreanor & Nairn, 2002). Kendall (2006) prompts the research world to turn its eyes from problems and deficits to resilience and privilege and to ask the following questions:

- How can research be conducted as a means of interrogating white privilege?
- If we broaden the question beyond race, how can the researcher

interrogate those dimensions of diversity associated with unearned privilege that serve to sustain the status quo?

In asking such questions, researchers and evaluators also need to interrogate their own motives for working against discrimination and oppression.

Chilisa (2005) addresses the issue of social justice in research within the context of an HIV/AIDS prevention program in Botswana that made use of a Eurocentric belief system and the associated cost of ignoring indigenous languages and belief systems:

> That the HIV/AIDS epidemic in Botswana is escalating amidst volumes of research may be an indication that ongoing research is dominated by Eurocentric research epistemologies and ethics that fail to address the problem from the researched's frame of reference. Creating space for other knowledge systems must begin by recognizing local language and thought forms as an important source of making meanings of what we research. . . . Given the HIV/AIDS epidemic in Sub-Saharan Africa, the need for diversity in research epistemologies has become not a luxury of nationalism of the African Renaissance, but rather an issue of life and death. (p. 678)

Maori researchers' dissatisfaction with mainstream researchers has led to an increased desire and capacity for "by Maori, for Maori, with Maori" research (Cram et al., 2004). Maori researchers ask such questions as:

- How do we decolonize research so that it serves us better?
- How do we create research spaces that allow our stories to be told and heard?
- How do we use research to destabilize existing power structures that hold us in the margins? (Smith, 2004).

Such questions, along with critical reflection, serve as catalysts to the production of research that has transformative potential for the Maori, the researchers, and, by gaining such wisdom, to wider society.

Amsden and VanWynsberghe (2005) work in the area of youth-led participatory action research. They believe that the focus of other research approaches on deficits rather than assets has led to services that either treat young people as problems that need to be solved or simply fail to reflect their realities. Instead, these researchers stress the need to recognize and respect the inclusion of those who have a stake in decision making at community and policy levels. They write:

Young people need to be included in local and broader planning and decision-making processes so that their needs are addressed and their assets mobilized. . . .

Including youth in local decision making requires going beyond traditional adult-run structures, such as committee tables and one-off consultations, to develop processes that engage their unique energy and expertise. Such processes need to offer a fulfilling process and lead to meaningful results. Participatory Action Research (PAR) is a methodological framework that can fill the need for meaningful and engaging approaches to community planning. (p. 358)

Participatory action research is one example of an approach that is compatible with the transformative paradigm when it is applied to the goal of social justice. The next section explores specific examples of transformative research and evaluation work.

Examples of Transformative Research and Evaluation

The principles and implications of the transformative paradigm for the social justice agenda are illustrated by these examples.

- The Talent Development (TD) Model of School Reform (Boykin, 2000) is designed to explicitly address the strengths in students and their communities primarily in underresourced urban schools serving low-income students, most of whom are African American (Thomas, 2004). Guided by the TD model, Howard University's Center for Research on the Education of Students Placed at Risk (CRESPAR) developed an evaluation framework based on transformative principles that seeks to provide information that will enlighten and empower those who have been oppressed by, or marginalized in, school systems. The center recognized the alienation felt by many of the poor and African American students from mainstream schooling and took deliberate steps to engage the community in the planning and implementation of the evaluation in such a way that their cultural experiences were highlighted in a positive manner.

- Irwin (2005) used a peace polling strategy to address possible solutions to the troubles in Northern Ireland that have burdened that country with civil unrest for hundreds of years. He developed a series of surveys, involving members of historically acrimonious groups, to find strategies for peace that, although not ideal to any one group, were satisfactory to all. The results of his peace polling were used as a basis for the peace agreements that led to a significant decrease in violence in that part of the world.

• The American Educational Research Association Commission on Research in Black Education edited a volume entitled *Black Education: A Transformative Research and Action Agenda for the New Century* (King, 2005). Contributors provide an internationally based critique of black education, as well as directives and examples of transformative, culturally sensitive research in the service of advancing the social justice agenda for this population. The authors explicitly acknowledge the need to put the issue of racism on the research agenda as one means to improve the educational experiences of black students in the United States and the world.

• Chilisa's (2005) work in Botswana on HIV/AIDS promotes the use of local understanding of research concepts related to the prevention of this disease, rather than depending on the Western definitions that are not shared by the Botswana population most at risk. Her critique provides insight into possible reasons underlying the failure to stop this epidemic. Subsequently, she has received a grant from the U.S. National Institutes of Health to study prevention of HIV/AIDS in Botswana youth using an indigenous cultural understanding as a basis for development of an intervention (2007, personal communication).

• Elze (2003a) examined the comfort levels of lesbian, gay, bisexual, and transgender youths in schools and determined that the majority of these students experience verbal and physical abuse. She used her results to recommend changes in policies and practices in schools, as well as to examine specific ethical implications of research methodologies with this population (Elze, 2003b, 2005).

Examples of Shifting Paradigms

Feminists, Women, and Development

Feminists have struggled to include a specific focus on women's issues in international development activities for a very long time. Initially, their efforts were rewarded when a women-in-development (WID) strategy was included in the agendas of many international donor agencies that treated women's issues as separate concerns. Subsequently, a gender-and-development (GAD) approach was developed in which gender relations were analyzed in terms of power differentials between women and men (March, Smyth, & Mukhopadhyay, 1999). Mukhopadhyay (2004) notes that GAD has had the result of mainstreaming gender, as evidenced by the strategy adopted at the U.N. Fourth World Conference of Women in Beijing to promote the gender equality agenda within development institutions. Using case studies from her work in South Asia and Southern Africa, Mukhopadhyay expressed concern that this mainstreaming of gender normalizes the political project of gender in a way that is ahistorical, apolitical, decontextualized, and technical, and that leaves the prevailing and unequal power relations intact. She suggests that in repositioning gender in development policy and practice, we need to consider how to get back to the political project while not abandoning the present mode of engagement with development institutions. She suggests a shift in focus to gender as a political project that involves working on rights and citizenship issues within development institutions and on the outside to create a "voice" of the most marginalized.

Lesbian, Gay, Bisexual, Transgender, and Queer

Much research done on issues of relevance to the lesbian, gay, bisexual, transgender, and queer (LGBTQ) population does not ask about sexual orientation, gender, and gender identity, and hence conceals identities in a way that may reinforce the cultural hegemony of those who wield power (Dodd, 2009; Mertens et al., 2008). Queer theory has emerged as a way to challenge the two-dimensional separation of male or female—a very imprecise measure of meaning and identity. Such lack of clarity is intensified by a lack of critical reflection on how meaning making involves not only context but also the socially constructed identity of the individual in the setting. For the LGBTQ community, persistent internalized homophobia can conceal discrimination to the degree that subtle degrading manipulation is not even acknowledged or those demeaned feel powerless to challenge the question (see, e.g., Kahn, 1991). By establishing a transformative approach and reaching out to concealed communities, researchers have the opportunity to engage voices that have been traditionally unrecognized or excluded.

Disability Populations

In the disability community, there is a growing movement toward understanding the sociocultural basis of this population's experiences (Gill, 1999; Mertens & McLaughlin, 2004; Seelman, 2000; Wilson, 2005). The social model of disability challenges the medical perspective by allowing people with disabilities to take control over their own lives by shifting the focus onto social, rather than the biological, factors in understanding disability. Box 1.1 summarizes the paradigm shift in the disability community.

BOX 1.1. Paradigm Shift in the Disability Community

Underrepresented Groups and Research and Evaluation

- ❑ For example: People with disabilities have been framed in terms of a variety of paradigms, including:

  - ❑ The medical/deficit model: People who have a disability have a "problem" and they must be fixed.

  - ❑ The sociocultural model: People with disabilities form a cultural group that has been systematically discriminated against and oppressed by society. The "problem" is not "in" the people with a disability; rather it is in the inadequate response from society to accommodate their needs.

- ❑ Researchers and evaluators have used a variety of paradigms to conduct systematic inquires on/for/with people who are pushed to the margins of society.

  - ❑ The transformative paradigm is the approach that most closely parallels the sociocultural view of people with disabilities, as well as people occupying less privileged positions in society who therefore experience discrimination and oppression.

Intersection of Disability and International Development

When disability is coupled with an additional layer of complexity—that is, working with people with disabilities in an international context—the paradigm shift from a medical/deficits model to a sociocultural participatory model gains another perspective (Wilson, 2005). People with disabilities in developing countries have historically been denied basic social services by their governments and have had to rely on overseas charitable organizations for education, job training, and basic health care. Poor governments, straining to meet the needs of entire populations, typically disregard the needs of their disabled populace and encourage the benevolent contributions made by foreign organizations. Social and participatory action research are a means through which people with disabilities can be heard, empowered, and moved to action to lobby for inclusion in all aspects of society. The U.N. (2003–2004) report on its first 50 years of addressing the needs of people with disabilities provides this picture of the life of a disabled person in the developing world:

> Not surprisingly, many of the disabled are poor. The overwhelming majority— perhaps 80 per cent—live in isolated rural areas. Almost that many live in areas where the services needed to help them are unavailable. Too often their

lives are handicapped by physical and social barriers in society which hamper their full participation. Because of this, and in all parts of the world, they often face a life that is segregated and debased, and without help, many will live in isolation and insecurity. (United Nations, 2003–2004)

Wilson (2005) conducted mixed-methods studies in deaf communities in Africa, the Caribbean, and South America. This research became the catalyst for social changes for the deaf participants and their advocates. Wilson took several unique factors into account when conducting research in deaf communities. Because most foreign agencies view deaf people as dependent and disabled, the agencies have focused on the medical impact of deafness rather than on the social impact. As a result these agencies have donated hearing aids, audiology equipment, and vaccines that prevent deafness, and they have supported oralism[6] in the schools they have built, rather than honor the existing indigenous sign languages. By looking at deafness as a medical problem, rather than considering the social barriers that deaf people face because of their inability to communicate easily within the greater community, deaf people have been prevented from developing a political framework with which they can locate and share their experience of having a unique culture and language.

Positive Psychology and Resilience Theory

Another shift is evident within the field of psychology with the emergence of positive psychology and resilience theory (Seligman, 2006; Seligman, Steen, Park, & Peterson, 2005). Positive psychology as a theoretical framework changes the focus from one of mental illness to one of mental health. To date, psychology as a discipline has done well at defining "abnormal behavior" and working to improve the lives of individuals who are suffering. However, psychology has much to learn about making happy people happier and studying such constructs as gratitude, wisdom, and finding meaning in life. Szarkowski (2002) conducted a study based on the positive psychology movement and focused on finding positive features within a challenging experience. She describes the ways in which hearing parents of deaf children learn to "make the most" of the situation they have been handed. Many of them come to cherish their child and their experience of raising a deaf child, indicating that it has changed their lives for the better. Their challenges have led to greater meaning and awareness in their lives. This example highlights the use of the transformative paradigm in understanding a situation commonly believed to be "difficult." In Szarkowski's study, hearing parents of deaf children were asked about the *positives* associated with their experiences of raising deaf children. The parents not only defined positive experiences, they also relished the opportunity to think about their children from a new, or often not discussed, perspective. Data from parent journals and interviews revealed that a focus on the positive, rather than the problem-focused discussions to which they had become accustomed, was beneficial to them.

Critical Race Theory

Another example of a shift in theoretical understanding is provided by critical race theory (CRT) in race-based research (McCaskill, 2005). CRT provides the basis for an analytical model that focuses on the failure of the U.S. education system to adequately educate the majority of culturally and racially subordinated students. CRT shapes data collection within a framework of five broad themes: (1) oral narrative, (2) racism, (3) educational inequity, (4) differential treatment, and (5) interest convergence. CRT posits that the experiential knowledge base of people of color is legitimate and provides them with a forum for sharing and voicing their experiences.

CRT and Intersection with Deafness

McCaskill (2005) recognizes that the voices of black deaf Americans are rarely heard in the literature. She conducted a mixed-methods research study with black and white deaf, hard-of-hearing, and hearing pariticpants. The CRT framework allowed acknowledgment of the legitimacy of their voices and provided a forum in which their voices could be heard. CRT argues that racism is common throughout society, and racism was clearly a salient factor in the way that white administrators interpreted and administered official policy for black deaf and hard-of-hearing students. School funding is an obvious reflection of educational inequity. Black deaf residential schools suffered with inadequate funding to provide quality education to their students. The most serious and threatening form of racism was evidenced in the differential treatment in deaf schools. Finally, as the interest convergence principle maintains, the white administrators promoted racial advances for black deaf students only when those advances also promoted white self-interest.

Need for the Transformative Paradigm and Scholarly Literature

The need for transformative research and evaluation is evident in scholarly literature that addresses experiences of marginalized groups from a perspective of access to appropriate services. For example, the National Center on Low-Incidence Disabilities (NCLID) conducted a needs assessments for people who are deaf, blind, or have severe disabilities and they documented needs in the areas of access, literacy, and teaching personnel (Ferrell et al., 2004). They noted critical shortages in personnel to serve low-incidence students, challenges in accessing the general curriculum, and definitions of literacy that emphasize reading and writing and that consequently do not accurately reflect literacy that would encompass alternative modes of understanding and communication.

Two summaries of literature in the personnel preparation area were produced as part of the Center on Personnel Studies in Special Education project. Harold Johnson (2003) addressed the knowledge base and research needs for U.S. deaf education teacher preparation programs, and Anne Corn and Susan Spungin (2003) addressed the personnel crisis for students with visual impairments and blindness. There is a severe shortage in the number of trained teachers available to serve deaf or blind students. Corn and Spungin report that the situation is even more serious for deaf–blind students, as only six programs were operating in 1999, and the percentage of the faculty time in these programs, added together, equaled only four full-time equivalent (FTE) faculty.

If we add the dimension of social and cultural diversity to the low-incidence disability population, we see many other issues. Gerner de Garcia (2004) directed the Literacy for Latino Deaf and Hard of Hearing English Language Learners: Building the Knowledge Base Project. The goal of the project is "to create a scientific review of relevant research literature in deafness, special education, and the education of hearing English Language Learners, as well as Latino children and their families" (p. 7). Her conclusions reveal that many Latino families seek professional help with their deaf children; however, the schools often lack staff with the linguistic and cultural skills to make parent participation a reality. My colleagues and I reached similar conclusions in a national study that focused on parents' descriptions of their early experiences with their deaf and hard-of-hearing children (Meadow-Orlans et al., 2003). We attempted to disaggregate parent experiences based on a number of characteristics, such as if the child was deaf or hard of hearing, was from a racial/ethnic minority group, had a disability in addition to a hearing loss, or if the child's parents were deaf.

Voices: Scholarly Literature and Community Members

The sources I cite support the need for research and evaluation with people from disenfranchised groups. Scholarly literature from representatives of indigenous communities provides another source of support. Duran and Duran (2000) wrote:

> The problem of irrelevant research and clinical practice would not be so destructive to Native American people if institutional racism did not pervade most of the academic settings for research and theoretical construction. These institutions not only discredit thinking that is not Western but also engage in practices that imply that people who do not subscribe to their worldview are genetically inferior. (p. 93)

Chilisa (2005) added:

> In research, definitions of terms are first referenced to dictionaries and then operationalized. It is also important to make reference to local meanings attached to experiences. Proverbs, folklore, songs, and myths should be part of the literature review and source of problem identification and meaning making as well as assisting in legitimizing findings. Proverbs, for instance, represent "cultural theories or models of experience, evaluative assertions from a moral perspective, generalized knowledge that can be applied to the interpretation of particular events, and a point of view or certain ways of looking at problems." (Tippens, Veal, & Wieseman, 1995, p. 2)

Lest we think that the raising of indigenous voices as a critique of Eurocentric thought is a recent phenomena, Henderson (2000) provides a historical perspective by citing a Cherokee in 1777 who commented:

> Much has been said of the want of what you term "Civilization" among the Indians. Many proposals have been made to us to adopt your law, your religion, your manners and your customs. We do not see the propriety of such a reformation. We should be better pleased with beholding the good effects of these doctrines in your own practices than with hearing you talk about them or of reading your newspapers on such subjects. (Hill, 1994, as cited in Henderson, 2000, p. 31)

My students at Gallaudet University read a cartoon from the *Wizard of Id* series that depicted the king's crier announcing that a new poll showed that the king had "high ratings." The king smirked and said, "There's a lot to be said for owning your own station." Cultural note for those readers unfamiliar with this U.S.-based cartoon: The king in the *Wizard of Id* is a tyrannical despot, not a benevolent leader. In response to their interpretation of the cartoon, the graduate students presented their thoughts in the class discussion board as to why they think we need rigorous research and evaluation for educational and social programs. Their comments were deep and profound and exceeded my expectations. Consider one student's response in which she indicated that the cartoon illustrated an example of what frequently happens in research and evaluation.

Student Perspective: Importance of Rigor in Research and Evaluation

There is a desired result or opinion that the commissioner of the study seeks to prove, and he sets out to prove it through manipulation of the research. The researcher filters the information through his/her own lens and presents it as though it is valid and reliable. . . . Certainly research takes on many forms, and while the king does well in his opinion polls through manipulation and ownership of the study, the question arises as to who the people are who the research is purported to represent. And . . . what would be the impact on the people affected by the results?

In the Mertens (2005) text, we see that there is a lack of stakeholder input into the research and that this will unduly influence the results to skew and cater to those in powerful positions. Certainly, this is not the first time that those with power have undertaken a study to take yet more power from those without it. The comic strip emphasizes this point effectively.

Interestingly enough, just as in real life, the less powerful may not be aware that this manipulation has taken place, or they feel powerless to address it. In this case, this is a king, not an elected president. To me, this underscores how little powerless subjects are enabled to change the results of ill-completed research, yet must contend with the results. . . . The comic strip suggests that the king is so well liked, he will never have to change the way he behaves in leadership. . . . This comic strip illustrates that we must have valid research so that the king can be forced to look out the window at his subjects rather than at a mirror in arrogance. Without research, we cannot know the true state of affairs for us or for others, and without research, change is impossible.—Risa Briggs (2004)

These comments suggest that we need good research and evaluation because there are real lives at stake that are being determined by those in power. The voices of those who are disenfranchised on the basis of gender, race/ethnicity, disability, or other characteristics remind us of the issues of power that surround so much of the public sphere, even those supposedly neutral and objective worlds of research and evaluation. In my own work, I have witnessed many occasions in which issues of power were used to attempt to obscure the real problems that were facing individuals who are deaf, as noted in Box 1.2.

BOX 1.2. Power and Sexual Abuse

A study of sexual abuse in a deaf residential school provides one poignant example of the misuse of power (Mertens, 1996). I was contacted by a consulting firm to collect data for a contract they had received from a state's Department of Education. The consulting firm did not mention sexual abuse in our initial communications; however, I discovered the allegations when I asked for a copy of the request for proposals (RFP) and the proposal. The first line in the RFP stated: "Because of serious allegations of sexual abuse at the residential school for the deaf, an external evaluator should be brought into the school to systematically study the context of the school." When I mentioned this serious issue to the consulting firm contact person, they acknowledged it was a problem but suggested that we could address it by asking if the curriculum included sex education and if the students could lock their doors at night. I indicated that I thought the problem was more complex than that, but I was willing to go to the school and discuss the evaluation project with the school officials.

Upon my arrival, I met with the four men who constituted the upper management of the school. For about 30 minutes they talked about the need to look at the curriculum and the administrative structure. They did not mention the topic of sexual abuse. So, I raised the topic, saying, "I'm a bit confused. I have been here for about a half hour, and no one has yet mentioned the issue of sexual abuse, which is the basis for the Department of Education requirement of an external evaluation." After some chair scraping and coughing, one school administrator said, "That happened last year, and I am sure if you ask people, they will say that they just want to move on." The administrators were correct that the incidents resulting in the termination of the superintendent's contract and the jailing of two staff members had happened in the spring of the year, and I was there in the fall. I assured them that it was indeed quite possible that some people would say that they would prefer to move on, but it was important for me to ask a wide range of people two questions: What were the factors that allowed the sexual abuse to happen? What would need to be changed in order to reduce the probability that it would recur? I found that there were many answers to these questions, one of which was a desire to not talk about it and move on. However, allowing those with power to frame the questions would have resulted in a continuation of an overall context that had permitted many young deaf people to be seriously psychologically and physically hurt. A different approach to research and evaluation is needed to address the needs of those who have not been adequately represented in these contexts.

Need for the Transformative Paradigm and Public Policy

In the United States the requirements set forth in the No Child Left Behind (NCLB) legislation increased awareness of the need for good research and evaluation. The NCLB sets the use of standardized tests and randomized designs, using the scientific method as the desired approach to demonstrate a program's effectiveness (*www.ed.gov/nclb/methods/whatworks/whatworks.html*). The privileging of standardized tests and randomized control group designs presents challenges in assessing the effectiveness of interventions in culturally complex communities (and in less complex communities as well).

The American Evaluation Association (AEA) (2003) takes the position that there is not one right way to evaluate the effectiveness of a program. In response to the U.S. Department of Education's requirement for the scientific method, the AEA stated:

> While we agree with the intent of ensuring that federally sponsored programs be "evaluated using scientifically based research . . . to determine the effectiveness of a project intervention," we do not agree that "evaluation methods using an experimental design are best for determining project effectiveness." (*www.eval.org/doestatement.htm*)

AEA (2003) is joined by other organizations, such as the National Education Association (NEA), in providing commentary on NCLB. The NEA communicated with the U.S. Secretary of Education, Rod Paige, cautioning that we need to use an approach other than the scientific method to demonstrate effectiveness of programs. The position specifically advocates that "(1) the evaluation approach used be appropriate for the problem or question the program itself seeks to address; (2) that the evaluation definition and set of priorities used are not so narrow that they effectively preclude the funding of worthwhile programs; and (3) that the Department continue to recognize the importance of third party, independent evaluators" (*www.eval.org/doe.nearesponse.pdf*).

One of the potentially positive aspects of NCLB is the accountability requirement and the report card. The report card shows how minority groups are faring, and we are finding, not surprisingly, that their levels of achievement are very low. Such data force all of us—educators, parents, researchers, evaluators, and others—to find out why these children are not succeeding and implement changes to make sure that no child is left behind. In order to do this, we need to conduct research about effective practices and evaluate the programs. We need to identify specifically what we need to evaluate, not just the program as a whole. With so much visibility given to research and evaluation in the NCLB, this is a propitious moment for those concerned with the children who are historically left behind to raise the issue of their experiences in the school system and to propose appropriate ways to capture the complexity of this experience that can lead to higher achievement levels for all.

The American Psychological Association (2008a) maintains a Public Interest Government Relations Office for the specific purpose of supporting its members in researching and advocating for programs in the public interest that relate to children, individuals with disabilities, ethnic minority populations; HIV/AIDS; aging; lesbian, gay, bisexual, and transgender issues; socioeconomic status; and women's issues. American Psychological Association members are called upon to participate in conversations about public policy as a civic responsibility that is enriched by their particular expertise.

Complexities That Challenge

What challenges are associated with the planning and conducting of research and evaluation in culturally complex communities? How are these challenges exacerbated by corruption, bribery, and war? What challenges are associated with research that meaningfully includes people who are male or female, able-bodied or disabled, members of racial/ethnic groups, and/or those associated with more or less privilege?

The NCLID leadership (Ferrell et al., 2004) identified a number of complexities associated with conducting research and evaluation with people with low-incidence disabilities. Although the NCLID places the issues within this context, many of these complexities are more broadly applicable to other communities who are pushed to the margins of society. For example, there is a lack of systematic empirical methods that are tailored to address the needs of such communities, and there are particular problems associated with the use of control groups determined by random assignment. The educational programs for students with low-incidence disabilities are set forth in an individualized education plan (IEP), one of the legislatively mandated tools designed to identify appropriate accommodations and educational strategies for people with disabilities. The IEP has in its name the term *individual*, thus indicating that this person requires a unique program in order to receive early intervention services or a free appropriate public education. Tensions exist between the legislative mandate to serve persons with disabilities with individually designed services and that of the

NCLB legislation that places priority on random assignment to experimental and control groups, as is illustrated in the following questions.

- Given the individual nature of such a person's needs, how can "treatment" be determined by random assignment?
- How can these students be placed in a control group, which means that they will be denied the carefully identified services that constitute the IEP?
- What are the ethical implications of random assignment when a child's case has been carefully studied to determine strengths and areas in need of improvement, and a small number of personnel with highly specialized skills and knowledge were determined to be needed in order to provide an appropriate educational experience for this child?
- What generalizable concerns arise in working with other communities that are pushed to the margins of society?

Box 1.3 summarizes the complexities that face researchers and evaluators who work with people with disabilities, as well those from other underrepresented groups.

Other challenges arise because of the need to use multiple measurements, observations, and ongoing assessments. While many good instruments have been developed for use in educational settings, their appropriateness for people from diverse cultural groups, such as those with low-incidence disabilities, must be determined on a case-by-case basis. The highly idiosyncratic characteristics of low-incidence populations also introduces challenges related to rigorous data analysis due to possibly small samples and restricted or highly variable ranges. The uniqueness of the population also creates problems with attempts to replicate findings. Replication makes an assumption that similar people in similar circumstances can be used to demonstrate the generalizability of results. The assumption may not be met in such a population.

The context surrounding research with people who have low-incidence disabilities adds another layer of challenges. For example, the low-incidence population is, by definition, heterogeneous. People who are deaf, blind, or have severe disabilities differ on those dimensions as well as many others, including sex, race/ethnicity, home language, communication preferences, presence of additional disabilities, to name a few. The fact that these are *low-incidence* disabilities means that the affected population involves small numbers of people across large geographic areas.

BOX 1.3. Complexities That Challenge

Researchers and evaluators are challenged to employ . . .

- ☐ Systematic, empirical methods
- ☐ Controls, random assignment
- ☐ Different conditions, evaluators, observers
- ☐ Multiple measurements, observations, and studies
- ☐ Rigorous data analysis
- ☐ Replication
- ☐ Peer review

When they encounter . . .

- ☐ Heterogeneous populations
- ☐ Populations with low-incidence disabilities
- ☐ Geographic dispersion
- ☐ Little federal funding
- ☐ Unsophisticated designs
- ☐ Inability to replicate
- ☐ Few researchers

Finally, small numbers of children with low-incidence disabilities (a redundancy, I know) means that there are a small number of professionals who serve them. Of this small number, much is asked. Adding the conduct of research and evaluation may seem an impossible burden. In addition, the small numbers also mean fewer dollars to support research and evaluation with such populations.

Ethical Impetus

Professional associations in the human sciences have a long history of developing ethical codes to guide research and evaluation studies that involve human participants. In the United States, the National Commission for the Protection of Human Subjects of Biomedical and Behavioral Research (1979) issued the Belmont Report that provides guidance for institutional review boards (IRBs; the legal entities charged with the protection of participants in research). The three ethical principles identified include:

1. Beneficence: Maximizing good outcomes for science, humanity, and the individual research participants and minimizing or avoiding unnecessary risk, harm, or wrong.

2. Respect: Treating people with respect and courtesy, including those who are not autonomous (e.g., small children, people who have mental retardation or senility).

3. Justice: Ensuring that those who bear the risk in the research are the ones who benefit from it; ensuring that the procedures are reasonable, nonexploitative, carefully considered and fairly administered.

The Belmont Report also identified six norms to guide scientific research:

1. Use of a valid research design: Faulty research is not useful to anyone and is not only a waste of time and money, but also cannot be conceived of as being ethical in that it does not contribute to the well-being of the participants.

2. The researcher must be competent to conduct the research.

3. Consequences of the research must be identified: Procedures must respect privacy, ensure confidentiality, maximize benefits, and minimize risks.

4. The sample selection must be appropriate for the purposes of the study, representative of the population to benefit from the study, and sufficient in number.

5. The participants must agree to participate in the study through voluntary informed consent—that is, without threat or undue inducement (voluntary), knowing what a reasonable person in the same situation would want to know before giving consent (informed), and explicitly agreeing to participate (consent).

6. The researcher must inform the participants whether harm will be compensated.

Personally, I cannot argue against any of these principles and norms. In fact, as I am looking over the landscape of ethics, these seem to be quite useful. However, in the conduct of research and evaluation, issues of an ethical nature arise that are not clearly addressed in these principles and norms. In my experience, some ethical issues will surface differently or not at all, depending on the researcher's or evaluator's paradigmatic stance. For example, Chilisa (2005) suggests that research ethics narrowly defined as protection of the individual fail to protect the researched in important ways. Referencing research ethics in the Third World, she highlights the need to consider ethics in light of respect for and protection of the integrity of the researched communities, ethnicities, societies, and nations: "Researched communities should validate research findings, which are generalized or extrapolated to them. Such an exercise will enable the researched to have full participation in the construction of knowledge that is produced about them" (p. 678).

The revision of the AEA's (2004) Guiding Principles provides one example of how the use of a different lens to view this code of ethics yields different issues. For example, the original version contained five categories of principles: systematic inquiry, competence, integrity/honest, respect for people, and responsibilities for general and public welfare (see Box 1.4). The original principles were accompanied by a statement that recognized that they were part of an evolving process of self-examination by the profession and should be revisited on a regular basis. When the review process was complete, the categories were essentially unchanged. However, changes did appear in the statements that amplify the meaning of each overarching principle. For example, the following statement was added to the 2004 version of the Guiding Principles under the Competence category:

> To ensure recognition, accurate interpretation and respect for diversity, evaluators should ensure that the members of the evaluation team collectively demonstrate cultural competence. Cultural competence would be reflected in evaluators seeking awareness of their own culturally-based assumptions, their understanding of the worldviews of culturally-different participants and stakeholders in the evaluation, and the use of appropriate evaluation strategies and skills in working with culturally different groups. Diversity may be in terms of race, ethnicity, gender, religion, socio-economics, or other factors pertinent to the evaluation context. Retrieved October 14, 2005, from *www. eval.org/Guiding%20Principles.htm*.

The establishment of a causal link between the transformative paradigm and this change in language is not possible. Nevertheless, this change in language arose because evaluators who work in a spirit compatible with the transformative paradigm provided feedback to the association. Hence, this change in language is one example of what happens at the borders and crossroads of research and evaluation paradigms.

Revisions of professional association codes indicate a greater awareness of the need to consciously incorporate principles of cultural competence as a salient dimension of their ethical codes, for example, the ethical codes of the American Psychological Association, American Educational

---

BOX 1.4. AEA's Guiding Principles

A. **Systematic inquiry:** Evaluators conduct systematic, data-based inquiries about whatever is being evaluated.

B. **Competence:** Evaluators provide competent performance to stakeholders.

C. **Integrity/honesty:** Evaluators ensure the honesty and integrity of the entire evaluation process.

D. **Respect for people:** Evaluators respect the security, dignity, and self-worth of the respondents, program participants, clients, and other stakeholders with whom they interact.

E. **Responsibilities for general and public welfare:** Evaluators articulate and take into account the diversity of interests and values that may be related to the general and public welfare.

Retrieved February 11, 2008, from *www.eval.org/Guiding%20Principles.htm.*

Research Association, American Evaluation Association, American Sociological Association, American Anthropological Association, and the United Nations. Researcher and evaluator guidelines are also available from indigenous communities that provide insights into ethical grounding of research. The ethical implications of these codes and guidelines are discussed further in Chapter 2 in the section on the axiological assumptions of the transformative paradigm.

Striving for Improved Validity

Validity in data collection is generally defined as using an instrument that actually measures what it is intended to measure,[7] but *validity* also has broader meanings. Kirkhart (1995, 2005) and Lincoln (1995) provide leadership in the discussion of the integral connection between the quality of the human relations in research and evaluation settings and the validity of the information that is assembled. Kirkhart (2005) proposes specific consideration of what she terms "multicultural validity,"[8] which she describes as referring to the "correctness or authenticity of understandings across multiple, intersecting cultural contexts" (p. 22). She outlines five justifications for multicultural validity:

1. Theoretical: The cultural congruence of theoretical perspectives underlying the program, the evaluation, and assumptions about validity.
2. Experiential: Congruence with the lived experience of participants in the program and in the evaluation process.
3. Consequential: The social consequences of understandings and judgments and the actions taken based upon them.
4. Interpersonal: The quality of the interactions between and among participants in the evaluation process.
5. Methodological: The cultural appropriateness of measurement tools and cultural congruence of design configurations. (Kirkhart, 2005, p. 23)

Additional arguments for the value of placing our work within the transformative paradigm rest on the criteria for quality in research and evaluation identified by Lincoln (1995) and presented in Box 1.5.

Is it easy to address issues of social justice through transformative research and evaluation? We can take inspiration from those who took on this charge during the civil rights era in the United States, as well as from members of indigenous communities who remind us of the need for courage, as illustrated in these quotations:

• "You cannot be afraid if you want to accomplish something. You got to have the willin', the spirit and, above all, you got to have the get-up" (National Public Radio, Hidden Kitchens, March 4, 2005). This quotation is from Georgia Gillmore, who was fired after speaking against the white bus driver who kicked her off his bus in 1956 in Alabama. She opened her own "kitchen," sold food to raise funds for the civil rights movement, and died 25 years later—still cooking.

• In another sense, courage is about Maori researchers themselves embracing the margins that they have found themselves occupying, including being marginal to mainstream research institutions and marginal because they are the arbiters of research findings that unsettle the status quo (L. T. Smith, 2004).

• It also takes courage when we are confronted by the day-to-day hardship that many of our people are experiencing, even if this is what makes us so determined that their voices should be heard and that any research ethic must be about social justice (McIntosh, 2004; Pomare et al., 1995, as cited in Ormond, Cram, & Carter, 2004, p. 164).

BOX 1.5. Criteria for Quality in Research and Evaluation

AUTHENTICITY

Authenticity refers to the presentation of a balanced view of all perspectives, values, and beliefs (Lincoln & Guba, 2000). It answers the question, has the researcher been fair in presenting views? Among the criteria identified by Lincoln and Guba to judge the authenticity of investigations are the following:

Fairness—This criterion answers the question, to what extent are different constructions and their underlying value structures solicited and honored in the process? To be fair, the researcher must identify the respondents and how information about their constructions was obtained. Conflicts and value differences should be displayed. There should also be open negotiation of the recommendations and agenda for future actions.

Ontological authenticity—This criterion refers to the degree to which the individual's or group's conscious experience of the world became more informed or sophisticated as a result of the research experience. The presence of this type of authenticity can be determined by checking with members of the community to determine their changed understandings or by means of an audit trail that documents changes in individuals' constructions throughout the process.

Catalytic authenticity—This criterion refers to the extent to which action is stimulated by the inquiry process. Techniques for determining the extent to which this type of authenticity occurred include respondent testimony and documentation of actions that were taken during and after the study.

POSITIONALITY OR STANDPOINT EPISTEMOLOGY

Lincoln (1995) describes the inherent characteristic of all research as being representative of the position or standpoint of the author. Therefore, researchers should acknowledge that all texts are incomplete and represent specific positions in terms of sexuality, ethnicity, and so on. Texts cannot claim to contain all universal truth because all knowledge is contextual; therefore, the researcher must acknowledge the context of the research.

COMMUNITY

Research takes place within, and affects, a community (Lincoln, 1995). The researcher should know the community well enough to link the research results to positive action within that community.

(continued)

BOX 1.5. *(continued)*

ATTENTION TO VOICE

Lincoln (1995) cites the question that bell hooks (1990) has asked in her writing: Who speaks for whom? Who speaks for those who do not have access to the academy? The researcher must seek out those who are silent and must involve those who are marginalized.

CRITICAL REFLEXIVITY

The researcher must be able to enter into a high level of awareness that understands the psychological state of others to uncover dialectical relationships (Lincoln, 1995). The researcher needs to have a heightened degree of self-awareness for personal transformation and critical subjectivity.

RECIPROCITY

The researcher needs to demonstrate that a method of study was used that allowed the researcher to develop a sense of trust and mutuality with the participants (Lincoln, 1995).

SHARING THE PERQUISITES OF PRIVILEGE

Researchers should be prepared to share in the royalties of books or other publications that result from the research. Lincoln (1995) says: "We owe a debt to the persons whose lives we portray." In her closing remarks at the annual meeting of the American Educational Research Association, Lincoln (1995) envisioned a different set of criteria for judging the quality of research from what is currently used in most academic settings: "Try to imagine an academic world in which judgments about promotion, tenure, and merit pay were made on the basis of the extent of our involvement with research participants, rather than on our presumed distance."

Based largely on Lincoln (1995).

Summary

✓ The prism is used as a metaphor for transformative research and evaluation because of its multiple facets and the resulting unique outcomes that reflect ever-changing contextual factors.

✓ The purpose of this text is to make explicit the underlying assumptions and methodological implications of working from the transformative paradigm, which prioritizes the furtherance of human rights and social justice.

✓ The transformative paradigm is put forward as a metaphysical umbrella that covers research and evaluation that is designed to challenge the status quo.

✓ The need for the transformative paradigm is discussed in terms of societal inequities; movement from a deficit-based to a resilience-based perspective; examples of transformative study outcomes; and the shifting paradigms evidenced in various contexts, including international development, feminism, disability rights, and critical race theory.

✓ The need for the transformative paradigm is also explored in terms of scholarly literature, which documents the needs of particular populations, as well as public policy, which contains implications for research and evaluation that are culturally responsive.

✓ This chapter also discusses the complexities that challenge researchers and evaluators who work in culturally diverse communities.

✓ A growing awareness of the need to reframe ethics and validity to encompass cultural competence is the final topic addressed in Chapter 1.

MOVING ON TO CHAPTER 2 . . .

Following a general discussion of the meaning of paradigms in research and evaluation, the basic beliefs of the transformative paradigm are explained in detail along with examples of theories that are commensurate with transformative work.

 If you twist a prism hanging in the window on a sunny day, you can see changing patterns of light. If you use your imagination, you can see the colors dancing around the room.

Notes

1. For more about how prisms work, see Appendix A.
2. At the moment, the world of research and evaluation is operating with several competing paradigms: the post-positivist, the constructivist, the pragmatic, and the transformative. Research and evaluation methods texts are available that explore the first three paradigms and very few that explore all four paradigms (Mertens, 2005).
3. Readers interested in further exploration of similar philosophical treatments of transformation are referred to Habermas's (1981, 1996) communicative action theory and Foucault (1980), Lyotard (1984), and Todorov (1995) on the academic rhetoric supportive of institutional forms of power, values, domination, and control.
4. Disability rights activists have suggested the term *temporarily able-bodied*, as we all go through periods of our lives when we are disabled in some respect. For example, I may be able-bodied now, but at times my back goes out. Then I am temporarily disabled. Also, many deaf people prefer to be thought of as part of a cultural group, rather than as part of a group with a disability.
5. The Nuremburg Code provides a historical basis for the protection of human participants in research and evaluation. It is discussed further in the section on ethics in this chapter.
6. Oralism is an approach to communication for deaf people that emphasizes speech training, lip reading, and technology (e.g., hearing aids and cochlear implants) to enhance residual hearing. While this approach is successful for some people with hearing loss, exclusive use of oral-based communication has had a detrimental effect on deaf people who benefit more from visual communication strategies, such as sign languages. This emphasis on oral strategies has been a source of much acrimonious debate for centuries.
7. This concept is further explored in Chapter 8 on data collection.
8. Kirkhart first introduced the term *multicultural validity* in 1995; she expanded the concept considerably in her 2005 chapter.

CHAPTER 2

The Transformative Paradigm

Basic Beliefs and Commensurate Theories

The wide variety of approaches that are available to evaluators of any development initiative today is an expression of the influence of a combination of differing theoretical assumptions, philosophical premises, practical objectives, and contextual appraisals. The set of profound beliefs that each evaluator holds as his or her worldview about the nature of reality (ontology), the nature of knowledge (epistemology), and the nature of human nature (axiology), is reflected in the approaches he or she chooses to employ in practice—knowingly or unknowingly, consciously or unconsciously. Given the paramount influence that the worldview perspective that any individual evaluator brings to bear in any particular exercise of evaluation, it is not only regrettable when the issue of perspectives remains unaddressed, but also grossly negligent. If indeed, as Stufflebeam (2001) argues, any evaluation is a study that is designed and conducted to assist some audience to assess an object's merit and worth, then explicit attention must be paid to foundational assumptions about the nature of worth and value, and to how these can come to be known in any given contextual situation, if it is to be an ethically defensible practice.

—BAWDEN (2006, p. 38)

IN THIS CHAPTER . . .

▼ The basic beliefs of the transformative paradigm are explained and illustrated, including:

   ▼ Axiology—the nature of ethics

   ▼ Ontology—the nature of reality

   ▼ Epistemology—the nature of knowledge and the relation between the knower and that which would be known

   ▼ Methodology—appropriate approaches to systematic inquiry

▼ Theories that are commensurate with the transformative paradigm are discussed, including feminist theories, CRT, postcolonial theory, and queer theory.

▼ Issues of power and privilege are explored in relation to the paradigmatic assumptions.

This chapter focuses on understanding the transformative paradigm and the basic beliefs that underlie it. What does it mean to identify your own worldview or, in research/evaluation language, to identify your paradigm? We need to look at the word *paradigm* and see what it means.

A woman is doing a crossword puzzle and wants to know if her husband can tell her what a paradigm is. He shrugs and says, "Twenty cents?"

Some background knowledge is assumed in order for this joke to be funny. You have to know that in U.S. currency, there is a coin called a *dime* and that it is worth 10 cents. If I have a pair of dimes, then it is worth 20 cents. The reader needs to know that the concept of paradigm has a meaning that is not defined as a monetary value. Also, this humor is based on the phonological similarity of "pair of dimes" and "paradigm," which requires that the reader be able to hear the similarity of the sounds. If the reader is deaf, this necessitates a somewhat detailed explanation. If the joke is presented visually, then it either needs to be translated into Braille or read aloud with a description of what is happening for blind people to have access to the information.

In this moment in time we are not talking about monetary worth; we are talking about a paradigm—which is a metaphysical construct associated with specific philosophical assumptions (basic beliefs) that describe a worldview. However, I use this joke as a way of introducing the concept of paradigm because it illustrates the fact that members of a dominant culture sometimes use terms that are familiar within their world of experience without realizing that the cultural influence inherent in the use of that language can preclude access to the information for those who are not part of the dominant culture.

Paradigms and Basic Belief Systems

As noted, four basic belief systems are relevant to defining a paradigm in a research/evaluation context:

- Ethics (axiology)
- Reality (ontology)
- Nature of knowledge and relation between knower and that which would-be-known (epistemology)
- Appropriate approach to systematic inquiry (methodology)

The axiological assumption asks the question: What is considered ethical or moral behavior? As presented in Chapter 1, three basic principles underlie regulatory ethics in research and evaluation: respect, beneficence, and justice. Ontologically speaking, how do we know that something is real? I don't mean a table or a computer, which I can touch. I mean the realities that we can know only at a conceptual level. For example: When is an environment least restrictive? When is literacy real? In the ontological sense, we have an assumption about what is real when we decide what type of evidence we will accept to establish that someone is indeed literate, has a learning disability, or has any other socially constructed conceptual characteristic.

Epistemologically speaking, we ask ourselves: What is the nature of knowledge and how do I come to know that the knowledge is "true"? Is knowledge absolute or relative (i.e., defined in a context of power and privilege)? If I am to learn if something about certain people is real, how do I need to relate to those people from whom I am collecting data? The knower is the researcher or evaluator and the "would-be-known" is the subject or participant in the study. Should I become close to the participants in order to really understand their experiences, or should I maintain distance between myself and them so that I can remain "neutral"? This question raises the definition of objectivity as it is operationalized in a research or evaluation context. Methodologically, I have choices that go beyond quantitative or qualitative or mixed methods to include how I collect the data about the reality of a thing in such a way that I can feel confident that I have indeed captured its reality.

The world of research and evaluation is operating on several competing paradigms: the post-positivist, the constructivist, the transformative, and the pragmatic (Mertens, 2005). Each paradigm is associated with its own philosophical assumptions about ethics, reality, relationships, and methodology. Box 2.1 contains an example of how basic belief systems underlie various paradigmatic perspectives.

BOX 2.1. Basic Belief Systems and Paradigms: Santa Claus

In the United States, a country with roots in Christianity and a deep involvement with the commercial sector, a tradition is to have children visit Santa Claus to tell him what they want for Christmas. Santa Claus supposedly brings gifts only to good girls and boys. Hence, it is not unusual at this time of year to see little boys and girls sitting on Santa's lap as he asks them, "Have you been a good little girl or boy?" How does the child answer? If the child knows the "deal," he or she will say "Yes," because that is the way to get presents under the tree on Christmas. But suppose you have a Santa who is interested in obtaining empirical evidence of the little girl's "good" behavior? What would Santa do? That would depend on his worldview and the paradigm from which he conducts his research.

The concept of paradigm in a research and evaluation context allows us to formalize the way in which we discuss the worldviews that influence us. Suppose that the little girl answered that she wanted to know if Santa means that, to be good, she must conform to the stereotypical image of a passive subservient female? Santa suddenly decides that he would rather not do the research or evaluation study; instead, he'll go work in gift wrap! Before we allow Santa this easy "out," let's see how his story here can illuminate the concept of paradigms.

Suppose: You have a program that is supposed to teach little girls to be good. You want to evaluate the program to see if the girls in the program are indeed good. What you see on Santa's lap is a "graduate" of the "good girl program."

Ontologically speaking, good can be defined in a numeric sense—that is, we could give a checklist to Santa (or a teacher) and say, "Check off the behaviors of this little girl, and we'll see if we have a 'good girl' here." The list might contain qualities such as being quiet, obedient, and not causing any trouble, depending on who created the checklist. If you believe that a good girl should fit the passive, subservient stereotype, then anyone who answers in a way that fits that stereotype will be considered good. (The others will not be considered as good or may even be deemed "bad.") If you set up a checklist to define a good girl—and you do not consider that contextual factors might require multiple definitions of that "good girl" reality—then you are working in the post-positivist paradigm. If you say, "Wait a minute, there might be multiple realities and no one definition of good girl," then you have to consider the definition of good girl from the perspective of the girl, Santa, and maybe others in the setting—and then you are working from the constructivist paradigm. Meanwhile, the pragmatist would say, "Which definition would be best for me to use in this situation to get the information I need?"

If you say, "Hmmmm, it is possible to have different definitions, but some of the definitions might result in harm to the little girl if she accepts them, so I have to think of issues of power when constructing the definition of the concept," then you are choosing to work in the transformative paradigm. For example, the transformative paradigm would suggest that passive subservience might result in a girl who does not speak up for herself in school, does not believe she can do the "hard" subjects of science and math, does not challenge others in an appropriate way, and that such behaviors have harmful conse-

(continued)

BOX 2.1. *(continued)*

quences attached to them. Girls do not take the classes they need to advance academically and do not prepare for the higher-paying positions (not that money is the definition of success . . .). Nevertheless, passive subservience is associated with worse economic conditions, a greater likelihood of being a victim of abuse, lack of participation in the governance process that makes the rules that affect lives, and other consequences (Mertens, 2005). Therefore, the transformative researcher/evaluator would critically examine the definition of good girl from the perspective of which definitions might lead to more harm to the most vulnerable.

Epistemologically speaking, how would the researcher or evaluator relate to the people in the setting in order to get an accurate picture of the girl's behavior and Santa's interpretation of her response? From the post-positivist paradigm, you would want to remain neutral and "distant" from the girl and Santa because you don't want to influence them in the way you answer. You might ask someone who does not interact with the girl at all to rate her behavior to avoid interjecting your own bias into the ratings. From the constructivist paradigm, you might interview both Santa and the girl (and maybe some of their significant others in the context) to determine their viewpoint regarding "good girl." As a pragmatist, you might say "What is the best way to interact in this situation to get the information that I need?"

From the transformative paradigm, you would need to interact with Santa and the girl as well as consider who else might have power in this context to influence the definitions. You would need to understand the societal influence in the definition. You might challenge both Santa and the girl to think about the consequences of their definitions.

Methodologically speaking, in the post-positivist paradigm you would use an instrument that would allow you to remain neutral, to ask the questions exactly the same way to each person, and to analyze the data into a numeric value with a margin of error. In the constructivist approach, you would establish rapport with the people in the study through sustained contact and incorporate multiple definitions in the words of the persons with the lived experience. Pragmatically, you would suggest what makes sense in this situation. In the transformative approach, you would need to acknowledge that there is a power differential between you and the people in the study. You would need to understand the community through some kind of sustained involvement, such that they would trust you to give you accurate information. You would end up with a critically examined definition of "good girl," along with recommendations for social action associated with the definitions. You might encounter resistance if you challenge the assumption, encouraged by commercial interests, that many gifts on Christmas indicate the goodness of the child or the love of the parent or a way to assuage guilt for not spending time with a child (an assumption supported by values of greed and duplicity).

The Transformative Paradigm and Its Basic Belief Systems

These are the characteristics that define the transformative paradigm:

- Places central importance on the lives and experiences of communities that are pushed to society's margins (e.g., women, racial/ethnic minorities, people with disabilities, those who are poor, and more generally, people in nondominant cultural groups).
- Analyzes asymmetric power relationships.
- Links results of social inquiry to action.
- Uses transformative theory to develop the program theory and the inquiry approach.

The basic beliefs of the transformative paradigm are presented in Box 2.2. The assumptions associated with the transformative paradigm include:

- *Axiology:* Ethical choices in research and evaluation need to include a realization that discrimination and oppression are pervasive, and that researchers and evaluators have a moral responsibility to understand the communities in which they work in order to challenge societal processes that allow the status quo to continue.

- *Ontology:* The transformative ontological assumption rejects cultural relativism in the sense that multiple definitions of reality are possible. It also investigates issues of power that lead to different definitions, acknowledging that multiple realities are socially constructed, and that it is necessary to explicitly identify the social, political, cultural, economic, ethnic, gender, and disability values that underlie definitions of realities.

- *Epistemology:* Knowledge is neither absolute nor relative; it is constructed in a context of power and privilege with consequences attached to which version of knowledge is given privilege. In order to know a community's realities, it is necessary to establish an interactive link between the researcher/evaluator and the participants in the study. Knowledge is socially and historically located within a complex cultural context.

- *Methodology:* A researcher can choose quantitative or qualitative or mixed methods. However, there should be an interactive link between the researcher and participants in determining the definition of the problem; methods should be adjusted to accommodate cultural complexity; power

BOX 2.2. Basic Beliefs of the Transformative Paradigm

Axiology: assumptions about ethics	Ethical considerations include respect for cultural norms of interaction; beneficence is defined in terms of the promotion of human rights and increase in social justice
Ontology: assumptions about the nature of what exists; what is reality	Rejects cultural relativism and recognizes the influence of privilege in determining what is real and the consequences of accepting one version of reality over another; multiple realities are shaped by social, political, cultural, economic, ethnic, gender, disability, and other values
Epistemology: assumptions about the nature of knowledge and the relationship between the researcher/evaluator and the stakeholders needed to achieve accurate knowledge	Recognizes an interactive link between researcher/ evaluator and participants/co-researchers/evaluators; knowledge is seen as socially and historically situated; issues of power and privilege are explicitly addressed; development of a trusting relationship is seen as critical
Methodology: assumptions about appropriate methods of systematic inquiry	Inclusion of qualitative methods (dialogical) is seen as critical; quantitative and mixed methods can be used; interactive link recognized between the researcher/evaluator and participants in the definition of the focus and questions; methods are adjusted to accommodate cultural complexity; and contextual and historical factors are acknowledged, especially as they relate to discrimination and oppression

First presented in Mertens (1998) and further developed in Mertens (2005).

issues should be addressed explicitly; and issues of discrimination and oppression should be recognized.

Axiological Assumption

The transformative axiological assumption promotes the principles of respect, beneficence, and justice on several fronts. Respect is critically examined in terms of the cultural norms of interaction in diverse communities and across cultural groups. Beneficence is defined in terms of the promotion of human rights and an increase in social justice. An explicit connection is made between the process and outcomes of research and evaluation studies and the furtherance of a social justice agenda.

The codes of ethics from relevant professional associations and organizations provide guidance for researchers and evaluators as to what constitutes ethical practice. As mentioned in Chapter 1, those codes of ethics have been critically reviewed and revised to reflect a greater concern for principles that reflect the axiological assumptions of the transformative paradigm. The American Evaluation Association modified its guiding principles to include an explicit principle related to the role of cultural competence in ethical evaluation practice. The American Psychological Association revised its ethics code in 2002 to strengthen protection of participants in research that involves deception (Fisher, 2003). Research ethics in psychology have been extended by Brabeck's (2000) application of feminist principles. In addition, the American Psychological Association has published several guides for working with and researching in the LGBTQ community as well as for writing in ways to avoid heterosexual bias (American Psychological Association, 1991a, 1991b, 2000b).

Two subgroups of the American Psychological Association also developed ethical guidelines relevant to the transformative paradigm. The Council of National Psychological Associations for the Advancement of Ethnic Minority Interests (CNPAAEMI) is composed of the presidents of the five national ethnic/racial minority professional associations: Asian American Psychological Association, Association of Black Psychologists, National Hispanic Psychological Association, Society for the Psychological Study of Ethnic Minority Issues (Division 45 of the American Psychological Association), and the Society of Indian Psychologists, as well as the president (or his or her designee) of the American Psychological Association (2002). The CNPAAEMI published "Guidelines for Research in Ethnic Minority Communities," and the American Psychological Association's Joint Task Force of Division 17 (Counseling Psychology) and Division 45 (Psychological Study of Ethnic Minority Issues) published "Guidelines on Multicultural Education, Training, Research, Practice, and Organizational Change for Psychologists" in 2002.

The American Psychological Association organized the multicultural guidelines by citing basic principles of ethical practice from the scholarly literature, from which they derived one principle specifically focused on research. They then derived implications for practice from the principles and guideline (see Box 2.3). Applying this guideline to our work as researchers and evaluators suggests that we must be wary of the deficit models that place the blame for social problems in the individual or culture, rather than in the societal response to the individual or cultural group.

BOX 2.3. American Psychological Association's Guidelines for Multicultural Research

PRINCIPLES

1. Recognition of the ways in which the intersection of racial and ethnic group membership with other dimensions of identity (e.g., gender, age, sexual orientation, disability, religion/spiritual orientation, educational attainment/experiences, and socioeconomic status) enhances the understanding and treatment of all people. . . .

2. Knowledge of historically derived approaches that have viewed cultural differences as deficits and have not valued certain social identities helps psychologists to understand the underrepresentation of ethnic minorities in the profession, and affirms and values the role of ethnicity and race in developing personal identity. . . .

3. Psychologists are uniquely able to promote racial equity and social justice. This is aided by their awareness of their impact on others and the influence of their personal and professional roles in society. . . .

These principles led to the following guideline for research:

Guideline #4: Culturally sensitive psychological researchers are encouraged to recognize the importance of conducting culture-centered and ethical psychological research among persons from ethnic, linguistic, and racial minority backgrounds.

IMPLICATIONS FOR METHOD

Related to the research question is choosing culturally appropriate theories and models on which to inform theory-driven inquiry. . . . Psychological researchers are encouraged to be aware of and, if appropriate, to apply indigenous theories when conceptualizing research studies. They are encouraged to include members of cultural communities when conceptualizing research, with particular concern for the benefits of the research to the community. . . .

From American Psychological Association (2002). Copyright 2002 by the American Psychological Association. Reprinted by permission.

The Guidelines for Research in Ethnic Minority Communities contains the following description of the researcher's ethical responsibilities:

> As an agent of prosocial change, the culturally competent psychologist carries the responsibility of combating the damaging effects of racism, prejudice, bias, and oppression in all their forms, including all of the methods we use to understand the populations we serve. . . . A consistent theme . . . relates to the interpretation and dissemination of research findings that are meaningful and relevant to each of the four populations[1] and that reflect an inherent understanding of the racial, cultural, and sociopolitical context within which they exist. (American Psychological Association, 2000b, p. 1)

The concept of cultural competency is explored further in Chapter 3 on human relations in research and evaluation. Interestingly, the CNPAAEMI describes the role of the psychologist as an agent of prosocial change; this is reflective of the axiological assumption of the transformative paradigm that ethical research and evaluation are defined by their furtherance of social justice and human rights, all the while being cognizant of those characteristics associated with diverse populations that impede progress on these fronts. There are other ethical guidelines associated with various professional associations, government agencies, and donor agencies (see Mertens & Ginsberg, 2009). Researcher guidelines are also available from indigenous communities that provide insights into the ethical grounding of research and evaluation from that perspective. For example, Cram (2001, as cited in Smith, 2005, p. 98) provided guidelines for researchers from the Maori people. These include:

- Respect for people, meaning people are allowed to define their own space and meet on their own terms.
- Meet people face-to-face: Introduce yourself and the idea for the research before beginning the research or sending complicated letters or other materials.
- Look and listen: Begin by looking and listening and understanding in order to find a place from which to speak.
- Sharing, hosting, being generous: These form the basis of a relationship in which researchers acknowledge their role as learners with a responsibility to give back to the community.
- Be cautious: Harm can come from a lack of political astuteness and cultural sensitivity, whether the researcher is an insider or an outsider.

- Do not trample on the dignity of a person (*mana*): Inform people without being patronizing or impatient. Be wary of Western ways of expression such as wit, sarcasm, and irony.

- Avoid arrogant flaunting of knowledge: Find ways to be generous with sharing your knowledge in a way that empowers the community.

Ontological Assumption

The ontological assumption of the transformative paradigm holds that what we can know of what exists, or the reality that we accept as true, is socially constructed. In addition, the transformative sense of ontology embraces a conscious awareness that certain individuals occupy positions of greater power and that individuals with other characteristics may be associated with a higher likelihood of exclusion from decisions about the accepted definition of what exists. This assumption has implications for the determination of the focus of a study, the development of guiding questions, and other methodological aspects of the inquiry. The transformative ontological assumption rejects a perspective of cultural relativism and recognizes the influence of privilege in determining what is real and the consequences of accepting different perceptions of reality.

Ontological assumptions rooted in positivist philosophy have been criticized by many groups who have been pushed to the margins in the scholarly decolonization literature. A critique from Native American communities notes that "production of meaning from a Eurocentric perspective does not capture any 'truth' of Native and tribal lives but also infiltrates Native lifeworlds in the form of 'epistemic violence'" (Spivak, 1988, as cited in Duran & Duran, 2000, p. 96). Furthermore:

> Social scientists have been rewriting tribal canonical texts (i.e., ritual) via anthropology and other disciplines since first contact and therein have produced meaning that has changed and distorted tribal understandings or forced them underground. Clinical psychology as well as research-oriented psychology is extremely narrow-minded. The assumptions of these fields are based on a utilitarian worldview. . . . Western empirical research is based on the illusion of objectivity, with a transhistorical, transcultural orientation. It operates within an a priori essentialist Cartesian model of a unified, rational, autonomous subject, the construction of which is problematized in the work of French poststructuralism and German critical theory. (Duran & Duran, 2000, p. 96)

The ontological assumption asks the question, what is real? In a research or evaluation context, those conducting the work identify variables and measure aspects of those variables in an attempt to locate objective truth, what is real within some level of defined probability, or truth as defined within a complex cultural context. A transformative lens focuses the ontological question on an explicit acknowledgment that reality is socially constructed and that specific characteristics associated with more or less power determine which version of reality is accepted as "real." Power issues pervade the choice of variables and their definitions, determining what is "researchable" or "evaluable." Power is implicit in decisions about which interpretations of reality will be accepted. This point is illustrated in the power associated with explanations of the achievement gap between minority and majority students in the United States, as well as in the power to label others as having a "deficit," as noted in the following student's thoughts.

Student Perspective: The Picture of a Deficit View

It does make a huge difference whether one supports the deficit perspective or the transformative paradigm since they are two very different and opposite views. If one supports the deficit perspective, that means they are focusing on deafness as a defect and it needs to be "fixed" . . . in any way possible. It seems that those who support the deficit perspective frown on the deaf. One looks down upon the deaf in society as human beings with defects. If one supports the transformative paradigm, they understand that deafness is not a defect and recognize that the deaf have their own language and culture. One accepts the deaf as equals among society.—Matt Laucka (September 2004)

O'Connor and Fernandez (2006) describe the results of a National Research Council (NRC) report that explains the impact of poverty as the basis for the overrepresentation of minority youth in special education. They critique this explanation as oversimplifying the concept of compromised development associated with being poor, and underanalyzing the effect of culture and the organization of schools that situate minority youth as academically and behaviorally deficit, thus increasing the probability that they will be placed in special education. The NRC recognized that children in high-poverty districts attend schools with less-qualified teachers, a higher degree of teacher bias, and lower funding. The NRC concludes that these variables contribute to the higher incidence of disability. In contrast, O'Connor and Fernandez describe a different reality based on the evidence:

It is schools and not poverty that place minority students at heightened risk for special education placement. . . . There is nothing about poverty in and of itself that places poor children at academic risk; it is a matter of how structures of opportunity and constraint come to bear on the educational chances of the poor to either expand or constrain their likelihood of achieving competitive, educational outcomes (O'Connor, 2002). Disproportionality, then, is the structured probability with which minority youth are more likely to be "documented" as disabled. (p. 10)

Ladson-Billings (2006) makes a similar argument in her explanation of the "achievement gap" between minority and disadvantaged students and their white counterparts. She suggests that a significant amount of research on the poor, African American, Latina/o, American Indian, and Asian immigrant students has led to very few solutions. A long history of educational research and evaluation studies has given privilege to the explanation that race/ethnicity and/or poverty are to blame for a lack of academic achievement. Might we better explore the historical, economic, sociopolitical, and moral debt in the United States that results in poor opportunities for quality educational experiences for those pushed to the margins? "What we need is a serious investigation of the costs of segregation and the costs of equitable funding. We need to use our research and evaluation skills to understand that "a cumulative effect of poor education, poor housing, poor health care and poor government services create a bifurcated society that leaves more than its children behind" (Ladson-Billings, 2006, p. 10).

Another ontological example is seen in the common assumptions that are made by hearing people unfamiliar with deaf culture who have the power to define reality for deaf people. Consider these assumptions (Harris et al., 2009):

- All deaf people can be cured by the use of a cochlear implant or a hearing aid, and all deaf people want to be cured.

- Having an interpreter is sufficient for the hearing person if he or she does not know the culture or the language, and all interpreters are good.

When deaf people are in a position to define reality for themselves, these false assumptions and beliefs will be challenged. Discourse systems, according to Ladd (2003), contain their own "unspoken rules as to what can or cannot be said and how, when and where. Each, therefore, constructs canons of 'truth' around whatever its participants decide is 'admissible evidence,' a process that in the case of certain prestigious discourses, such as those found in universities, medical establishments and communication medias, can be seen as particularly dangerous when unexamined, for these then come to determine what counts as knowledge itself" (p. 76).

As mentioned in Chapter 1, Maori scholars write about decentering whiteness (Cram et al., 2004), and deaf researchers describe a parallel process of decentering hearingness. Consider one student's views.

Student Perspective: Decentering Hearingness

Hearingness is the way hearing people see the world. We need to decenterize that to allow for everyone to be able to see the world from the lens of different people and cultures. For example, at the TISLR 9 [9th Theoretical Issues of Sign Language Research] conference in Barcelona, I was aghast to see that the conference was held in a darkly lit, very narrow and long hallway, with church-style wooden stiff benches and elaborate and dizzingly painstaking painting from bottom to the ceiling. How were we as deaf people able to see/ watch the interpreter in this kind of setting? It was awful and exhausting on my eyes. The conference organizers were obviously looking at this conference from a hearing center—not thinking from "deaf eyes."—Raychelle Harris (February 26, 2006)

Epistemological Assumption

The epistemology of the transformative paradigm describes the nature of knowledge and the type of relationship between the researcher/evaluator and the participants that are needed to achieve an understanding of what is valid knowledge within a transformative context. Transformative epistemology is characterized by a close collaboration between researchers/evaluators and the participants of the study, including both community leaders and members. Communication is achieved by use of the participants' language of choice. The research or evaluation purpose, design, implementation, and utilization are developed and implemented with appropriate cultural sensitivity and awareness. Researchers and evaluators require collaboration with the host(s) of the community—not necessarily the leaders but people of the community. The relationship is interactive and empowering.

The epistemology of the post-positivist stance is reflected in the early work of Donald Campbell, in which he envisioned an "experimenting society" that would lead to incremental reform as knowledge was gained through random assignment to alternative treatments (Campbell & Stanley, 1966). This approach included the notion that researchers and evaluators should be value neutral in order to produce scientifically valid knowledge. Christians (2005) criticizes this post-positivist notion that "a morally neutral, objective observer will get the facts right" (p. 148). He asserts that ethical behavior must be cognizant of power relations associated with gender, sexual orientation, class, ethnicity, race, and nationality. (I would add disability and other dimensions of diversity associated with less power, depending on context.) What do we gain or lose in our struggle for ethical behavior by allowing the perspectives of feminists, and others who are steeped in multivocal and cross-cultural representation, to raise questions and proffer different considerations in the ethical domain? What do we gain by having these conversations at the borderlands of ethics in research and evaluation?

The epistemological assumption raises the issue of the relationship between the researcher/evaluator and the participants in the study. In the transformative paradigm, understanding the culture and building trust are deemed paramount. There are complications associated with this assumption, however. For example, suppose a researcher or evaluator is studying people who do violence to gay men or lesbian women, or studying a white supremacist group. What does it mean to understand culture and build trust in such a context? This is another tension that surfaces in transformative work. A partial answer comes from an understanding of the notion of privilege and the investigation of unearned privilege.

Kendall (2006) explains:

> The superiority of whiteness is a social construct, created by some white men but in all our names. This construct informs both the past and the present and affects each of our lives daily. All of us who are white receive white privileges. . . . We can use [these privileges] in such a way as to dismantle the systems that keep the superiority of whiteness in place. One of the primary privileges is having greater influence, power, and resources. . . . As white people, we keep ourselves central, thereby silencing others. . . . If we look at race in North America as only a black–white construct, we miss the true purpose of the system. We must be aware of how the power holders oppressed all people of color to shape the country as they wanted it. Racism is one of several systems of oppression. Others are class, sexism, heterosexism, the institutionalized primacy of Christianity, and able-bodiedism. These systems work toward a common goal: to maintain power and control in the hands of the wealthy, white, heterosexual, Christian, able-bodied men. Examining the intersections is essential to understanding the intentional and finely crafted nature of the system. Finally, this system is brilliant but not impervious to change. We can dismantle it if we know it well and work together toward that goal. (pp. 62–63)

Another source of epistemological tension is introduced when members of nondominant cultural groups study members of the dominant culture. One student's thoughts follow.

Student Perspective: Research and the Other

Interesting reading about the word research being one of the dirtiest words in the indigenous world's vocabulary (Denzin & Lincoln, 2005, p. 1). It made me realize that research is mostly about "others"—thus all the paradigms or theories categorize "others"—like feminists, Marxists, ethnic groups, cultural groups, and queers. Are there any studies conducted on the super white male?—Heidi Holmes (January 29, 2006)

Heron and Reason (2006) ask these important questions:

Isn't it true that people can fool themselves about their experience? Isn't this why we have professional researchers who can be detached and objective? The answer to this is that certainly people can and do fool themselves, but we find that they can also develop their attention so they can look at themselves— their way of being, their intuitions and imaginings, their beliefs and actions— critically and in this way improve the quality of their claims of knowing. We call this "critical subjectivity"; it means that we don't have to throw away our personal, living knowledge in the search for objectivity, but are able to build on it and develop it. We can cultivate a high-quality and valid individual perspective on what there is, in collaboration with others who are doing the same. (p. 149)

Epistemology and Indigenous Peoples

Gordon (1990) writes about the necessity of considering African American epistemology in educational theory and practice. Wright (2003) supports the notion of understanding epistemology within the context of the African American experience when he cites the work of Scheurich and Young (1997, 1998) on "coloring epistemologies," Delgado Bernal (1998) on Chicana feminist epistemology, Ladson-Billings (2000) on an "ethnic epistemology," and Dillard (2000a, 2000b) on an "endarkened feminist epistemology" (p. 198).

Dillard's "endarkened feminist epistemology" (2000a, 2000b) is based on the intersection of race, gender, nationalism, and spirituality as it forms a sociocultural identity rather than a biological conception of race and gender. She explicitly acknowledges research as a political and utilitarian tool associated with an obligation to the black community and as an intervention to disrupt the white hegemonic research paradigm. She speaks of "*research as a responsibility* answerable and obligated to the very persons and communities being engaged in the inquiry" (Dillard, 2000a, p. 663, emphasis in original). She calls for a "transformation at the epistemological level if education research is to truly change or transform" (p. 663). The concept of endarkened feminist epistemology brings with it a change in the role of the researcher as a supportive and reflective activist in the community, as well as one who challenges the prevailing research establishment (Dillard, 2000a, as cited in Wright, 2003, p. 202).

Methodological Assumptions

Methodological assumptions create the philosophical basis for making decisions about appropriate methods of systematic inquiry. Inclusion of a qualitative dimension in methodological assumptions is critical in transformative research and evaluation as a point of establishing a dialogue between the researchers/evaluators and the community members. Mixed-methods designs can be considered to address the informational needs of the community. However, the methodological decisions are made with a conscious awareness of contextual and historical factors, especially as they relate to discrimination and oppression. Thus, the formation of partnerships with researchers/evaluators and the community is an important step in addressing methodological questions in research and evaluation.

Research and evaluation in the transformative paradigm involve multiple approaches, methods, and techniques, as well as different theories. The transformative paradigm does not have a specific set of methods or practices of its own. Richardson and St. Pierre (2005) use the concept of crystallization as a guiding metaphor for the inclusion of different perspectives, such as fiction, field notes, and scientific articles, because a crystal is composed of many facets. Researchers and evaluators get more out of their study by listening to and valuing each member's "voice" (facet) so that crystallization occurs, not triangulation and its limited three-sided perspective. Rather, several possible approaches to the interpretation of the study are welcomed. The concept of crystallization deconstructs the traditional idea of validity in social science research and conveys the prismatic nature of transformative work.

Methodologically, the transformative paradigm leads us to reframe not only the understanding of our worldviews but also our methodological decisions. Sampling needs to be reframed to reveal the dangers of the myth of homogeneity, to understand which dimensions of diversity are important in a specific context, to avoid additional damage to populations by using labels such as "at risk" that can be demeaning and self-defeating, and to recognize the barriers that exist to being part of a group that can contribute to the research and evaluation results. The transformative paradigm also leads us to (1) reconsider data-collection decisions so we are more inclined to use mixed methods; (2) become consciously aware of the benefits of involving community members in the data-collection decisions and the appropriateness of methods in relation to the cultural issues involved; (3) build trust to obtain valid data; (4) make the modifications that may be necessary to collect valid data from various groups; and (5) tie the data collected to social action.

QUESTIONS FOR THOUGHT

"Little Red Riding Hood" is a fairy tale that is popular in the United States and is familiar worldwide. It involves a little girl, Red Riding Hood, who visits her grandmother in the woods. To make a short story even shorter, a wolf comes and eats the grandmother, but a woodsman comes and chops open the wolf and the grandmother appears unharmed. The wolf, obviously, is not so lucky. Remember that the ontological assumption asks, what is reality? The story of Little Red Riding Hood ends with the familiar phrase: "They all lived happily ever after." Many people read that book as a child, or maybe their parents read it to them. I know my parents read it to me many moons ago, and I read it to my children. A common response to the ending in my house, and I expect in others, was the acceptance that they lived happily ever after because the grandmother was saved and the wolf was killed. Right? Well, what if the wolf were reading the story? Would the wolf agree that the ending was happy? Well, that depends on which definition of happiness you accept. Box 2.4 provides an opportunity to reflect on these questions as they are examined within the context of this popular fairy tale.

Trust as Link to Social Action

The transformative paradigm emphasizes the need for trust between the researcher/evaluator and the participants. This challenge of building trust and using research and evaluation findings to further justice is exemplified here by a graduate student at Gallaudet University.

Student Perspective: Building Trust

There is an energy created from people giving their opinions, but there is also a common downside as well. Many times, people ask for feedback simply for the sake of asking. It is more of a public relations tool in this sense, with the decision being reserved for those with administrative power. If this is the case, which happens often, it will actually undermine the energy created as people feel used and judge their time in giving the feedback worthless. This causes a lack of trust in the process of feedback in general . . . and lack of desire to participate in any other feedback-giving sessions because their ideas are never implemented. Therefore, if an administrator intends to solicit this information, he or she must implement some of the strategies suggested, or a larger mess will be left behind than when the person started.—Risa Briggs (2004)

Similar critiques have appeared in scholarly literature from Africa (Chilisa, 2005) and New Zealand (Smith, 2005). These are explored further in Chapter 3.

Validity

Gaventa and Cornwall (2006) argue for the need to evolve new concepts of validity in participatory research, ones that measure the quality of participation as well as the quality of knowledge:

> This implies a new understanding of participatory ethical concerns regarding such things as confidentiality and protection of research subjects, to ask questions about who participates in and benefits from research processes, how information is used and by whom, and how the process transforms or

---

BOX 2.4. Basic Beliefs and Various Paradigms: Little Red Riding Hood

The post-positivist paradigm assumes that there is one reality that can be known within a certain level of probability. If we want to measure the level of happiness at the end of the story, we might use an instrument called "The Scale of Happiness." This scale was developed with a norm group of human beings to measure general happiness. We could read the story of Little Red Riding Hood to a group of forest dwellers and then ask them to indicate how happy they feel at the end of the story by taking the Scale of Happiness. We could then compare their responses to the norm group to see if they are indeed happy, within a certain probability level. In the transformative paradigm, we would agree that happiness is a socially constructed concept, but we would want to recognize that the reality of happiness is influenced by social, political, cultural, economic, ethnic, gender, and disability values. So, we might ask what influences each character in Little Red Riding Hood as he or she pursues happiness. Has the forest been clear-cut so that the wolves no longer have access to their natural prey? Instead of killing the wolf, should thought be given to reforestation or moving the wolves to better hunting grounds? And, then there is a pragmatic approach: You are happy if you feel happy, and feeling happy is good, so don't question it.

supports power relations. How to evolve such quality standards, and how to use them to hold differing actors and institutions to account, represents one of the most important challenges facing participatory research today. (p. 80)

Chilisa (2005) furthers the conversation about the need for Eurocentric epistemologies, especially the post-positivist ones, to honor their cherished value of multiple realities and to extend it to Third World research contexts. For instance, whose validity is privileged when there are multiple realities? If validity is achieved through triangulation, which elements are triangulated? In countries where the written text was produced by the First World researchers, how much of it validates invalidity and perpetuates stereotypes about the "other"? Ethics in research should thus include creating space for other knowledge systems, including the use of local knowledge as archival sources to identify research problems and to legitimize research findings.

The concept of validity enters the axiological arena as a critical dimension in the pursuit of ethical research and evaluation practice. To establish the validity of social science research and program evaluation through a cultural lens, researchers and evaluators need to address the cultural diversity through appreciation, awareness, respect, and engagement. As mentioned in Chapter 1, multicultural validity refers to "the authenticity of understandings across multiple, intersecting cultural contexts" (Kirkhart, 2005, p. 22)—hence the importance of this dimension of validity in research and evaluation that involves researchers' understanding of and responsiveness to culture. The embedded biases of researchers and evaluators toward culturally diverse peoples threaten validity. In contrast, validity is enhanced by cultural responsiveness.

The use of triangulation in traditional qualitative research allows researchers to validate their findings through different methods: some combination of interviews, documents, field notes, and member checks, among others. Richardson and St. Pierre (2005) argue that researchers in creative analytical ethnographies do not use triangulation because they do not recognize three sides. Moreover, the metaphor of the prism (crystal) in the transformative paradigm conveys the central point that knowledge is multifaceted, and therefore a triangle is not adequate to the task. Crystallization includes an "infinite variety of shapes, substances, transmutations, multidimensionalities, and angles of approach" (p. 963). Triangulation suggests limits, whereas a crystal is a prism that grows, changes, and alters. Acting from such a transformative stance requires consideration of cultural competency, a topic addressed later in this text.

Theories Commensurate with the Transformative Paradigm

Feminist Theories

Madison (2005) describes feminist theory as being concerned with women's inclusion and access to institutions that historically denied them, as well as to transform the exclusionary structures relative to discrimination practices at multiple levels (e.g., women, family, race, sexuality, economic inequities, and the environment) with a goal of making them more just and society more equitable. Feminist theory emphasizes the divisions of labor and the distribution of wealth both nationally and internationally, as well as how meaning and value (relative to freedom and opportunity) are constituted globally.

Feminist researchers and evaluators problematize systematic relations of power in the social construction of knowledge, recognizing the centrality of gender in such power relations. Feminists make explicit the social construction of gender with its accompanying power structures and institutional and interpersonal relations, which translate difference into hierarchy and power asymmetries and privilege male over female. Feminists also recognize the multiple identities that women have and the resultant susceptibility to interlocking discrimination in their lives. For example, women of color, lesbian women, and women with disabilities encounter multiple layers of discrimination because of their sexual orientation, race/ethnicity, and disability. Feminists often disclose their biases, feelings, choices, and multiple identities in terms of their own location within the research process (Maguire, 2006, cited in Reason & Bradbury, 2006b).

Abbott, Bievenue, Damarin, and Kramarae (2007) brought a feminist lens to their review of research on gender equity in the uses of technology, and the impact that the integration of information technology into curricula and course management has had on male and female students' interest and engagement at each level of the educational continuum and teacher preparation. They reported that parity in access to technology exists for males and females in the United States, but that gaps still exist based on race/ethnicity and socioeconomic status. They did uncover differential uses of technology resulting in limitations for females regarding their future education and career options. Specifically, they examined the reasons why significantly more males than females take classes in computer science and programming in terms of the male-dominated computer culture, societal gender bias, and gender bias in computer software.

Sielbeck-Bowen, Brisolara, Seigart, Tischler, and Whitmore (2002) presented the following principles of feminist evaluation as they are derived from Western research literature:

- The central focus is on gender inequities that lead to social injustice; every evaluation should be conducted with an eye toward reversing gender inequities.
- Discrimination or inequality based on gender is systemic and structural.
- Evaluation is a political activity; the contexts in which evaluations operate are politicized, and the personal experiences, perspectives, and characteristics evaluators bring to evaluations lead to a particular political stance.
- The evaluation process can lead to significant negative or positive effects on the people involved in the evaluation.
- The evaluator must recognize and explore the unique conditions and characteristics of the issue under study; critical self-reflection is necessary.
- There are multiple ways of knowing; some ways are privileged over others.
- Transformative knowledge that emanates from an experiential base is valued.

Interestingly, when I shared these principles with evaluators from Africa who were designing evaluations to address the United Nations' priorities for women in Africa, they found them useful but were resistant to using the term *feminist* to describe the work they would do in the name of women's rights (Whitmore et al., 2006). In that context, *feminist* is a word associated with exclusion rather than inclusion. It is seen as reflecting the concerns of white women rather than the concerns of African women of color. The evaluators preferred to use the term *gender responsive* to describe their work.

Critical Race Theory

Parker and Lynn (2002) note that the roots of CRT are embedded in African American, Latino/Latina, and Native American critiques of social thought. Demands for an acknowledgment of racism in society have led to demands for examination of racism in the research and evaluation community. However, different perspectives on the character and appearance of racism in society can lead to different responses to this call to action. If racism is understood solely as a willful act of aggression against a person based on skin color or other phenotypic characteristics, then the discussion may not examine the deeply embedded racism in U.S. society. One goal of CRT is to make visible the implicit structural and less visible forms of racism as a system of oppression. Parker and Lynn (2002) note the following goals of CRT:

1. To present storytelling and narratives as valid approaches through which to examine race and racism in the law and in society;
2. To argue for the eradication of racial subjugation while simultaneously recognizing that race is a social construct; and
3. To draw important relationships between race and other axes of domination. (p. 10)

Queer Theory

Plummer (2005) locates the emergence of queer theory in the mid- to late-1980s in North America as a reflection, in part, of the academy's recognition of the legitimacy of lesbian and gay studies. Queer theory examines and addresses concerns of lesbian, gay, bisexual, transgender, and gender queer people, challenges the binary conception of male–female in identifying sex or gender, and abandons the view that some forms of sexuality are deviant.

Postcolonial and Indigenous Theories

Battiste (2000b) explains indigenous theories based on Native American scholarship; Kawakami, Aton, Cram, Lai, and Porima (2008) do so for Native Hawaiian and Maori cultures; and Chilisa (2005) contributes to this theoretical perspective from her location as an African scholar. Of great import to indigenous and postcolonial scholars is the recognition of their connection with each other and the world in historical, spiritual, and physical terms. The power to determine what is investigated, how the research and evaluation are conducted, and how the results are interpreted and used rests with the indigenous community members. This approach requires culturally appropriate and ongoing communications among the researchers/evaluators and community members, often with community members assuming the role of lead researcher/evaluator.

Additional theoretical viewpoints have much to offer the transformative researcher and evaluator, including symbolic interactionism, phenomenology, ethnomethodology, neo-Marxism, and semiotics. The *Sage Hand-*

book of *Qualitative Research* (Denzin & Lincoln, 2005) contains several chapters that explicate these theoretical perspectives.

Politics and Power

What about power relations in research and evaluation? Suppose that two female coworkers are talking, and one of the women, who is about to have a baby, wants to know if she'll have to continue to work overtime after the baby arrives. Her older, more experienced friend assures her that she will still be expected to carry on, as usual. However, doing so will call her priorities into question. The young mother-to-be recognizes the pending tension between motherhood and career that our society often imposes. She wonders if the mothers can ever win. Her friend sagely acknowledges that nothing will change until we get "more of our people on the committee."

What does this vignette suggest about who is "at the table"? What are the consequences of being at the table or not being at the table? How could a transformative perspective enter into a study, both in terms of program design and research and evaluation, associated with that issue? Here are the thoughts of one student.

Student Perspective: Issues of Power

The paradigm filters the world for us into understandable components. Therefore it is everything when considering that a researcher filters the data and transforms them into information. The idea of subjectivity now concerns me as I wonder who can be absolutely objective when interpreting data. Are we not a product of our upbringing, culture, experiences, and education?

As a minority, this especially concerns me as researchers make assumptions about my racial identity and tie it to certain factors regarding the success that I am or am not afforded in school and life. Indeed many of the researchers, often coming from privileged backgrounds do not ascertain the complexities causing the minority to have a more difficult ascension to a life the privileged are simply born into. Then I am to subscribe to myself and my people the understanding that a privileged researcher has filtered through a lens that I will never see nor comprehend. Certainly, who measures success but the researcher based on some arbitrary understanding that she/he picked up somewhere other than in my culture?—Risa Briggs (2004)

The political dimension of research "affirms people's right and ability to have a say in decisions which affect them and which claim to generate knowledge about them. It asserts the importance of liberating the muted voices of those held down by class structures and neo-colonialism, by poverty, sexism, racism and homophobia. The "pedagogy of the oppressed," to borrow Freire's term, must be matched by a 'pedagagy of the privileged': inquiry processes which engage those in positions of power, and those who are simply members of privileged groups—based on gender, class, profession, or nation" (Reason & Bradbury, 2006b, p. 10).

Research knowledge authorizes views and perceptions about the researched. An accumulated body of knowledge on the researched becomes the point of reference for legitimizing new knowledge (Chilisa, 2005). The problem of giving legitimacy to research knowledge is that most of the accessible research was not carried out by the researched. "Even in cases where there is a collaborative research between the First World researchers and Third World researchers, the First World researcher's voice is dominant and imposes the foreign categories of research, hence determining what type of knowledge can be produced" (Chilisa, 2005, p. 676).

Power is reframed by feminists as energy, strength, effective interaction, and access to resource mobilization for other and self, rather than as domination of others, whether by money, force, or the cult of personal leadership and ego (Hartsock, 1974, as cited in Maguire, 2006, p. 67). A key influence on research and evaluation is the restructuring of the power dynamics of the inquiry process itself. Based on lived experience, feminists redefined power in inquiry from their work with the poor and marginalized in adult education, community development, and development assistance (Maguire, 2006, p. 67). This issue is further explored in Chapter 3.

QUESTIONS FOR THOUGHT

Reflect on your own ideas regarding where you stand in terms of the transformative paradigm of research and evaluation. Contemplate the following questions:

- How have you experienced depiction of people who are pushed to the margins of society in your own life, in the media, or, specifically, in research/evaluation contexts?

- What evidence have you seen of the deficit perspective with regard to people who are pushed to the margins?

- What evidence of the transformative paradigm have you seen in the world?

- What difference does it make if you hold a deficit or resilience view of people who are pushed to the margins and the social systems that surround us?

A Deeper Reflection

Reflect on your position in reference to the transformative paradigm and indicate any changes (growth) you feel you have experienced by reading and reflecting on this paradigm. Specifically, consider:

- How does the concept of paradigm further your understanding of the experiences of people who are pushed to the margins of society?

- To what extent do you find yourself intrigued by, or comfortable with, the transformative paradigm? Do you find yourself somewhat in the middle? Are you withholding judgment until you know more?

- Use the words *axiology, ontology, epistemology,* and *methodology* in your explanation. Discuss your position and give your reasons.

- Discuss methodological challenges you anticipate would be associated with the transformative paradigm.

Summary

✓ The meaning of the concept of paradigm is explained in terms of four basic belief systems: axiology (ethics), ontology (reality), epistemology (knowledge), and methodology.

✓ The meaning of the transformative paradigm is explained in terms of these four belief systems.

  ✓ Axiology—emphasizes human rights and social justice.

  ✓ Ontology—rejects cultural relativism and acknowledges the influence and consequences of power and privilege in what is deemed real.

  ✓ Epistemology—advocates culturally competent relations between the researcher/evaluator and community members.

  ✓ Methodology—employs culturally appropriate mixed methods tied to social action.

✓ The importance of trust, validity, and power issues foreshadows further discussion of these topics in Chapter 3.

✓ Commensurate theories such as feminist theories and CRT are presented.

MOVING ON TO CHAPTER 3 . . .

In the following chapter, issues related to the establishment of trust in research and evaluation relationships are explored. This process begins with the development of self-understanding by the researcher or evaluator and moves to the development of relationships with community members that focus on creating conditions for transformative work to occur.

 A prism is grown. Isaac Newton did not understand the intricacies of prisms because he used too wide a spectrum of light to study them. Scientists who followed Newton applied a more refined method of study that yielded insights into the missing bits of information.

Note

1. The American Psychological Association developed guidelines for four specific groups: Asian American/Pacific Islander populations, persons of African descent, Hispanics, and American Indian participants.

CHAPTER 3

Self, Partnerships, and Relationships[1,2]

I see having some version of self-reflective practice as a necessary core for all inquiry. For example, anyone engaging in collaborative research needs robust, self-questioning discipline as their base.
—MARSHALL (2006, p. 335)

In the absence of detailed conceptual and methodological guidance from existing approaches to evaluation, therefore, this last part of the project in India is very much a work in progress. And at its heart lies a difficult conundrum: For our team of evaluators to assist in the development and judgement of criteria related to the transformation of worldviews to accommodate profoundly systemic perspectives on the world—essentially the facilitation of stakeholder development as "systemic beings"—we ourselves need to undergo such an epistemic transformation as a precondition.

The logic presented here, I believe, dictates that such a competency is imperative in the face of the complex challenges of epistemic transformation for systemic development.
—BAWDEN (2006, p. 45)

IN THIS CHAPTER . . .

▼ The role of human relations in the process of conducting transformative research and evaluation is examined as a means to enhance validity and develop respectful partnerships that prioritize ethics and reciprocity.

▼ Methods that facilitate critical self-reflection in a social justice context are explored, with specific emphasis on the roles of power and privilege.

▼ Knowing yourself in relation to the community is discussed in terms of potential bias, membership in the community (or not), and cultural competence as an essential disposition in conducting transformative work.

▼ Strategies for developing relationships and partnerships are presented, with a focus on the concept of trust.

▼ Challenges associated with building respectful and effective partnerships and relationships are discussed, including issues of language, the will to engage, ethics, and capacity building.

Honest and respectful relationships among human beings involved in any inquiry are essential to achieve the goals of transformative research and evaluation. The development of effective relationships is a multifaceted endeavor. Establishment of effective relations is fraught with challenges, including securing the time needed to develop a relationship, dealing with variations in levels and types of power, addressing mismatched or conflicting priorities, and accommodating differences on key characteristics between researchers/evaluators and participants. The importance of working through these challenges is critical to the conduct of valid research and evaluation within the transformative paradigm.

As the opening quotations of this chapter make clear, self-knowledge is an essential part of establishing effective partnerships and relationships, as well as for clarifying worldviews. Self-knowledge alone is not sufficient, however; personal transformation is a necessary part of social transformation. Combining self-knowledge with cultural knowledge and skills in effective partnering facilitates (1) the development of the research or evaluation focus and identification of questions; (2) the development of interventions; and (3) making decisions about design, measures, samples, data collection, analysis, interpretation, and use that are in keeping with the philosophical assumptions of the transformative paradigm. Later chapters address these specific aspects of the partnership relationship. In this chapter, enhanced validity is discussed as the basis for justifying a focus on understanding self and self in relation to community, as are strategies to enhance knowledge of self, culture, and the synergistic factors intrinsically involved in human relationships—all of which are essential for the establishment of effective partnerships and relationships.

QUESTIONS FOR THOUGHT

• What is the place of self-reflection and human relations in research and evaluation?

• What are the ramifications of sharing some salient characteristic of the community in which I am researching or evaluating?

- What are the ramifications of being an "outsider" to that community?
- How do power and privilege affect relations in research and evaluation?
- How can I gain the self-knowledge required to respectfully engage with participants?
- How can I come to understand a community in its full complexity?
- What are my options if time constraints prevent a prolonged and sustained involvement with the community?
- How can I create the will to engage in self-reflection, honest understanding of cultural complexities, and trusting partnerships?
- How can I facilitate the development of transformative partnerships?

Human Relations as Factors Contributing to Research Validity and Rigor

As mentioned in Chapter 1, Kirkhart (2005) and Lincoln (1995) provide arguments that support the integral connection between the quality of the human relations in research and evaluation settings and the validity of the information that is assembled. In this chapter, the relevant justifications for focusing on human relations are explored further as a basis for enhanced validity, especially Kirkhart's "interpersonal justification" (i.e., the quality of the interactions between and among participants in the inquiry process), and Lincoln's (1995) standards for quality in research and evaluation that relate to the notion of community and the need to understand the community and the effects of the study process and findings on the community.

Kirkhart (2005) notes that "evaluators' personal characteristics, orientations and identifications, life histories, academic training, and cultural experiences are inescapably woven into the theoretical understandings they put forth for consideration" (p. 25). Definitions of validity used in the world of research and evaluation are themselves culturally constructed constructs. Based on Kvale's (1995, as cited in Kirkhart, 2005) critique of the cultural boundaries of validity as a social construction, Kirkhart discusses the gatekeeping function that validity plays in determining what is seen as legitimate knowledge. If this gatekeeping is used to exclude the views of the nonmajority communities, then it serves to support the status quo and disallows challenges to power distributions. Hence, culturally unexamined constructions of validity can serve as collaborators of oppression and discrimination. Kirkhart (2005) defines validity as "an overall judgment of the adequacy and appropriateness of evaluation-based inferences and actions and their respective consequences" (p. 30). In relation to this inclusive definition, validity is strengthened by critical self-reflection, especially directed at assumptions that emanate from a position of majority privilege.

Lincoln's (1995) standards for rigor in research include the assertion that the researcher should know the community "well enough" to link the research results to positive action within that community. This standard raises the question, what does it mean to know a community *well enough*? The work of indigenous research scholars provides insights into possible answers to this question.

When Maori people discuss the meaning of having researchers come into their community, they emphasize the need to consult with appropriate people and to learn the basic principles of interacting in a trustworthy way within their culture (Cram et al., 2004). Researchers who want to work within the Maori community need to behave in ways that reflect:

- *Whakapapa*—Research begins with revealing where you come from and who your family is; what are your family connections?

- Telling it like it is, to the right people—Researchers must identify people in the community to engage in the research process and be honest throughout the research endeavor.

- The importance of both *kanohi kit e kanohi* (being present) and *kanohi kitea* (the seen face)—Researchers must be present and face-to-face with the people.

- Being knowledgeable about the history of research in this community—Researchers need to be aware of the history of legislation, policy, discrimination, and oppression, as well as the community's cultural legacy.

McKenzie (2001) adds the following concepts from the Maori culture:

- *Whakaiti* means being humble, not standing out from the crowd (a belief held so strongly by many Maori students that they will disguise their abilities rather than be treated above their peer group)—Researchers should acknowledge that their knowledge is limited and they are eager to learn from the community members.

- *Whakahihi* is the opposite, being boastful and bragging—Researchers should not appear to be boastful or self-praising.

Smith (1999) added to this list:

- *Aroha kit e tangata*—show respect for people.
- *Titiro, whakarongo . . . korero*—Look, listen . . . speak.
- *Manaaki kit e tangata*—Share and host people; be generous.
- *Kia tupato*—Be cautious.
- *Kaua e takahia te mana o te tangata*—Do not trample over the *mana* of the people.
- *Kaua e mahaki*—Don't flaunt your knowledge.

These Maori scholars provide us with a way of entering a community that has the potential of enhancing the validity of our work by engaging respectfully with the community members. Reciprocity is a key element in establishing research and evaluation partnerships that can yield valid information for all concerned because it helps to address power differentials that can diminish a willingness to share life experiences in an open way.

Reciprocity and Validity

Broom and Klein (1999) posit that reciprocity is necessary for healthy, trusting relationships. People need to feel that they are receiving as much valuable energy as they are giving. Determining reciprocity is a complex matter because people's ideas of equity and fair exchange usually involve varying ideas of right and wrong (or the rules that we use to determine what is fair or unfair). People usually respond positively if they feel they are getting enough in return for what they are giving. They may respond angrily when they feel they are facing bias, unfairness, or injustice. A successful exchange depends on an ability to identify the stakes for all the players. To this end, we can ask the participants: "What kinds of outcomes do you want for yourself in this exchange?" (p. 85). Broom and Klein describe six basic types of exchange currencies first proposed by Uriel and Edna Foa (Foa & Foa, 1974). These include money, tangible goods, intangible service, positive regard, prestige, and sexual gratification. These are more closely associated with the traditional notion of beneficence than the transformative notion; this issue is further explored in Chapter 7 in the section on beneficence.

Native American populations have developed research review processes that involve the participating tribes and place a premium on participatory and collaborative research that balances the needs of the community and the needs of the researchers (Caldwell et al., 2005). When this balance is upset, trust may be broken, resulting in problems with the research study. Authentic partnerships are viewed as give-and-take relationships and require that both researchers and participants initiate the research and frame the focus of that research. Establishing an equal partnership requires reciprocity: that is, if a researcher takes participants' ideas and time, he or she is expected to give back in the way of resources, skills, employment, or training. Caldwell et al. (2005) explain:

> It is customary for researchers to describe the anticipated benefits, risks, and costs of the research when preparing grant proposals and in submissions to IRBs. Prior to tribal control of research, discussions of anticipated research benefits in Indian Country tended to be abstract. Requiring researchers to explicitly outline concrete costs and benefits to the participating tribe(s) tends to clarify thinking and make assumptions and expectations explicit. In our experience, this process is beneficial to all parties involved. (p. 9)

Caldwell et al. note that there can be conflicting perspectives on the benefit of the research to the tribe, based on differing positions within the tribe and the attitudes of tribal members toward change. Involvement of diverse members of the tribe in the process can yield improved study acceptance and benefit; however, it is also possible that the research will become mired in conflict and abandoned. Or, if the research is carried out without taking the time to explore and respond to differences, the results of the study may be rejected.

Ethical Considerations

Cram et al. (2004, p. 158) provide a valuable perspective that integrates ethical principles with what you need to know about yourself and the community. A process of writing, reflection, presentation, and community participation (*hui*, or Maori ceremonial gathering) was used to develop a research protocol for doing research that is *tika* or right. Three themes emerged from this process:

- The importance of researchers knowing themselves.
- The importance of knowing yourself in relation to your community.
- Growing in one's ability to function in a culturally competent manner.

These themes provide a reasonable structure for the remainder of this chapter.

Knowing Yourself

Researchers and evaluators must be critically self-reflexive and able to enter into a high-quality awareness to understand the psychological state of themselves and others thereby enabling participation in dialectical relationships (Lincoln, 1995). This heightened self-awareness is necessary for personal transformation and critical subjectivity. Self as instrument is a topic of discussion in much of the qualitative research literature (Marshall, 2006). In keeping with the acknowledgment that there are no value-free interactions between two human beings, knowledge of self is a requirement for doing any type of valid research or evaluation work, no matter what methods are used. In the spirit of full disclosure, my story is included as Appendix B, in which I describe my journey along the road of discovery that led to my immersion in the transformative paradigm. An explanation of my journey can be seen in a more succinct way in the illustration of me with my mentor Eleanor Roosevelt (in spirit) (Box 3.1).

Cram et al. (2004) contribute the Maori perspective on the importance of knowing yourself in terms of the social, cultural, and political context in which the research or evaluation is conducted. Specifically, researchers and evaluators need to be aware of their own expectations and assumptions and their competence in communicating these to participants in the inquiry process.

Symonette (2004) examined the importance of self as instrument and provided guidance in how to increase self-awareness in culturally complex research and evaluation settings. She wrote:

> Culture is dynamic and ever changing, so becoming multicultural is a lifelong process. Standing still in one's current repertoire of sociocultural knowledge, skills and insights automatically starts a downward slide. Complacency in current understandings breeds and fuels a creeping intercultural incompetence. This "self-in-dynamic-context" learning and development journey is without end in that it summons ongoing personal homework: notably, ever deepening awareness and knowledge of self-as-instrument and lifelong project in process. (pp. 96–97)

How we see ourselves or what we believe we bring to the situation is insufficient, and possibly inaccurate, self-knowledge. Symonette (2004) calls

BOX 3.1. Eleanor Roosevelt and Working Together

Eleanor Roosevelt died in 1962 and was buried in Hyde Park next to her husband. Her contributions to the cause of peace and the welfare of people was expressed clearly by Adlai Stevenson, former ambassador to the United Nations, at the time of her death: "What other human being has touched and transformed the existence of so many? . . . She walked in the slums of the world, not on a tour of inspection . . . but as one who could not feel contentment when others were hungry. Her glow warmed the world . . . she embodied the vision and the will to achieve a world in which all men [sic] can walk in peace and dignity."

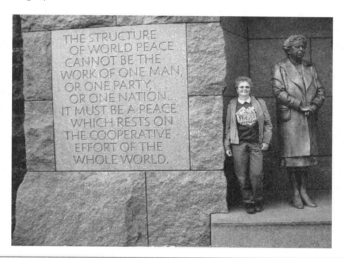

this unilateral self-awareness and suggests that multilateral self-awareness is even more essential:

> Even more important for the viability, vitality, productivity and trust-building capacity of a transaction and relationship cultivation is multilateral self aware-ness: self in context and self as pivotal instrument. Who do those that one is seeking to communicate with and engage perceive the evaluator as being? . . . Regardless of the truth value of such perceptions, they still rule until authenti-cally engaged in ways that speak into the listening. (p. 100)

Bell (2001) developed a modified Johari Window[3] to enhance self-awareness of social justice educators. I modified the context and probing questions to fit the research/evaluation context. Bell used the following graphic to depict the relevant quadrants:

Johari Window		
	Things I know about myself	Things I don't know about myself
Things others know about me	Open area	Blind area
Things others don't know about me	Hidden area	Unknown area

The *open area* is our comfort zone—I know such-and-such about myself, and I am comfortable sharing it with others. The open area allows for personal growth through self-disclosure and receiving feedback from others. You can use the following questions to expand your open area:

- How open am I about my own process of learning about social justice and my own socialization?
- What kinds of things about myself do I share easily with others?
- How do I use myself and my experiences in my research?
- What is open for discussion in my interactions with others?

The *hidden area* represents self-knowledge of which I am conscious but that I choose not to disclose to others. I may have very good reasons to keep some personal things private about myself. However, Bell encourages us to think about what we choose not to disclose by asking ourselves these questions:

- What do I avoid disclosing about myself? Why?
- What are my motivations for not disclosing certain things?
- What do I hide that I might want to disclose?
- What do I hide that I think could interfere with good research or evaluation? Is my rationale clear and conscious?

The *blind area* holds great potential to impede our ability to work within the transformative paradigm because it contains those things about ourselves of which we are not conscious but that others notice about us.

These are the things that may be hidden from us by normative socialization, cultural blindness, and assumptions of privilege. Bell suggests these questions for this area:

- What am I likely not to perceive due to my own social positioning?
- What have I learned that was previously in my blind area?
- How open am I to feedback and how do I respond when others give me feedback?
- What important insights/learning have I gained from inviting feedback in the past?

Kendall (2006) discusses the blind area in the context of imbalances of power and privilege. The potential for miscommunication is great and may result in damage to relationships and suspicion in further contacts. White people often find it difficult

> to accept that a person of color would automatically be suspicious of any white person they are talking to, just as someone who is nonprivileged in other areas of identity would be—people with disabilities of able-bodied people; women of men; lesbian, gay, bisexual, or transgender people of heterosexuals; poor people of wealthier people. Because so many white people see ourselves as individuals and as relatively good people, we have a hard time imagining that we pose a threat to someone we work with or are talking to. We see ourselves as entering into conversations as just us; usually, the person of color sees us as a representative of our race, our gender, and our class. (p. 129)

Such a blind spot can lead to good intentions that are belied by behavior that does not have the desired impact.

The *unknown area*—of which neither we nor others are aware—represents a large unexplored area. Bell suggests that this area can be reduced by self-exploration, education, psychotherapy, and broadening of life experience. This ongoing self-exploration may reveal reasons for triggers, provide a deeper understanding of our own socialization and personal psychology, uncover unexplored potentialities, and reveal motivations, fears, and expectations related to social justice issues. Questions to ask:

- What was previously unknown to me (and to others) which I now know about myself?
- How did I become aware of this?
- What other puzzles intrigue me and call me to further exploration?

The Johari Window provides a method for reducing our blind area by inviting feedback from others, reducing the hidden area as we decide to disclose things that would be appropriate, and reducing the unknown area through a process of self-exploration. Symonette (2004) summarizes:

> The deepest and richest insights emerge from authentic communications and deliberations across relevant diversity divides. Again, such communications require more than facts-and-figures knowledge and skills or do's-and-taboos checklists—especially when they are associated with making evaluative judgments about merit, worth, value, congruence, etc. Like any other social relations, it matters who is carrying what and how in determining the extent to which assessment and evaluation processes are embraced as a resource or suspiciously tended to in a perfunctory way. (p. 101)

Self-Checks Built into the Self-Knowledge Process

Guzman (2003) recognizes that evaluators have emotional reactions to the participants and the community members in their projects. She suggests that evaluators build a process check into their evaluation plans that would allow the evaluators to have constant discourse with members of the evaluation team and the community. In this way, evaluators can share their feelings about their experiences with the participants and obtain feedback from community members as to how to interpret their own and the participants' emotions.

Marshall (2006) also emphasizes the importance of knowing yourself in terms of taking time to notice how you perceive, make meaning, frame issues, and make choices to speak or not to speak. She calls this process the inner arc (p. 335) and recommends that researchers pay attention to their assumptions, repetitions, patterns, themes, dilemmas, and key phrases that are charged with energy or that seem to hold multiple meanings. To this end, she suggests the use of journaling to capture inner streams of inquiry. She uses different-colored pens and pencils to reflect additional insights that she gains throughout the duration of her research. She then describes her reflective processes in terms of exploring outer arcs; that is, by pursuing understandings outside of herself in some way. "This might mean actively questioning, raising issues with others, or seeking ways to test out my developing ideas. Or it might mean finding ways to turn issues, dilemmas or potential worries into cycles of (explicit-to-me) inquiry into action, perhaps seeking to influence or change something and learning about situation, self, issues and others in the process" (p. 336). She recommends trying to keep notes on what people are saying, as verbatim as possible, at least of key phrases and ways of formulating meaning. Selective attention is a known limitation in all research; therefore, this act of writing, reflecting, and acting becomes a cyclical engagement throughout the research process as ideas emerge and evolve.

Autoethnography

Autoethnography is one approach with which researchers or evaluators can come to terms more explicitly with who they are in the inquiry context. The definition of *autoethnography* ranges from memoir to recollection to personal journals to stories, and ethnographic accounts (Charmaz, 2006). Anderson (2006) identifies five key features of autoethnography:

- The researcher is a complete member of the group that he or she is studying. However, the researcher plays a dual role as group member and researcher; hence the necessity of being consciously aware of conversations and behaviors while simultaneously engaging in those conversations and behaviors.

- Reflexivity has long been a hallmark of qualitative work, and involves understanding the reciprocal influence between the researcher and his or her settings and informants. Autoethnography focuses on trying to understand both self and others through a reflective examination of one's actions and perceptions in dialogue with others.

- The researcher is a highly visible social actor in the written text, including his or her feelings and experiences and how they changed as vital data that contribute to understanding the social world being described.

- As the autoethnographic researcher is trying to understand a phenomenon in a complex world, it is important that data be collected through dialogues with others.

- Analysis of the data should go beyond representation of this single case toward building theories about the phenomenon.

Charmaz (2006) raises the issue of adding fictional elements to the narrative as a way of telling the story in order to say something about the human condition. However, the introduction of fictional elements into a data-based narrative is problematic. To what extent is the narrative rendering an accurate description of the experience versus one that claims verisimilitude? To what extent has the author taken other perspectives into account? To what extent do researchers move beyond their own experiences when they engage with members of the studied world? Charmaz suggests that autoethnography can serve to reify stereotypes if the researcher does not learn of varying perspectives from his or her engagement with others.

Spry (2007) describes authoethnography as a means to achieving personal transformation when researchers/evaluators place their experiences within the larger context of society. Autoethnography invites transformation when it is undertaken as critical self-reflection and as a means to subvert an oppressive dominant discourse. Stimulus questions might include:

- What transformative moments in my own life do I recall?
- How do those experiences illuminate my experiences in relation to others?
- What was I thinking? What was I feeling?
- How do I relate to those experiences now? How do I feel now?

Spry illustrates the power of autoethnography as a tool in research on many sensitive topics, including the death of a child, parenting a teenage boy, alcohol or drug abuse, and sexual assault.

Self-Awareness of Power and Privilege

How does sitting in a position of power and privilege influence one's ability to develop relationships in a research context? Nairn and McCreanor (1991) recognized the potential blindness created when those of privilege try to understand the experience of those with less privilege. Symonette (2004) also addressed this issue:

> Most important is the extent to which the meaning-making transactions and interpretations are perceived and received as on-target and appropriate by those on the other side(s) of relevant diversity divides. Those who stand and sit on the privilege- and power-connected sides of diversity divides typically have not a clue regarding these dynamics or their implications for social relations and outcomes. As Kaylynn TwoTrees (1993) puts it, "privilege is a learning disability." Consequently, one may look but still not see, listen but still not hear, touch but still not feel. In contrast, those not so situated within the power-and-privilege hierarchy maintain high consciousness nearly all of the time because such consciousness enhances opportunities for access and success and more fundamentally enables survival. Such divergent realities often manifest in persons vigorously talking past each other even when seemingly using the same words. (2004, pp. 100–101)

Unearned Privilege and Personal Work

Kendall (2006) notes that addressing issues of privilege (whether based on skin color or other characteristics associated with differences in privilege) is challenging. Many people with privilege (such as myself) find it incredulous when someone initially points out that they do have privilege. My self-image included a lot of different perspectives, but power and privilege had not risen to a conscious level for me. Only upon concentrated self-reflection and interaction with critical friends was I able to begin to address this issue at a personal level. Kendall acknowledges that there is a need for clarification as to why we would pursue an undertaking that is difficult and uncomfortable. When asked why, Kendall (2006) replies: "For many people the most immediate answer is that it is the right thing to do. If we do not work to change ourselves and our systems, we continue to be complicit in the oppression of others whether we mean to or not. We do this exploration because our lives depend on it—our physical, psychological, spiritual, and economic lives" (p. 23). Bennis and Thomas (2002) call opportunities for transformative experiences that allow an individual to come to a new or altered sense of identity "crucibles." As the word *crucible* implies, pain can be associated with this transformative process.

The basic beliefs of the transformative paradigm explicitly recognize the role of power and privilege in the definition of what is real, the interactions between the researcher/evaluator and the community, and in the choice of methods for data collection.

The words *power* and *privilege* have been increasingly associated with negative connotations in the world of those who seek social justice. For example, Symonette (2004) reminds us that "evaluators need enhanced understandings of related systemic processes of asymmetric power relations and privilege, not simply awareness and knowledge of difference and diversity. . . . How and to what extent is sociocultural diversity associated with patterned differences in access, resource opportunities, and life chances?" (p. 108).

Some people think of power in terms of a dichotomy, such that organizations and experts have power and the oppressed, grass-roots, marginalized do not (Gaventa & Cornwall, 2006). Broom and Klein (1999) acknowledge that when power is viewed as finite, it sets up a situation wherein one person's winning means another person's loss. However, they propose the conceptualization of power as an infinite game (i.e., any set of activities that has rules and participants) in which win–win is a possible outcome. The purpose of playing a win–win game is to continue and maintain the game, thus neither self-esteem nor identity is at stake. Rather playing the game is motivated by curiosity, a love of learning and creativity, and a valuation of differences. In Broom and Klein's (1999) words:

> In a world operating from the infinite perspective, gender and racial differences would be viewed not only as spicy additions to the essential sameness of humankind but also as integral factors in improving the human condition. The contributions that women and people of color would make if invited to participate fully with men and whites in the game of power would certainly be remarkable. Moreover, the mutual learning produced by this perceptual shift would act as a vital key unlocking the harmonic potential of technologies, organizations, societies, and perhaps the entire world. We would see how differences can form harmonic relationships and how conflict can move toward resolution; in this way, we would appreciate the beauty of diversity just as we might appreciate the beauty of music, its forms comprising tonal differences linked in concordant ways. However, as the infinite view is eminently practical, we would most appreciate the transformative power of creating harmony from differences—the real improvements that can result. (p. 19)

For effective partnerships to evolve, the issue of power differences needs to be recognized. Chilisa (2005) comments on inequity in power relations:

> Collaborative research between First and Third World researchers invariably begins with a contract that positions each researcher within a hierarchical structure. . . . First World researchers are invariably referred to as team leaders, lead researchers, or research co-coordinators. They bring certain methods to be learnt and applied by the Third World. As leaders they are also assigned the responsibility of producing the final document. The assumption is that they are better researchers in comparison with the "other" because their educational background is superior in comparison with the . . . "other" and also because research is communicated in their language at which they are masters and of which the "others" should be masters. The framework goes back to established colonial times, when the colonized were regarded as empty vessels to be filled. But it also indicates the colonial ideology that seeks to fashion the world into sameness. The draft of the contract agreement between the First World researchers and the Third World researchers was clear on who was producing and controlling knowledge. (p. 676)

The contract read thus: "Any and all intellectual property including copyright in the final and other reports arising from the work under this agreement will be property of the University of X." Chilisa (2005) describes her growing self-awareness that was sparked by these contractual terms as well as by the conflicts she felt between the Western-based research methods and their results and her knowledge and lived experience of Botswana culture. She writes:

> I . . . describe my journey into the empire and back as one who has studied in the Western centers. Returning to my own communities, cultures and languages brings me to realize the gap between my training and my culture. I therefore wish to reflect and narrate on the lessons I learnt as an indigenous, Western educated intellectual, co-opted into the dominant First World epistemologies on HIV/AIDS and participating in the naming and description of the "other." The discussion is based on a critique of research studies that I conducted, along with researchers from the so-called First World. I found myself troubled by the standard topics and language in the research on HIV/AIDS because they trivialized the core values that define my identity such as the totem and taboos that I continue to practice without question. Worse still, these topics and languages are in most cases further entrenched through data-gathering instruments such as the questionnaire survey that makes it impossible to escape from Western perceptions on HIV/AIDS. (p. 668)

Recognition of power differentials in the research and evaluation context contributes to the process of knowing yourself as a researcher or evaluator. It also adds credence to a view of power as productive and relational (Foucault, 1979). Gaventa and Cornwall (2006) extend Foucault's conception of power to include the effect of power on those who are relatively powerful and those who are relatively less powerful: "Power can exist in the micro-politics of the relationship for the researcher to the researched, as well as in broader social and political relationships; power affects actors at every level of organizational and institutional relationships, not just those who are excluded or at the bottom of such relationships" (p. 73). Thus, Gaventa and Cornwall suggest a need not just to study the "pedagogy of the oppressed" (Freire, 1970b), but also the "pedagogy of the oppressor" and the relation between the two. Questions to consider include:

- How do we understand the dynamics of the power when participatory methods are employed by the powerful?
- Whose voices are raised and whose are heard?
- How are these voices mediated as issues of representation become more complex with the use of participatory methods in larger-scale planning and consultation exercises?

Knowing Yourself in Relation to the Community

This section explores the issues of power and privilege in relation to indigenous perspectives, and touches on ways to enhance methodological rigor through the development of partnerships. Questions arise: What if I am a member of the researched or evaluated community? What if I am not a member of the community? To what extent is there a need to reflect the demographic characteristics of the community in the person of the researcher/evaluator? Is the validity of research/evaluation work threatened if it is conducted by a member of the community? (I find it mildly amusing that the question of allowing researchers' or evaluators' personal biases to sway perception and judgments arises in the context of indigenous researchers, when my perception tells me that there are no value-free interactions between two human beings. So, I'll add the question: Is the validity of research/evaluation work threatened if it is conducted by someone who does *not* share salient characteristics of diversity with the participants in the study?)

The term *insider research* is something of a misnomer in most circumstances as even if researchers belong to the community they are researching, they are obliged, within a relationship ethic, to establish and maintain a role as a researcher (Smith, 2004, as cited in Cram et al., 2004, p. 162). For example, when Cram returned home (New Zealand) to do her dissertation research, she experienced conflicts; she did not fit in at home at this point, whereas she did fit in the academic community where she had spent several years. She realized the importance of reconnecting with the people in her home community through visits, talk, and sharing in the everyday rituals of drinking and eating. Even though she was from this community, she needed to spend time reestablishing relationships over a 2-year period in a Maori-respectful way before she could proceed with her research.

A critical and implicit concept in the journey to understanding self in terms of community is the notion of respect. Smith (2004, as cited in Cram et al., 2004) noted that misinterpretations in partnerships sometimes result from clashes in cultural views as to the meaning of respect. Respect in research and evaluation in U.S. contexts means respect for the individual and his or her autonomous decision-making capacities. In Maori culture, respect in a research context is conveyed by how you greet someone, how you choose to dress, and how you spend a few months establishing a relationship.

The evaluation framework developed at the Howard University Center for Research on the Education of Students Placed at Risk (CRESPAR) and the Talent Development (TD) Model of School Reform includes direct recognition of the importance of matching salient characteristics of the evaluation team with the participants. Butty, Reid, and LaPoint (2004) cite Frierson, Hood, and Hughes (2002) in their discussion of the self as instrument and the need for shared vantage points in order to obtain quality data. They state:

> Therefore, an instrument (or individual) that is an improper measure provides invalid data. In other words, if those who are collecting and recording the data are not attuned to the cultural context in which the program is situated, the collected data could be invalid. As individuals with a shared racial background with the stakeholders, TD (Talent Development) project team members went into the urban school context with an increased level of sensitivity and awareness to the plight and lived experiences of the various stakeholder groups. (p. 44)

In the evaluation of a school-based family, school, and community partnership program (part of the TD CRESPAR initiative), LaPoint and Jackson (2004) also identified the deliberate matching of similarities between the evaluation team and the school community as a facilitating factor in the establishment of a trusting relationship. They attempted to match race, ethnicity, gender, age, social class, and cultural similarity or familiarity between the evaluators and the participants. They also indicated that the evaluation staff had several years of experience in working with low-income, black participants in research, policy, program, and advocacy activities in a variety of settings.

Thomas (2004) affirmed the benefits associated with the sharing of salient characteristics between researcher/evaluator and the participants in the evaluation of an urban school setting in which many of the students were African Americans from low-income homes. At the same time, she recognized that diversity goes deeper than race in such situations, citing dimensions such as social class, education level, gender, status, and needs that relate to power differentials in the setting.

Heron and Reason (2006) suggest the following procedures as a means of removing the distortion of uncritical subjectivity from the various ways of knowing that emerge:

- *Research cycling.* Participants should be prepared to go through the inquiry process several times, cycling between action and reflection, thereby refining their understandings and reducing distortions.

- *Divergence and convergence. Convergence* is a strategy that allows participants to revisit the same research focus several times;

divergence means that the group moves on to a new research focus as a result of what they learned in earlier cycles of the inquiry process.

- *Authentic collaboration.* The inquiry group needs to develop an authentic form of collaboration based on egalitarian relationships. People need to sustain their involvement in the group throughout the cycles of research, in a way that allows every group member to express his or her views and be heard.

- *Challenging consensus collusion.* Any group member can challenge the assumptions that underlie the knowledge being created or any part of the process by which it is created.

- *Managing distress.* The group needs to develop mechanisms that allow distress to surface and that process the distress in a respectful way.

- *Reflection and action.* A balance between reflection and action is necessary so that participants can move through the cycle of action and reflection.

- *Chaos and order.* Balance needs to be maintained and restored as necessary, given that divergence of thought is encouraged. Yet, an inordinate degree of confusion and ambiguity may result in stalling a group's progress. Thus groups need to be prepared to deal with differences in a constructive manner, without exercising premature closure for the purpose of maintaining peace.

Who Can Research or Evaluate Whom?

bell hooks (1990) raised this question of voice by asking: Who can research whom? Who speaks for whom? Who speaks for those who do not have access to the academy? The researcher/evaluator has an obligation to seek out and involve those who are silent or pushed to the margins.

Spivak (1988) framed the question of voice in this way: "Can the subaltern speak?" (p. 217). Chilisa (2005) notes that the subaltern does speak with a discourse of resistance. And, if research or evaluation excludes the indigenous ways of knowing, it is likely to fail to come up with results that can enhance the quality of life of the communities. Feminists raised the question of who can research whom many years ago. Can women only study women? Men only men? Extending the idea: Africans only Africans? Deaf only deaf? Maori only Maori?

The argument that one must share a particular salient characteristic to do research or evaluation with a community has merit. This merit persists, despite examples of individuals who do not share such characteristics who have contributed to our understanding of discrimination and oppression in the context of furthering social justice. Jonathon Kozol (2005) comes to mind as a white, hearing, able-bodied man with a degree from a prestigious university who chooses to teach in the poorest county in the United States and writes books that graphically depict the conditions of life under which children who live in poverty are expected to learn. Hence, sharing a salient characteristic has the potential to add validity to a study; however, this is not the only possible strategy for transformative research and evaluation.

Bias: Everyone Can Have It

Tensions are created in a complex cultural context when researchers and evaluators attempt to be part of the process of social change. Accuracy in representation is critical. The outsider supposedly looks at things with an objective, neutral eye. The insider supposedly looks at things with a higher degree of cultural sensitivity and can thus yield data of higher validity. This tension has been discussed and debated for many years. The resolution of the tension seems to lie in the notion of partnership and methodological rigor. The topic of partnership is addressed in this chapter; the topic of methodological rigor is the essence of this entire book. As a foretaste of things to come, consider Thomas's (2004) advice on triangulation in Box 3.2. Heidi Holmes (personal communication, 2006) suggested the addition of multicultural triangulation that would include language, race/ethnicity, and socioeconomic status (SES).

Cultural Competence

Cultural competence is an integral concept for those working within the philosophical assumptions of the transformative paradigm (Mertens, 2005). Multiple definitions of cultural competence exist in the scholarly literature (see Box 3.3). Some of these definitions were developed by professional associations and others by scholars working in indigenous communities.

Cultural competence is a critical disposition that is related to the researcher's or evaluator's ability to accurately represent reality in culturally complex communities. Symonette (2004) makes explicit the implication that culturally competent researchers and evaluators must understand

BOX 3.2. Veronica Thomas's Advice on Triangulation

Investigator triangulation: Create a research/evaluation team of members with shared interests in a topic and diverse perspectives and areas of expertise regarding the topic (e.g., a multidisciplinary study team including a sociologist, anthropologist, social worker, and psychologist).

Multiple operationalism: Use different ways to measure a single concept in an effort to gather multiple perspectives and a deeper understanding of the issue (e.g., measure student achievement in terms of standardized test scores, grades, and teachers' ratings).

Methodological triangulation: Use more than one method or data-collection technique that may assess different dimensions of a problem (e.g., quantitative and qualitative).

Target-person triangulation: Collect data from more than one person on a particular issue (e.g., gathering student behavioral data from students, family members, and teachers).

Analysis triangulation: Use more than one strategy or statistical technique to analyze the same data.

Adapted from Thomas (2004, p. 14). Raychelle Harris asked: "Should there also be ethnicity triangulation? Linguistic triangulation? SES triangulation? Is there a term that incorporates all those? Transformative triangulation?!!!!" (February 24, 2006).

themselves in relation to the community in question. Cultural competence is not a static state. It is a journey in which the researcher/evaluator develops increased understanding, through self-reflection and interaction with members of the community, of the reality of differential access to power and privilege (Symonette, 2004; Sue & Sue, 2003). The benefits of cultural competence and culturally responsive evaluation approaches include, but are not limited to, the ability to transform interventions so that they are perceived as legitimate by the community (Guzman, 2003), and the ability to serve as an agent of prosocial change to combat racism, prejudice, bias, and oppression in all their forms (American Psychological Association, 2000b). To this end, the culturally competent researcher or evaluator is able to build rapport across differences, gain the trust of community members, and self-reflect and recognize one's own biases (Endo, Joh, & Yu, 2003).

QUESTIONS FOR THOUGHT

- In your world of experience, how would you define cultural competence in research and evaluation?
- How would you modify the meaning of cultural competence as presented here to capture a more particular meaning in your context?
- What is the importance of understanding the meaning of this concept in the context in which you do research and evaluation?
- How can improved understandings be linked to social justice?

Additional questions that community members and researchers or evaluators can ask when considering the development of a partnership are listed in Box 3.4.

BOX 3.3. Definitions of Cultural Competence

❑ "Cultural competence refers to an ability to provide services that are perceived as legitimate for problems experienced by culturally diverse populations. This definition denotes the ability to transform knowledge and cultural awareness into interventions that support and sustain healthy participant-system functioning within the appropriate cultural context" (Guzman, 2003, p. 171).

❑ Many health and evaluation leaders are careful to point out that cultural competence cannot be determined by a simple checklist, but rather it is an attribute that develops over time. The root of cultural competency in evaluation is a genuine respect for communities being studied and openness to seek depth in understanding different cultural contexts, practices, and paradigms of thinking. This includes being creative and flexible to capture different cultural contexts, and a heightened awareness of power differentials that exist in an evaluation context. Important skills include: ability to build rapport across difference, gain the trust of community members, and self-reflect and recognize one's own biases (Endo et al., 2003).

❑ Cultural competence in evaluation can be broadly defined as a systematic, responsive inquiry that is actively cognizant, understanding, and appreciative of the cultural context in which the evaluation takes place; that frames and articulates the epistemology of the evaluative endeavor; that employs culturally and contextually appropriate methodology; and that uses stakeholder-generated, interpretive means to arrive at the results and further use of the findings (SenGupta et al., 2004).

BOX 3.4. Questions Communities and Researchers/Evaluators Can Ask in a Proposed Partnership

Questions for the community

1. As a community member, have you been adequately informed about the focus of the proposed study?
2. As a community member, have you been invited to assist in the design of the project and is that project likely to benefit your community?
3. Has consideration been given to how the study can be designed so that the results are more likely to be directly applicable to pressing problems of concern to the community?
4. As a community member, have you been invited to participate in an equal way in all of the steps in the research or evaluation cycle—from the development of the focus to the application of the findings to addressing current problems?
5. What are the consequences of the research or evaluation on the community and its members?
6. What are important priorities for the community that researchers/evaluators may need to understand and work with?
7. What are all of the community's assets and liabilities?
8. What are the constraints on the research/evaluation from the community's perspective?

Questions for the researcher/evaluator

1. What questions should you ask yourself before beginning a study with underserved groups?
2. How do you access community resources and information? Are you planning to do so without involving community members or leaders?
3. What benefits might result from working with community members when you conduct a study? What obstacles might be overcome?
4. What ethical issues should you take into consideration before doing a study?
5. Do you want to achieve a well-balanced, well-designed questionnaire and implementation plan?
6. What are the community's cultural traditions?
7. What impact will the research/evaluation have on the community?
8. Will the benefits apply to the community or only to researchers/evaluators?
9. Will you expect positive or negative changes in the community? Will the community experience bias, stigma, or prejudice because of the research/evaluation?

Based on Kret (2006).

Strategies for Developing Partnerships/Relationships

Kendall (2006) describes the importance of developing an alliance as a form of partnership, noting:

> Allies are committed to the never-ending personal growth required to be genuinely supportive. . . . Allies are able to articulate how various patterns of oppression have served to keep them in privileged positions or to withhold opportunities they might otherwise have. For many of us, this means exploring and owning our dual roles as oppressor and oppressed, as uncomfortable as that might be. . . . Sharing the power of decision making about what will happen is essential. (pp. 150–151)

Broom and Klein (1999, pp. 134–135) offer a five-step method to building effective partnerships:

1. Make your primary goal the building of a relationship of high mutual equity.
2. Check out your assumptions about other people (i.e., have a conversation that starts with checking on assumptions as a way to clear the air and revise assumptions to be in line with expressed positions).
3. Seek to increase other people's equity before increasing yours. (Be curious about, interested in, and appreciative of other people's feelings, assumptions, and goals).
4. Get clear about what you want and ask for it (don't *not* ask for fear of being ignored, the object of anger, or otherwise being made more vulnerable).
5. Discuss and negotiate, discuss and negotiate until you reach a resolution that will lead to high equity for all parties. Use patience, passion, and persistence.

Box 3.5 provides a glimpse into the importance of forming partnerships in school reform initiatives.

If one considers that researcher/evaluators' relationships with community members may not be characterized by full trust on either side, and that both sides may have a reason to withhold full disclosure, the question arises, what strategies can be used to foster a will to engage in a trusting transformative partnership?

BOX 3.5. Reflections on Forming Partnerships

Transforming a school to be more responsive to students' needs requires a culture change in which both teachers and students believe they are valued. In the midst of significant change toward school improvement, the rate of accepting change will vary from teacher to teacher, and differences in approaches and teaching philosophies will come to light. When teachers are involved in decision-making, they develop greater ownership and the partnership necessary to sustain the effort begins to unfold.

From Academy for Educational Development—Middle Start Initiative, March 2003, www.WKKF.org.

Trust

Reina and Reina (2006), in *Trust and Betrayal in the Workplace*, have provided a comprehensive framework for trust-building work along with a battery of assessment instruments for individuals, teams, and organizations. They identify transactional (interpersonal) trust components as contractual trust (trust of character), competency trust (trust of capability), and communication trust (trust of disclosure). Contractual trust means that we will do what we say we will do—provide a service, share information, attend a meeting. This type of trust is facilitated by making expectations clear, establishing boundaries, appropriately delegating responsibilities, honoring agreements, and being consistent. Communication trust includes sharing information, being honest, admitting mistakes, maintaining confidentiality, giving and sharing feedback, avoiding gossip, and speaking openly and constructively about what is on our minds. Competency trust includes demonstrating respect for people's knowledge, skills, abilities, and judgments, involving others and seeking their input, and helping people learn the necessary skills.

These three components of transactional trust provide the basis for the development of transformative trust in organizations. Organizations have achieved transformative trust when they reach a critical point where trust between people takes on a dynamic energy and force of its own. People feel believed in and therefore they believe in what they are doing. When people feel acknowledged and respected, they continue to work together because they know what they are doing makes a difference. See Reina and Reina's website (*www.trustinworkplace.com*) and book for more information.

Promises Made

Part of trust is being aware of the consequences of making promises that we may not be able to keep, as illustrated in this passage:

Desires for social change usually have repercussions within a wider society and are often fought because they have resource implications. And so often it's around multiple levels of why we do research, being very clear about what research can achieve and being honest about why we may be committed to social change. Sometimes it's very difficult for research to achieve social change because when research challenges a power structure, it's invariably looked at really, really closely and unpicked by those who want to dispute the findings and the (resulting) request for social change. We've seen that time and time again. . . . So I think that it's a tricky thing that we do sometimes. I got over a long time ago ever promising anyone that research would result in change. (Fiona Cram, in Cram et al., 2004, p. 162)

Building Trust and Community

Cardoza Clayson, Castaneda, Sanchez, and Brindis (2002) provide an example of factors that need to be considered in building trust in the context of culturally diverse communities. They worked with members of a Hispanic community and saw their role as serving as interpreters between the native stakeholders and the mainstream stakeholders. This role involved much more than translating from Spanish to English; rather, it revolved around establishing communications that were viewed as trustworthy by all parties involved. They recognized the multilayered nature of trust while taking into consideration the participants' country of origin outside of the United States. They found that trust, for Latinos in the United States, is based on mutual support and fluctuates depending on the potential threat of deportation. The Latinos may trust the researchers or evaluators to discuss who watches their children or where they work, but they would not feel safe disclosing that they do not have documents to work in the United States. Cardoza Clayson et al. held this up as an example of how economic and political contexts within a particular cultural group define levels of trust.

According to Cram et al. (2004), a relationship ethic encompasses the notion of researchers and participants as journeying together in a spirit of reciprocity; of participants' control over decisions and processes affecting them; and of researcher accountability (p. 160). If you are not a member of the community, then it is critically important to consult with trustworthy community people who can facilitate entry, clarify the relationship ethic, and safeguard the researcher. These community people can adopt various roles, such as caretakers, mentors, teachers, and protectors.

Working with a community can bring challenges, as seen in Wilson's (2005) work in the deaf community in Jamaica, in which she started the explication of her research focus based on her personal experience in international contexts and the limited scholarly literature available about U.S.

organizations that provide assistance for programs for people with disabilities in developing countries. U.S. programs designed to assist people with disabilities are rare and even fewer of these programs are designed to assist deaf people. Although research focused on best practices for U.S. organizations working with deaf communities in developing countries was not available, Wilson derived seven factors from the literature on the effectiveness of such programs for the general field of disabilities and development. Prior to traveling to Jamaica, Wilson contacted four Jamaican organizations that provide assistance to deaf people in that country, as well as the leadership of the indigenous deaf association. She also consulted with a deaf Jamaican leader, identified by the deaf community, and an American hearing administrator who had resided in Jamaica for 4 years, to obtain the benefit of their wisdom before traveling to the country to collect data. This groundwork was necessary, not only because of the dearth of literature, but also because of the need to build trust with the significant informants. These early contacts allowed Wilson to shape her research focus in a way that was consonant with the life experiences of the Jamaican deaf community.

Language and Building Trust

Hall and Hood (2005) discuss the importance of language as a means to building trust amongst stakeholder groups as well as to unlock meanings that would remain inaccessible if underlying assumptions were not accurately shared. Variations in language use are important both across and within groups; researchers and evaluators should not make the mistake of assuming homogeneity within a cultural group. For example, Wilson (2005) is an advanced American Sign Language (ASL) user. She learned Jamaican Sign Language (JSL) in order to communicate with the deaf Jamaican participants. JSL is used widely throughout the island. It is based on American signs; native JSL users who know ASL estimate that 80–90% of JSL consists of American signs. That being said, this is not meant to imply that knowing a language is sufficient to ensure that culturally competent transformative studies will be conducted.

The Will to Engage

To address the willingness of communities to build partnerships, Symonette (2004) suggests a strategy that fosters a willingness in the community to believe that assessment and evaluation are worth the time and effort. In her work with the University of Wisconsin's Design for Diversity on

27 campuses in that system, she described the process of cultivating that willingness as the result of "a student-centered and campus-centered focus organized around perceived campus needs and values. We have aimed to maximize the natural utility of program data collection, evaluation and reporting as a campus staff resource" (p. 103).

Ethical Partnership Strategies

Silka (2005) notes that as communities become more involved in research, ethical dilemmas arise at each stage in the research. These dilemmas include questions such as who decides the research agenda, who has the power in the research relationship, how will a partnership be formed and how can it work fairly, and who owns the data? The Center for Family, Work and Community at the University of Massachusetts, Lowell, developed strategies for building participatory research partnerships between the university and underserved communities. They developed tip sheets as a part of workshops on ethical issues in partnership-based research. The topics of the tip sheets and their web accessibility are included in Box 3.6.

Types of Partnerships/Relationships

Research Partnership Model

Silka (2005) worked with a consortium of universities to develop the research partnership model as an approach that utilizes a research cycle with ongoing relationships in the community as opposed to one-shot studies. The importance of having such a model was evident as she worked in research partnerships with immigrants and refugees new to the United States. Representation of newcomers is often accompanied by such challenges as researchers' inability to speak the home-country language, and immigrants' limited resources, and immigrants' unfamiliarity with U.S. laws and protections.

Partnerships to Relationships: Group Processes as Research and Evaluation Venues

Indigenous peoples' traditional group gatherings have been held up as models for research and evaluation venues rooted in respect for human beings and their cultural norms. Native Americans place a high value on relationships that result from interactions with the group and with all of creation (Little Bear, 2000, p. 79). A strong sense of connection among all creatures

BOX 3.6. Ethical Partnership Tips

Initiating partnerships: Gathering the players. This is the initial step in the process of acting on a felt need, identifying others who share a concern in the community and in the research or evaluation world, finding appropriate ways to contact and communicate with potential partners, and planning to have a community meeting to discuss the potential partnership (Boyer, 2004).

Ethical considerations in participatory research: The researcher's point of view. Researchers need to be aware of the diversity of perceptions as to what constitutes ethical practice in various communities (Costello, 2004). The questions that appear in Box 3.10 further illustrate how questions about ethics can be asked at all stages of the research/evaluation process.

Questions to ask about community-based research partnerships. A modification of these questions to ask about community-based research partnerships is displayed in Box 3.4.

Partnership-based research: How the community balances power within a research partnership. Partnerships should be arranged so that both researchers and participants are recognized as having power in that context (Serait, 2004).

Everything you always wanted to know about IRBs. IRBs, Institutional Review Boards, were mandated by U.S. federal legislation for any organization that receives federal funds to do research (Chiev, 2004). Communities can institute IRBs of their own with membership from within their cultural group. Ethical review boards are discussed more extensively in Chapter 7.

Overcoming the roadblocks to partnership. Communities can ensure that they derive benefits from proposed research or evaluation by forming community advisory boards, actively participating in the planning process, and considering successful models of partnerships that might transfer to their own situation (Martinelli, 2004).

"Science shops" in Lowell?. The Southeast Asian Environmental Justice Partnership is provided as an example of how universities and communities can form ethical partnerships (Pharmer, 2004).

Knowledge creation in research partnerships. Work together to create knowledge in a manner that respects differences between and within groups (Garbani, 2004).

These tip sheets can be accessed at the website of the Center for Family, Work and Community at the University of Massachusetts, Lowell: *www.uml.edu/centers/CFWC/programs/researchethics/research_ethics1. htm*; the Center's home page is *www.uml.edu/centers/CFWC*.

of the earth speaks not just to the interchange of material goods but also, more importantly, to the strength to create and sustain "good feelings." Maintaining good feelings is one reason why a sense of humor pervades aboriginal societies. Sharing also brings harmony, which sustains strength and balance. Native American use of group processes is illustrated by their Medicine Wheel (Battiste, 2000b) and other approaches. The Maori have a group process called *hui*; in Botswana, the group process is called *kgotal* (gathering of community members by the chief).

The Maori see partnership ethics as necessary to counter the nonindigenous researchers' desire to conduct research on Maori. When Maori scholars describe "by Maori, for Maori, with Maori" (Kaupapa Maori) research, they speak of relationship ethics. The Maori recognize the importance of their people leading the way in the research context. The essence of relationship is *whakapapa*—or the notion that we are connected with each other by where we are from and who our people are, all the while recognizing similarities and differences between people. Each gathering to discuss research/evaluation would begin with a recognition of *whakapapa* as a means to establish a safe and comfortable place to speak. Maori scholars distinguish a *partnership between* the researcher/evaluator and the community from a *relationship among* participants and researchers or evaluators (see Box 3.7).

Conducting research or evaluation within the Kaupapa Maori framework does not mean that the academy of researchers is excluded from participation in indigenous research (see Box 3.8). Rather, it means that non-Maori researchers and evaluators conduct studies at the invitation of, and in partnership with, the Maori community. Many types of transformative partnerships are possible. The W. K. Kellogg Foundation supported the development of 10 university–community partnerships that took different forms, depending on the context (Parsons, Hammond-Hanson, & Bosserman, 1998). The overall goal of the partnerships was to improve family and community development practices using a values-driven agenda. The partnerships shared the characteristics of focusing on strengths (not deficits), emphasizing self-determination and responsibility, engaging community members in culturally appropriate ways that respected their values, and focusing on action-based results. The program evaluators identified the positive contributions such partnerships can make to social change, as well as some of the challenges in such partnerships.

BOX 3.7. From Partnership to Relationship

RELATIONSHIPS: BUILDING, MAINTAINING, FURTHERING

In research protocols, often developed to guide nonindigenous researchers wanting to undertake research with indigenous peoples, the term *partnership ethic* has been coined. More so than a partnership ethic, a *relationship ethic* guides those who do "by Maori, for Maori, with Maori" research. Whereas "partnerships . . . must be founded on mutual understanding and trust" (Association of Canadian Universities for Northern Studies, 1997), the essence of a relationship ethic is *whakapapa* (G. Smith, 1995). The question "No hea koe?" connects us together at multiple levels—where we are from, who our people are—while acknowledging both similarities and differences. Russell Bishop (1996, p. 152) describes this as "identifying, through culturally appropriate means, your bodily linkage, your engagement, your connectedness, and therefore unspoken but implicit connectedness to other people."

A relationship ethic also encompasses notions of researchers and participants journeying together, learning from one another in the context of participant control and researcher accountability.

Adapted from Cram, Ormond, and Carter (2004, pp. 159–160).

BOX 3.8. The Relationship between the Academy and Indigenous Researchers

I would emphasize the importance of retaining the connections between the academy of researchers, the diverse indigenous communities, and the larger political struggle of decolonization because the disconnection of that relationship reinforces the colonial approach to education as divisive and destructive. This is not to suggests that such a relationship is, has been, or ever will be harmonious and idyllic; rather, it suggests that the connections, for all their turbulence, offer the best possibility for a transformative agenda that moves indigenous communities to someplace better than where they are now. Research is not just a highly moral and civilized search for knowledge; it is a set of very human activities that reproduces particular social relations of power. Decolonizing research, then, is not simply about challenging or making refinements to qualitative research. It is a much broader but still purposeful agenda for transforming the institution of research, the deep underlying structures and taken-for-granted ways of organizing, conducting, and disseminating research and knowledge.

L. Smith (2005, p. 88).

Challenges in Partnerships/Relationships

Challenges are associated with partnerships/relationships in the context of research whether or not the researcher or evaluator is a member of the community. Ormond, for example, described challenges associated with working in one's home community, noting: "It's very hard working in your home community. . . . They really hold you to what you say and it's not just that they hold you, you hold yourself because you just have this real sense of responsibility. To do what is right for them, represent them in a way that is fine with them and fine with the institution. It's a lot of work in your mind to get that settled so that you're at peace with it" (Cram et al., 2004, p. 165).

Partnerships: Cultural Clash Solutions

Chiu (2003) conducted a study in which community health educators interacted with primary health care professionals in the delivery of cervical cancer screening services to women from eight minority language groups. During the fieldwork, the community health educators indicated that they were experiencing difficulties in forming effective partnerships with the professionals. The issue was brought to focus groups as part of this study and was resolved by directly addressing solutions to redress the underlying power imbalance between the educators and the professionals. These included disseminating a clear explanation of the educators' roles to all program participants, providing official badges for the educators, and providing assertiveness training to the educators. The result was an enhanced capacity on the part of the educators to negotiate a more equal relationship with the medical professionals in the clinic.

Kirkhart (2005) identified the following components of ensuring multicultural validity that are relevant to the establishment of transformative partnerships:

- It takes time to reflect multicultural perspectives soundly; many evaluations are conducted in compressed time frames and on limited budgets, thus constraining the ability of the evaluator to become aware of, and sensitive to, the complexity of multicultural dimensions.

- Cultural sophistication needs to be demonstrated on cognitive, affective, and skill dimensions.

- The evaluator must be able to achieve positive interpersonal connections, conceptualize and facilitate culturally congruent change, and make appropriate cultural assumptions in the design and implementation of the evaluation.
- The evaluator must avoid cultural arrogance that is reflected in premature cognitive commitments to a particular cultural understanding as well as to any given model of evaluation.

LaPoint and Jackson (2004) identified several challenges that arose in the human relations arena when transformative partnerships were integrated into an ongoing program evaluation effort in an urban school setting. Partnerships can be tested by conflicting agendas between program evaluators and school staff and changes in those agendas throughout the process of the study. Changes in personnel in urban school settings occur frequently and can be disruptive to a partnership. School-level participants (including parents) may have a history of negative experiences in the school setting, as well as with other program evaluation efforts. Strategies to address these concerns are described in this and subsequent chapters.

Recognizing the Complexity of Culturally Competent Work

Accurate and appropriate representation of stakeholders is not without its challenges, some of which have been discussed earlier in this chapter. Inclusion of multicultural constituencies may be accompanied by disagreements among the stakeholders, which may slow or derail the research or evaluation. Different cultural groups, by definition, hold different values and expectations. Thus, the search for common ground is a challenge. This issue also involves the complexity of the community with which the researcher or evaluator is working.

Exposing Incompetence

King, Nielsen, and Colby (2004) noted tensions when trying to provide accurate and balanced reporting and protection of human participants in a study that exposed incompetence or resistance to implementation of a program. How can an evaluator present a balanced report (identifying both strengths and weaknesses), treat stakeholders with respect, and avoid harming them when evaluating levels of competence? King et al. wrestled with this ethical dilemma in their evaluation of a multicultural education program that placed social justice issues in the foreground. As is typical in many such programs, a continuum in the implementation of the intervention was found. The evaluators identified these challenges: How can they report on the differences in implementation without attacking individuals? From a social justice perspective, what do they do with the anger that is expressed by some of the participants because they see some of their colleagues as choosing not to reform their instructional practices to incorporate the multicultural principles? What do they do with the demands of some of the stakeholders that names be made public, thereby exposing "their colleagues with the hope of bringing them into alignment with the initiative's goals" (p. 74). What do they do when the lead decision maker rejects their carefully crafted, inclusive, stakeholder representative data and instead asks for a one-page checklist that principals can use to "check off . . . ideas they should think about to raise the visibility of multicultural issues in the building. Something really short that won't make anyone mad" (p. 76).

King et al. (2004) provide this summary: "[Demonstrating] multicultural competence in evaluation necessarily involves [giving] explicit attention to articulation of stakeholder values, especially when they have the potential to conflict, and to the likely tensions and necessary trade-offs among propriety, utility, and feasibility, and social action concerns" (p. 78). They hypothesize that evaluators may be more successful if they give explicit attention to value differences and necessary trade-offs in the steering committee, coupled with purposeful conflict resolution or mediation.

Dilemma: Budget/Time Constraints

What about research/evaluation that is conducted under severe budget/time constraints? Based on their work with funding agencies that bring the researcher/evaluator into a country for a short period of time, Bamberger et al. (2006) addressed this challenge through the use of Real World Evaluations (RWEs). RWEs involve adapting research/evaluation designs to meet the constraints imposed by the funding agency while still being aware of the cultural complexities in the current research context. Bamberger et al. describe time-saving strategies to apply when an outside consultant is brought in to work with a local consultant. The local consultant can be commissioned to collect background data and conduct exploratory studies prior to the arrival of the outside consultant. This work might involve the preparation of initial reports on the social and economic characteristics of the target groups or communities, describing the key features of the programs to be studied, how they operate, and how they are perceived. The local consultant may also provide a list of potential key informants and participants for focus groups. Additional design and data-collection strategies for RWE are explored in later chapters.

Purposes of Partnerships

Partnerships/relationships can be implemented in a variety of ways for a variety of purposes. Community members can be chosen to sit on an advisory board, frame the research/evaluation and identify appropriate interventions, implement the intervention, interpret results, and provide implications for follow-up actions. In a study of the accessibility of court systems for deaf and hard-of-hearing people in the United States, representatives of a diverse range of deaf community members and their advocates were employed at all of these levels (Mertens, 2000). An advisory board included two deaf judges (one used a cochlear implant, the other read lips), deaf and hearing attorneys who worked with deaf clients, judicial educators, and members of various advocacy teams for deaf people, including interpreters employed by police departments. This group guided the selection of members for focus groups that would represent the diversity of the deaf and hard-of-hearing communities. The focus group data were used as a basis for designing training that was provided to judges, other court personnel, and deaf people. Members of the deaf and hard-of-hearing communities participated in videos that were part of the training and disseminated widely, and they also participated personally in the training sessions. Finally, court personnel and deaf community members and advocates were involved in the development and implementation of an action plan and in the evaluation follow-up data collection.

Examples of Points of Interaction in the Research Process

Interactions with community members can occur at any point in the research and evaluation work. As noted above, this might include identification of needs, development of an intervention, or reaching an understanding of the current status of a phenomenon, among others, as illustrated in Box 3.9.

Building Capacity

Smith (2005) emphasizes the importance of building indigenous research capacity by developing and mentoring researchers and providing spaces

---

BOX 3.9. Points of Interaction in the Research/Evaluation Process

Community feedback and input on:

- ❏ Research/evaluation planning
- ❏ Research/evaluation types or questions
- ❏ Research/evaluation implementation
- ❏ Evaluation of research or evaluation study (meta-evaluation)
- ❏ Research/evaluation findings or results

Based on Kret (2006).

---

and support for their involvement in research. This type of effort must be accomplished without co-opting indigenous ways of knowing and of constructing knowledge. Transnational and international conversations serve to inform indigenous groups around the world of methodologies that have arisen in a variety of contexts. Indigenous researchers need to be trained in such methodologies, work in research contexts to deepen their skills, and be given opportunities to participate in a variety of research projects that use different kinds of approaches and methods. The group processes and cyclical models of research and evaluation described in Chapters 4 and 5 further elaborate on capacity-building opportunities and strategies for strengthening indigenous peoples' presence in the world of research and evaluation.

Indigenous Research/Evaluation Teams: Native American

Caldwell et al. (2005) recognized the training and employment of tribal members as research or evaluation staff as being a facet of reciprocity in the research process. While the researchers set this as a priority for the research or evaluation that would occur in the tribal setting, they also identified potential problems with participant anonymity and confidentiality as a tension that needed to be addressed. In small communities, use of local researchers needs to be approached with great sensitivity to long-term personal relationships.

Summary

✓ Researchers and evaluators can enhance the validity of their results by engaging in critical self-reflection that not only examines their own personal biases and assumptions but also their relationship to the community.

✓ Issues of power and privilege need to be addressed explicitly in order to build trusting and respectful partnerships and relationships between researchers and evaluators and community members.

✓ Challenges inevitably arise in the development of such partnerships and relationships; researchers and evaluators can benefit from the wisdom of indigenous scholars and others who have worked in culturally complex communities in this regard.

MOVING ON TO CHAPTER 4 . . .

In Chapter 4 the development of the research and evaluation focus and questions is explored. The exercises in self-awareness, self in relation to community, and development of partnerships and relationships from Chapter 3 form a key link in the subsequent research or evaluation planning, implementation, and use. Useful questions to ask about the challenges inherent in partnerships at various phases of the research or evaluation are displayed in Box 3.10.

We are all multifaceted. How can we see our own multiple facets and those of the people around us in their rich complexity?

Notes

1. I am indebted to Hazel Symonette and Bagele Chilisa, who raised my consciousness about the importance of this topic as critical to the conduct of transformative research and evaluation. I also want to thank my graduate students at Gallaudet University, Raychelle Harris and Heidi Holmes, for their valuable feedback on earlier drafts of this chapter.
2. The specific regulations that govern the protection of human participants in research are embodied in the work of institutional review boards. The history, principles, and processes of IRBs are explained in Chapter 7.

BOX 3.10. Questions to Ask Ourselves about Partnership at Various Phases of the Research/Evaluation Study

In the project planning stages:

- ❏ At what point am I involving the community?
- ❏ How is the community approached?
- ❏ What's the benefit for the community?
- ❏ How are the cultures and traditions of the community respected?

In the information-gathering stage of the project:

- ❏ How are participants recruited?
- ❏ How (and by whom) are research/evaluation questions selected?
- ❏ How are the privacy and confidentiality of the involved individuals and communities protected?
- ❏ What kinds of methods are being used (and how are they chosen)?
- ❏ How is the information going to be used?

In the data-analysis stage:

- ❏ How is the information that is gathered going to be analyzed or interpreted?
- ❏ What input does the community have in the analysis process?

At the end of the project:

- ❏ Is any sustainable change going to be stimulated by research/evaluation results?
- ❏ What are the roles of researcher/evaluator and community in determining what change looks like?

Based on Costello (2004).

---

3. *www.12manage.com/methods_luft_ingham_johari_window.html.* The Johari Window was developed by Joseph Luft and Harry Ingham (hence: **Joseph & Harry** = Johari) in the 1950s when they were researching group dynamics. It is still used as a model to understand and teach self-awareness, for personal development, and to improve communications, interpersonal relationships, group dynamics, team development, and intergroup relationships.

CHAPTER 4

Developing the Focus of Research/Evaluation Studies

Racism contributes to local and international racial disparities. These disparities are commonly found throughout virtually all areas of health, education, income, imprisonment and the like. Given the magnitude of the gaping racial disparities both within and between nations, the question needs to be asked: Why is it that researchers, evaluators, program and policy planners and those who implement societal programs seeking to reduce today's *racial disparities* generally fail to include serious investigations of *racism* as a potential contributor to such disparities?
— BROOKS (2006)

IN THIS CHAPTER . . .

▼ Influences of a transformative worldview on strategies to gather a knowledge base to determine areas in need of research/evaluation are explored:

　▼ Funding agency priorities, traditional scholarly literature, and web-based resources available on many topics are illustrated in terms of potential sources, strategies for searching, benefits, and limitations.

　▼ Knowledge from the transformative theoretical framework, in the form of fugitive (grey) literature and lived experience, is highlighted as a source for understanding issues from the perspective of those who historically have not been in the privileged position of presenting their views.

　▼ Group and individual strategies are explained, including focus groups and individual surveys, as well as use of indigenous methods such as the Maori *hui* and the Native American medicine wheel.

▼ Examples of research/evaluation questions are presented from studies that use a transformative lens.

Brooks (2006) suggests that disparities on the basis of race in all areas of society are worthy of inclusion in research and evaluation studies. She further suggests that the social issues closely associated with racial disparities are often framed without a conscious inclusion of the concept of racism. In keeping with the transformative paradigm, identification of the research/evaluation focus inherently includes not only acknowledgment of racism, but also of sexism, classism, able-ism, and other dimensions of diversity that are associated with barriers to accessing privilege in society. See Box 4.1 for an example of how a researcher came to the decision that race needed to be a focal point in her study.

In many research and evaluation texts, this chapter might be called Literature Review and Research/Evaluation Questions and include an introductory question: What is the research or evaluation problem? In the transformative mode, this view of research and evaluation as being focused on a "problem" is reframed to suggest that research and evaluation serve the information needs of the community. Thus, instead of focusing on research or evaluation problems and limiting our search to scholarly literature, the focus shifts to identifying the pluralistic conditions that provide a justification for the conduct of the research and evaluation and the resources available to address those conditions. So, instead of using the word *problem*, we would say: What is the research or evaluation focus? What factor indicates a need for this research or evaluation? How does a researcher or evaluator delve into the relevance, importance, and nature of conditions that support the need for a research/evaluation study from a transformative stance?

In evaluation texts, considerable attention is given to the process of identifying needs in a community, as well as to methods of examining a program or project in its formative stages. A *needs assessment* (Altschuld, 1999; Witkin & Altschuld, 1995) involves a detailed process of determining a community's needs. *Formative evaluation*, a term coined by Scriven

---

BOX 4.1. Deciding That Race Should Be a Focal Point in Research

Williamson (2007) illuminates issues related to the transition of African American deaf and hard-of-hearing adolescents from high school through post-secondary education. Williamson chose this topic following her review of high school yearbooks of deaf residential schools and noticing that pictures of graduating classes rarely included African Americans. She developed a model of factors that contribute to success of deaf African Americans based on a qualitative study of individuals' perceptions of variables that contributed to their success, and the obstacles that confronted them and how they overcame them. She has worked with numerous school systems to identify strategies that they can implement to capitalize on those variables that foster resilience.

(1967), describes a type of evaluation conducted during the planning and early stages of a program or project for the purpose of providing feedback for changes during the course of the intervention. When used within a transformative context, the community's voices are critical to determining the focus of the needs assessment and the planning and use of formative evaluation data. The actual strategies employed in needs sensing and formative evaluations are similar to those described throughout this text, including literature review, use of extant data, surveys, small trials, and group processes such as focus groups.

Purposes for the Gathering of Information at This Stage of the Inquiry

A variety of information-gathering methods at this stage of the inquiry are discussed in this chapter. The following statement captures reasons for this step in the process through a description of a review of literature by Slavin and Cheung (2003):

> The purpose of this review is to examine the evidence on reading programs for English language learners to discover how much of a scientific basis there is for competing claims about effects of various programs. Our purpose is both to inform practitioners and policymakers about the tools they have at hand to help all English language learners learn to read, and to inform researchers about the current state of the evidence on this topic as well as gaps in the knowledge base in need of further scientific investigation. (p. 2)

This statement includes many of the reasons that researchers and evaluators begin their process by trying to understand what research and evaluation studies have already told us and what else needs to be done. In addition, the practitioners, policymakers, and community members can serve as the audience for reviews in terms of the available knowledge base on a topic.

Sources That Support the Need for Research and Evaluation

Research and evaluation needs can surface and be articulated through a number of means. The lines between these sources may overlap at times, but it is nonetheless useful to think about the type of information most likely to surface from the different approaches:

- Funding agencies can define research and evaluation areas that they deem to be worthy of investigation.

- Scholarly literature is accessible through a number of databases in the major disciplinary areas. These generally yield published research and evaluation articles. Published articles frequently end with the author's identification of areas in need of additional investigation.

- Theoretical frameworks that undergird the research or evaluation approach or that provide a basis for program development can lead to the formulation of research and evaluation foci.

- The World Wide Web can be searched to provide access to sources that might partially overlap with scholarly databases, but that certainly provide a wider scope of information.

- Grey (or fugitive) literature[1] is generally that which is not peer reviewed and is disseminated outside the traditional peer-reviewed journals or scholarly books. Such literature may be more difficult to find than the literature that is accessible via electronic databases or published journals. Examples include conference papers, research and evaluation reports, policy statements, standards, newsletters, magazines, newspapers, brochures, fact sheets, annual reports, and more.

- As noted in Chapter 3, individuals rooted in a community have the advantage of a cultural and historical heritage that can contribute to the understanding of areas in need of research and evaluation, especially when scholarly literature is not adequate. Strategies for building trust in a community (e.g., focus groups, individual interviews, social networks, and other indigenous methodologies) can be used with a transformative lens to understand the research/evaluation needs accurately within a culturally complex community.

Whatever the sources used during this information-gathering stage of research or evaluation, whether scholarly or grey literature, the lived experiences of community members, theoretical stances, or funding agency priorities, all must be critically examined to determine the presence of cultural biases embedded in them.

Funding Agency Priorities

An important question to ask when starting to determine a research or evaluation focus relates to funding. This question can represent a tension for the researcher or evaluator if his or her heart is in one place and the money is earmarked for other priorities. On the other hand, it is difficult to do research and evaluation when there is no financial support, and so one can hope that there will be a convergence between what the funding agencies want to support and what the researcher/evaluator, in conjunction with the community, deem as worthy of inquiry.

Major government agencies and foundations have web-based postings of their current grants and contracts, as well as announcements of those that are open or expected to open within a short period of time. Organizations or individuals can electronically find and apply for more than $400 billion in federal grants at *www.grants.gov*. This website is a single access point for over 1,000 grant programs offered by all U.S. federal grant-making agencies. Other agencies have their own web presence that you can access directly, such as the U.S. Department of Education's database of discretionary and formula grants made from 2003 to 2006 (*www.ed.gov/fund/data/award/grntawd.html*).

Having funds to support your research and evaluation activities is good, obviously. When funds are obtained based on funding agency priorities, however, it is possible that several strings will be attached, as seen in the examples of federal government agencies statements of funding programs in Box 4.2. Foundations also offer potential funding opportunities that sometimes come with a less prescriptive approach than those found in government funding opportunities. A gateway into the funding world can be found at *fdncenter.org*; the larger foundations can be found at this website. The information in Box 4.3 illustrates the type of statements issued by foundations. Foundations tend to have priority interest areas and are often approached through a letter of inquiry, rather than submission of a full proposal. Specific foundation requirements can be found at their websites.

Cheek (2005) suggests that before accepting funds, researchers and evaluators ask these questions to determine the expectations and assumptions of the funders:

- Who owns the data and what can you do with the data?
- What if the funder wants to suppress results of the study? Or, wants to exclude parts of the results?
- What exactly is the deliverable (e.g., product expected by the funder)?
- In what time frame?
- Reporting requirements?
- What if there is a disagreement about the way the research or evaluation should proceed?

BOX 4.2. Sample Funding Statements from U.S. Government Agencies

The . . . priority is for applicants serving children with limited English proficiency (LEP). The Secretary is especially interested in those applicants including a specific plan for the development of English language proficiency for these children from the start of their preschool experience. Among other components explained in the invitational priority, the Secretary encourages applicants to include in these plans intensive professional development for instructors and paraprofessionals on the development of English language proficiency. The Early Reading First program is designed to prepare children to enter kindergarten with the necessary cognitive, early language, and literacy skills for success in school. That success, in turn, often is dependent on each child entering kindergarten being as proficient as possible in English so that the child can best benefit from the formal reading instruction in English when the child starts school.

From U.S. Department of Education, Office of Elementary and Secondary Education, Early Reading First Program (2006; *www.ed.gov/programs/earlyreading/2006-359a.doc*). About 1,500 school districts have received $4.8 billion in Reading First grants. An independent report from the U.S. Department of Education's Office of Inspector General found that illegal and unethical standards were used to steer money to the Reading First program. The Secretary of Education has promised to investigate (Feller, 2006). The U.S. Department of Education released a report on May 1, 2008, that reported that students who used Reading First scored no better on reading tests than did students who had no access to the program (United States Department of Education, 2008). An article in the *Washington Post* quoted the director of the U.S. Department of Education's Institute of Education Statistics as saying: "There was no statistically significant impact on reading comprehension scores in grades one, two or three," although students in both groups made gains (Glod, 2008, p. A01). Congress is once again concerned about the financial ties between federal officials who oversee the program and the publishers of Reading First.

*   *   *

The Office for the Promotion of Human Rights and Democracy of the Bureau of Democracy, Human Rights and Labor (DRL) announces a call for Statements of Interest (SOIs) from educational institutions, humanitarian groups, and nongovernmental organizations to support the advancement of democracy and human rights inside Iran. The Bureau of Democracy, Human Rights and Labor (DRL) invites organizations to submit statements of interest outlining program concepts and capacity to manage projects that will address the following priorities: • Political Party Development: Projects that provide institutional capacity building. Projects should assist in developing competitive and representational political movements, help political movements participate effectively in elections and govern responsibly. Programs that establish structures of political parties to enable more representative internal democratic practices. Projects that work with political movements in their role as the opposition. • Labor: Projects should support basic human and labor rights by assisting workers in their efforts to gain a voice in the political system. Such programs should help unions' participation in the reform process and assist members in the promotion of transparency and political reform. • Civil Society: Projects should support NGO development, networking, advocacy as it pertains to democracy, political empowerment

(continued)

BOX 4.2. *(continued)*

and increasing overall citizen participation in the political process. Promote capacity build-ing and/or networks of women or women's organizations. Working with students/sup-porting student movements. • Human Rights and the Rule of Law: Projects that promote respect for human rights, including tolerance and the fight against discrimination in all its forms, advocacy training, monitoring and reporting on law enforcement abuses and com-bating law enforcement abuses. Projects that promote respect for women's rights and those of other disadvantaged groups.

From U.S. Department of State, Office for the Promotion of Human Rights and Democracy of the Bureau of Democracy, Human Rights and Labor, Grant: DRLPHD-06-GR-003-NEA-060301, March 2006 (*www. grants.gov/search/search.do?mode=VIEW&oppId=8214*).

* * *

The purpose of the Demonstration Grants for Indian Children program is to provide financial assistance to projects that develop, test, and demonstrate the effectiveness of services and programs to improve the educational opportunities and achievement of pre-school, elementary, and secondary Indian students. To meet the purposes of the No Child Left Behind Act of 2001, this program will focus project services on (1) increasing school readiness skills of three- and four-year-old American Indian and Alaska Native children; and (2) enabling American Indian and Alaska Native high school graduates to transition successfully to postsecondary education by increasing their competency and skills in chal-lenging subjects, including mathematics and science.

From Office of Elementary and Secondary Education; Overview Information; Office of Indian Education—Demonstration Grants for Indian Children (2006).

* * *

CDC's Procurement and Grants Office has published a new funding opportunity entitled, "Identifying Ground-Breaking Behavioral Interventions to Prevent Human Immunodefi-ciency Virus (HIV) Transmission in High-Risk Groups." Approximately $800,000 will be available in FY2006 to fund four awards to develop and pilot test "ground-breaking" behavioral interventions that reduce the risk for HIV transmission among high-risk popula-tions for whom few or no evidence-based interventions are identified. All interventions must include promotion of abstinence, faithful monogamy, and correct, consistent con-dom use (ABC).

From Centers for Disease Control and Prevention, February 23, 2006 (*www.grants.gov/search/search. do?mode=VIEW&oppId=8140*).

BOX 4.3. Priority Statements from Foundations

Demonstrating the effectiveness and feasibility of HIV prevention strategies by supporting large-scale prevention initiatives, both in countries with emerging epidemics such as India, and in countries with high HIV prevalence such as Botswana. Grants will be awarded to support innovative social science and community-specific research that is expected to lead to the creation of more successful HIV prevention efforts in Nigeria.

Poverty is an issue that cuts across all our areas of giving. Our home state of Washington has among the nation's highest rates of poverty, unemployment, and hunger. The Bill & Melinda Gates Foundation supports non-profit organizations in Washington state and Greater Portland, Oregon that provide human services to vulnerable children and families.

Through Community Grants, we invest in non-profit organizations that help disadvantaged communities access the resources they need to survive and thrive. Priority populations include at-risk youth, low-income women and families, communities of color, immigrants, and refugees.

From Bill and Melinda Gates Foundation, March 2, 2006 (*www.gatesfoundation.org*).

*   *   *

Ford's trustees and staff try to advance human welfare by making grants to develop new ideas or strengthen key organizations that address poverty and injustice, and also promote democratic values, international cooperation and human achievement. Within these broad aims, we focus our grants on fields within *Asset Building & Community Development, Peace & Social Justice* and *Knowledge, Creativity & Freedom*. . . . Once the board approves work in a substantive or geographic area, program staff consult broadly with practitioners, researchers, policy makers and others to identify foundation initiatives that might contribute to progress, specific work grantees would undertake, benchmarks for change, and costs. When the program officer has completed this analysis, he or she presents the ideas in a memorandum reviewed by peers, a supervisor and at least two foundation officers. When approved, the program officer begins to make grants within the broad parameters of the approved memorandum and a two-year budget allocation. Grant-making staff are encouraged to make tentative plans for about 65 percent of their budget allocation and to leave 35 percent free for unanticipated proposals. Staff regularly provide reports to the board about grants made and ongoing lines of work.

From Ford Foundation, Guidelines for Grant Seekers, March 2, 2006 (*www.fordfound.org/about/guideline. cfm*).

*   *   *

(continued)

BOX 4.3. *(continued)*

The W. K. Kellogg Foundation funds in the following categories:

- ❑ Cross Programming
- ❑ Special Opportunities
- ❑ Health
- ❑ Youth and Education
- ❑ Greater Battle Creek
- ❑ Southern Africa

- ❑ Kellogg Health Fellows
- ❑ W. K. Kellogg Foundation General
- ❑ Philanthropy and Volunteerism
- ❑ Food Systems and Rural Development
- ❑ Latin America and the Caribbean
- ❑ Learning Opportunities

Under "active projects," the following excerpt illustrates the problem sensing and direction of a grant funded under WKKF's Youth and Education category:

> Middle Start gave Parkside teachers a crack at retooling their methods and curriculum to connect with vulnerable students, and provided a venue for them to pull together as a school community. When teachers decided on a collective goal (to produce capable, confident readers) the school leadership team got busy researching teaching strategies and tools. Parkside's school-wide literacy program is the result. Now one class period each day is dedicated to improving literacy skills, and every teacher and student in the building participates.

From *www.wkkf.org.*

Bamberger, Rugh, and Mabry (2006) identify funding agency constraints (e.g., budget, time, data, political considerations) that factor into evaluators' decision making about whether or not to conduct an evaluation. They identify the following constraints and strategies for dealing with them:

- *Budget.* Funds for evaluation may not have been included in the original project budget. Thus, design and data-collection strategies need to be tailored to available resources.

- *Time.* Funders may not call for an evaluation until the program is well underway. Thus, collection of longitudinal data is eclipsed, and the evaluation may need to be conducted in a compressed time frame.

- *Data constraints.* Baseline data may not have been collected; funders may not be interested in collecting data from groups with whom they are not working (e.g., collection of data from nonparticipants as a comparison measure).

- *Politics*. Programs are conducted for the public good; expanding one project may mean reducing or cutting another project. Projects often serve to advance a political agenda for one group or another.

Scholarly Literature

The development of the research or evaluation focus can be based on the synthesis of what is known and not yet known about your topic of interest. These gaps in our knowledge can be substantiated by a review of published literature on your topic. Many funding agencies expect to see a review of the literature as evidence of your understanding of the topic at hand. Access to scholarly literature has become easier (at least in the developed world) with the use of searchable databases available anywhere an Internet connection is possible. People working at universities with electronic collections have the easiest access to such databases. Box 4.4 lists various databases of scholarly materials that are accessible through universities, and to the general population, usually for a small fee per document.

Several options are possible for searching such databases, such as by author, title, and key words in the abstract and full text, for some publications. Instructions for searching the various databases are available by clicking on icons or hot links at the database website. Some databases include only abstracts, others have the full text, but not the tables, and some are saved in a format that saves all the information just as you would see it in a published journal. Three sample review strategies are presented here.

Language-Minority Students

"Research assistants at the Center for Applied Linguistics (CAL) in Washington, D.C. searched ERIC and other databases for all studies involving language minority students, English language learners, and related descriptors. Citations in other reviews and articles were also obtained. From this set, we selected studies that met the criteria . . ." (Slavin & Cheung, 2003, p. 7).

Combining Quantitative and Qualitative Methods

Bryman (2004) conducted a literature review to investigate ways that quantitative and qualitative research is combined in published journal articles. Only published journal articles were included, not conference papers or books. The search process used the Social Sciences Citation Index (SSCI) using key words or phrases such as *quantitative* and *qualitative* or *multi-*

BOX 4.4. Scholarly Literature: Electronic Databases

PSYCHOLOGY

The American Psychological Association (APA) produces the following databases:

❑ *PsycARTICLES*. This database contains full text articles from 42 journals that APA and other related organizations publish. The dates of coverage vary; earliest articles are from 1988, but APA is developing PsycArchives, which promises nearly 100 years of content coverage.

❑ *PsycINFO*. This database indexes and abstracts over 1,300 journals, books, and book chapters in psychology and related disciplines (1887–present).

❑ *PsycBOOKS*. Textbooks published by APA and selected classic books from other publishers are found in this database.

❑ *PsycEXTRA*. This database adds access to literature that is outside the peer-reviewed journals included in the PsycARTICLES database.

❑ *PsycCRITIQUES*. This database contains book reviews of over 6,000 contemporary books and plans to make reviews accessible that date back to the 1950s.

SOCIAL SCIENCE

❑ *Social Science Journals (ProQuest)*. Social science journal articles published 1994–present.

❑ *Sociofile*. A subset of Sociological Abstracts, distinguished only by dates of coverage: 1974 to the present.

❑ *Sociological Abstracts*. The premier online resource for researchers, professionals, and students in sociology and related disciplines. Sociological Abstracts includes citations and abstracts from over 2,000 journals, plus relevant dissertation listings, abstracts of conference papers and selected books, citations of book reviews and other media, and citations and abstracts from Social Planning/Policy and Development Abstracts.

❑ *Social Work Abstracts*. Index to articles "from social work and other related journals on topics such as homelessness, AIDS, child and family welfare, aging, substance abuse, legislation, community organization, and more."

❑ *Education Complete (ProQuest)*. Indexes more than 750 titles on education, including primary-, secondary-, and university-level topics. Almost 500 titles include full text. Includes the indexing and abstracts from H. W. Wilson's Education Abstracts.

(continued)

BOX 4.4. *(continued)*

❏ *ERIC (Educational Resources Information Center)*. The premier bibliographic database covering the U.S. literature on education; a key source for researchers, teachers, policymakers, librarians, journalists, students, parents, and the general public. Accessible to the public at *www.eric.ed.gov*.

❏ *ProQuest Dissertations and Theses*. Dissertations and theses published in the United States and internationally.

GREY LITERATURE

❏ *PsycEXTRA*. A companion to the scholarly PsycINFO database. It supplies clinicians, information professionals, policymakers, researchers, and consumers with a wide variety of credible information in psychology, behavioral science, and health. Most of the coverage is material written for professionals and disseminated outside of peer-reviewed journals. Documents include newsletters, magazines, newspapers, technical and annual reports, government reports, consumer brochures, and more. PsycEXTRA is different from PsycINFO in its coverage, and also in its format, because it includes abstracts and citations plus full text for a major portion of the records. There is no coverage overlap with PsycINFO.

From *www.apa.org/psycextra.*

---

method or *mixed method* or *triangulation* that appeared in the title, key words, or abstract. Five fields were included: sociology; social psychology; human, social, and cultural geography; management and organizational behavior; and media and cultural studies. The search was limited to the years 1994–2003. Articles were excluded if they did not use a truly qualitative approach, e.g., articles that claimed to use both quantitative and qualitative methods, but only analyzed responses to open-ended questions as the qualitative part of the study. Results: 232 articles that were then content analyzed (Bryman, 2004).

Mixed-Methods Research and Evaluation Approaches

Niglas (2004) employed mixed methods in her methodological aspects of published literature review of research papers in education. The search used leading academic educational research journals where both qualitative and quantitative aspects of methodology were used in 1999–2001. A mixed-methods approach was used with purposeful sampling, resulting in a sample size of 145 research studies. Niglas used qualitative analysis to establish categories, and a follow-up quantitative analysis of the study's characteristics (Niglas, 2004).

Information needed to establish a focus for a research or evaluation study is rarely, if ever, accurately or completely reflected in the scholarly literature. For example, Chilisa's (2005) critique of a needs assessment that served as the basis for the development of an HIV/AIDS prevention program in Botswana illustrates the application of the transformative paradigm to an evaluation study in a culturally complex community. The leader and several members of the evaluation team, from a European university, were contracted to work in a collaborative relationship with in-country evaluators. (Chilisa is an indigenous Botswanan with a PhD from a U.S. university.) The needs assessment preceded program development and consisted of a literature review and a standardized survey. Chilisa provides numerous examples of ontological, epistemological, and methodological tensions that arose when indigenous knowledge was ignored by the evaluation and program development teams. For instance, the literature review included the statement: "A high acceptance of multiple sexual partners both before marriage and after marriage is a feature of Botswana society" (p. 676). Working from a transformative framework, Chilisa recognized that realities are constructed and shaped by social, political, cultural, economic, and ethnic values, and that power is an important determinant of which reality is given privilege. When she saw this statement in the literature review regarding the sexual promiscuity of people in Botswana, she notified the European evaluation team members that these statements were in conflict with her knowledge of the norms of the society. In response, the First World evaluators stated that they would not change the statement, but that they would add additional literature citations to support it. Chilisa asks: "which literature, generated by which researchers and using which research frameworks? . . . What if the researched do not own a description of the self that they are supposed to have constructed?" (p. 677). This example illustrates the depiction of reality when viewed from a transformative stance with that of a team of evaluators who choose to ignore the cultural complexity inherent in indigenous voices and realities.

World Wide Web

The World Wide Web has certainly revolutionized access to information, especially in the developed world. The major search engines make it possible to type in a word, a thought, a phrase, or a lengthy quotation, and find sources of information unimaginable just a decade ago. The major search engines of today may or may not be the major search engines of tomorrow. Nevertheless, the following are recognized as being major sources currently:

- Google (*www.google.com*). Google currently holds the distinction of holding the top position for web-searching sites. This is a service that searches across documents that are posted on the web. It also has search icons that allow you to seek out images, weather, news, discussion groups, and products with a click of a mouse.

- Yahoo (*www.yahoo.com*). Launched in 1994, Yahoo is also a search engine that organizes the listings for its main results. In addition to search results, you can use tabs above the search box on the Yahoo home page to seek images, telephone listings, or shopping sites. The Yahoo Search home page offers even more specialized search options.

How Do Google and Yahoo Differ?

Many searches that use both Google and Yahoo yield quite similar results. However, when a searcher is looking for more complex information, Yahoo may yield results that are more directly tied to the topic (Sherman, 2004). Both Yahoo and Google use similar algorithms, but Yahoo has considerably more experience filtering out spam because of its history in the e-mail business, and is more sensitive to keeping such unwanted sites out of the search results.

The reader needs to be critical about the information that is obtained online. Criteria such as the academic credentials of the author, the date of the posting, and the verifiability of the information are important to keep in mind when using information from the web.

Grey Literature

Much of what is accessible through the World Wide Web is considered to be grey literature. However, documents that do not make it onto the web still have the potential to provide insights into the development of a focus statement. For example, the American Psychological Association's list of grey literature is found in Box 4.5.

BOX 4.5. American Psychological Association Grey Literature

- ❑ Research reports
- ❑ Policy statements
- ❑ Annual reports
- ❑ Curricula
- ❑ Standards
- ❑ Videos
- ❑ Conference papers and abstracts
- ❑ Fact sheets

- ❑ Consumer brochures
- ❑ Newsletters
- ❑ Pamphlets
- ❑ Directories
- ❑ Popular magazines
- ❑ White papers
- ❑ Grant information

From www.apa.org/psycextra.

Community Members/Stakeholders

Attenborough (2007, p. 80) recommended the following set of questions to guide the identification of stakeholders in a community in the United Kingdom in which steel mills had closed:

Who are the main victims or beneficiaries?

What are their experiences and views? Their needs and aspirations?

Who will "do the doing," make things happen?

What are their experiences and views?

What possible transformation processes are there (i.e., input to output)?

What are all the steps in the process that transforms inputs into outputs?

What are the inputs, and where from?

What are the outputs, and what happens to them next?

Whose worldview are we talking about? Have I tried all possibilities?

What is my own worldview and what influence does it have here?

Who has the power to stop the process or situation? Could this change?

Can the owner(s) help or hinder?

What are the constraints, e.g., funding, legislation, time, power?

Through using this set of questions, Attenborough was able to identify a diverse set of stakeholders and establish a transformative focus, including:

Redevelopment of contaminated land

Reduction in unemployment

Reduction in youth trouble

Acquisition of new skills for workers affected by the closure of steel plants

Greater community control by transfer of some power to the community

Group Processes

Social scientists have developed a number of methods and processes that might help you formulate a research or evaluation focus and approach. Trochim, Milstein, Wood, Jackson, and Pressler (2004) list a number of strategies for group processes, such as: brainstorming, focus groups, and qualitative text analysis. Trochim also developed a method called *concept mapping*, which is especially useful at the early stages of formulation and illustrates some of the advantages of applying social-science methods to conceptualizing a research or evaluation focus.[2] The Open University in the United Kingdom has a course in systems thinking that includes examples of a variety of diagramming strategies, including spray diagrams, rich pictures, systems maps, influence diagrams, multiple-cause diagrams, and sign graphs (Open University, 2007). Interested readers are encouraged to go to the university's website (*systems.open.ac.uk*) to see examples of these strategies.

Balch and Mertens (1999) used focus groups with diverse groups of deaf and hard-of-hearing individuals as a basis for devising an intervention for judges to improve accessibility to court systems throughout the United States. The advantage to conducting these focus groups lay not only in getting the perspective of issues related to court access from the "voices" of those who had that lived experience, but also in the ability to witness group dynamics in the provision of information from the cultural perspective of deaf and hard-of-hearing individuals and court personnel.

Community/Indigenous Perspectives

As previously mentioned, individuals rooted in a community have the advantage of a cultural and historical heritage that can contribute to the understanding of areas in need of research and evaluation, especially when scholarly literature is not adequate. Strategies for building trust in a community (explained in Chapter 3; e.g., focus groups, individual interviews, demonstrating knowledge of cultural and social networks and indigenous methodologies that must be respected) can be used with a transformative lens to accurately understand the focus of the research/evaluation within a culturally complex community. Although accurately revealing the community's perspectives is very important, once again, this process should not be undertaken with an uncritical eye. Just because information comes from a community member does not make it de facto more valid than information from other sources. As discussed in Chapter 1, there is a need to not over-romanticize indigenous or community knowledge. It is possible that local knowledge is based on ignorance, misunderstanding, or lack of historical context of cultural standpoints (Kirkhart, 2005). Key considerations include who is included and under what conditions and with what group dynamics.

The transformative researcher/evaluator needs to be prepared to challenge the definition of the focus of the inquiry if it is apparent that those with power have framed the "problem" in a way that leaves those who could be negatively impacted by the study at a greater disadvantage. The sexual abuse study (Mertens, 1996) discussed in Chapter 1 provides an example of how those in power can try to divert attention from the central issue in an emotionally charged context. The consulting firm that initially got the contract suggested that I ask two questions concerning the sexual abuse episodes: Can the students lock their doors at night? And, do they have sex education in the curriculum? When I arrived at the school and met with the administrators, they suggested that I look at the quality of the curriculum as it compared to schools for hearing children and the administrative structure of the school. I insisted that the issue of sexual abuse was the reason that stimulated the need for my presence there and that I needed to address that issue directly. I also agreed to address other issues of curriculum and administration that they had requested, although as a secondary focus of my work.

Lowell, Massachusetts, has one of the largest Cambodian communities in the United States, as well as a significant Laotian community. Silka (2002) and her colleagues engaged in community conversations as a method of identifying concerns in the Cambodian and Laotian refugee communities to determine perceptions of environmental threats and effectiveness of environmental communications. Cambodians, Laotians, health care providers, and university researchers discussed the role of fishing in their lives as a way of bridging the gap they experience between the Lowell culture and the South East Asian culture. Participants told stories about their love of catching and eating fish. In addition, issues arose related to environmental risks and ways of communicating about those risks to fishing families. The university-based representatives learned that the Laotians commonly fished at night, making it difficult for them to read posted signs about environmental risks. Moreover, the signs were written in English so that even if the fishing families could see the signs, they most likely would not be able to read them. These conversations served as a starting point to identify research foci and to suggest potential avenues for the development of effective interventions.

Based on scholarly literature and community voices, Duran and Duran (2000) present a focus area for research in the Native American community by noting that most of the literature having to do with Native Americans continues to focus on the lack of relevant approaches to psychological treatment as well as to paint a very grim picture of the extent of the problems afflicting the Native American community. Most approaches implemented with Native people constitute ongoing attempts at gaining further hegemony over their aboriginal worldview. Alcoholism, chemical dependence, and high rates of suicide continue to plague these communities. Programs responsible for addressing these problems appear impotent in the face of such a Herculean task, although there are some isolated instances of treatment success.

Native American writers describe the centered awareness that characterizes their historical relationship with the world (Duran & Duran, 2000). They live in harmony with the world seen in their collective tribal way of life, as compared to the individualistic Eurocentric approach. Native Americans exhibit harmony through acceptance and being part of the mystery of existence, in contrast to the ongoing struggle to understand the world through a logical positivistic approach.

Community-based knowledge traditionally has been associated with spaces where dialogue can occur regarding the power relations between the facilitator and the participants (Chilisa & Preece, 2005). In most African societies, group gatherings such as the Botswana *kgotla* (village council or community assembly) take place in the main village where the facilitator of knowledge is the chief or the chief's assistance. In smaller villages, the *kgotla* is held with the headman as the facilitator. Other gatherings, occurring at lower levels, are facilitated by the headman's assistant or by an extended family, in which uncles and aunts have important roles to play. The process is community centered and democratic and allows for the identification, definition, and discussion of problems and solutions, as well as the dissemination of findings, through involvement of the entire community. The process involves a *pitso* (a call) and a *morero* (dialogue). The *pitso* is made by community-selected dignitaries and serves as an invitation to *morero*. Chilisa and Preece note that the *kgotla* serves a valuable purpose; however, it has traditionally excluded women and youths. In keeping with the transformative paradigm, they suggest that researchers look for ways to support the legitimate inclusion of women and youths in these group processes.

Cram et al. (2004) offer a note of caution when relying on community involvement for the identification of the research focus. To avoid having only the articulate express themselves in a gathering, they recommend that

> an interpretive framework be provided to readers or listeners so that voices will not go unheard or be misinterpreted. This insures that a diversity of voices are heard, rather than just the most articulate whose words can be left to stand on their own without analysis. If a person is articulate and speaks in a way the researcher expects, then that person's voice may be given greater attention as compared to the person with the real lived experience who is not used to articulating it in a way that the researcher is accustomed to. (p. 163)

Other group strategies are described in subsequent chapters on research and evaluation methodologies, such as the Maori *hui*, participatory action research conferences, and Native American talking circles.

Theoretical Frameworks

Depending on the depth and breadth of your background knowledge with regard to theories (such as those discussed in the previous chapter), you may encounter theoretical frameworks that strike you as having benefit for your inquiry. For example, Clarke and McCreanor (2006) explicitly set their research within the indigenous research theory known as Kaupapa Maori research (Smith, 1999), which legitimizes and values the articulation of experience in a variety of ways. As mentioned elsewhere, the Kaupapa Maori approach is a methodology that is "by Maori, for Maori, with Maori," with a positive outcome for Maori people as a goal. The theory leads to the telling of counter-stories that subvert the reality of the dominant group. This is a proactive theory that recognizes the history as well as the future for the Maori people, as explained by Smith (2003): "In moving to transformative politics we need to understand the history of colonisation but the bulk of our work and focus must be on what it is we want, what it is that we are about and to 'imagine' our future" (as cited in Clarke & McCreanor, 2006, p. 30). Thus, their research uses this theoretical framework as a way to build confirmatory and transformational knowledge for

Maori. When dominant theoretical frameworks are presented uncritically, they can do damage to the interests of groups who are pushed to the margins.

Student Perspective: Theory and Power

I believe we can find plenty of research that is hearing centered. For example, a dissertation on the applicability of the speech act theory to ASL was awfully hearing centered because it relied on English glosses as translations of ASL sentences and ended the paper with "yes, the speech act theory is applicable to ASL." Why does every theory invented by a hearing-centered person have to be "tested" on ASL? Why doesn't ASL have its own theory because it is obviously very different from English? There's also debate on a new theory of reading for deaf people because they obviously read differently than hearing people. It's typical and common for researchers to try to apply hearing theories to deaf people without thinking about the ramifications of doing so. It's like trying to put a cube into a circular peg.—Raychelle Harris (2006)

Theoretical frameworks can be derived from social science as well as lived experience (Kirkhart, 2005). If social science theory has been developed on the basis of a majority perspective, it is possible that it may systematically exclude cultural standpoints. Researchers and evaluators need to examine the assumptions that underlie social science theory for its cultural validity. Kirkhart suggests the following questions as examples of critically assessing the transfer of theory to programs: "How does a plausible solution or intervention strategy make the leap from controlled environment to culturally contextualized service delivery setting, replete with resources, constraints, and implementation challenges? As social science theory is translated into program theory, what is lost or gained in the translation?" (p. 28).

As discussed in Chapter 2, feminist theory can also be used as a productive framework to guide transformative research and evaluation projects. Clewell and Campbell (2002) examined four theories to explain differences in science, math, engineering, and technology (SMET) course taking, performance, degree attainment, and workforce participation between males and females, including test-taking theories, biologically based theories, social-psychological theories, and cognitive theories. Their review of research on this topic revealed that only small differences on national tests and college entrance exams between boys and girls were evident using 1999 data, suggesting that precollege experiences for boys and girls are not very different. However, women choose SMET college majors at less than half the rate of men—a rate that has remained fairly stable since 1989. The disparity is greatest in fields of engineering, physics, and computer science. They also noted that relatively few African American, Hispanic, and Native American students, male or female, graduate from high school with the necessary educational experiences to enter a SMET program in college. Based on feminist theory, they suggest that a critical examination of interventions and the context in which they are implemented can shed light on ways to reduce these disparities.

Critical race theory was also discussed in the preceding chapter as a compatible framework for transformative research and evaluation. Smith-Maddox and Solorzano (2002) conducted research designed to interrupt racism in teacher preparation programs. They list the benefits of using CRT as a theoretical frame in research on teacher preparation as follows:

- Foreground race and racism in the curriculum;
- Challenge the traditional paradigms, methods, texts, and separate discourse on race, gender, and class by showing how these social constructs intersect to affect communities of color;
- Focus on the racialized and gendered experiences of communities of color;
- Offer a liberatory and transformative method when examining racial, gender, and class discrimination;
- Use the transdisciplinary knowledge and methodological base of ethnic studies, women's studies, sociology, history, and the law to better understand the various forms of discrimination. (pp. 68–69)

Making Use of Sources

What do you do with the knowledge you've gained from identifying the focus of the research or evaluation?

1. First, summarize the knowledge gained through this search process in terms of both the areas in need of research and evaluation and promising methodological approaches.

2. Second, develop a statement of the research or evaluation focus.

3. Develop a theory as to how a program works or what is required to reach the desired goals (see Chapter 6 on methodologies associated with intervention research and evaluation).

4. Use sources of information to develop an intervention to address inequities (described in Chapter 6).

And, in a nonlinear way, as you are undertaking these steps, check your perceptions with members of the community, using their perceptions to make revisions along the way.

Analyzing Scholarly Literature

A variety of strategies can be used to analyze scholarly literature. Slavin and Cheung (2003) recommend the "best-evidence synthesis" approach (Slavin, 1986). In their study, they described the process as follows:

> This section focuses on research comparing immersion and bilingual reading programs applied with English language learners, with measures of English reading as the outcomes. The review uses a quantitative synthesis method called "best-evidence synthesis" (Slavin, 1986). It uses the systematic inclusion criteria and effect size computations typical of meta-analysis (see Cooper, 1998; Cooper & Hedges, 1994), but discusses the findings of critical studies in a form more typical of narrative reviews. This strategy is particularly well suited to the literature on reading programs for English language learners, because this body of literature is too small and too diverse, both substantively and methodologically, to lend itself to formal meta-analysis. (p. 7)

Strategies for Deciding Which Articles to Include and Exclude

Researchers and evaluators, in consultation with community members, need to develop criteria that provide guidance as to which studies to include and exclude from the synthesis. The following criteria were set for the Slavin and Cheung (2003) review:

1. Comparative studies of children in bilingual classes and in English immersion classes were required.
2. Random assignment to conditions or pretesting or other matching criteria with statistical controls for preintervention differences were used.
3. Only studies with premeasures before the treatment began were included.
4. All subjects must be English language learners in elementary or secondary schools in English-speaking countries.
5. Quantitative measures of reading were available, such as standardized tests and informal reading inventories.
6. Treatment duration had to be at least a year to be included.

Even with these criteria and their rigorous application, the researchers needed to acknowledge the limitations of their review. Their research studies did not include any qualitative or case studies. They focused only on improvement of reading scores, not on other possible measures, such as interest in reading or reading behaviors outside of school. Many of the studies were quite old, and social and political contexts around bilingual and immersion programs have changed over that time.

Research or Evaluation Proposal Development

Research and evaluation proposals commonly start with a concept paper that the researcher or evaluator (including students) writes to articulate first thoughts about the inquiry's focus. The concept paper can include a brief description of the paradigm and its assumptions, as well as ways the researcher or evaluator is interacting with the community in the development of the project. Knowledge gained from preliminary focus activities such as the literature review and group processes can be used to prepare the concept paper, which can then serve as a discussion starter to further develop research and evaluation ideas.

A proposal commonly starts with an overview of the research or evaluation focus, paradigm choice, and discussion of group processes that are used to bring focus to the inquiry. The sections that follow can include preliminary research or evaluation questions and ways to select and engage participants. A part of this process is to spell out how to address ethical concerns.

Student Perspective: Ethical Concerns in the Proposal

I think that having a separate section for ethics in the dissertation proposal is necessary—to justify the ethical questions that might arise in my study and to address the validity of my study as well. I want to cover all of the bases when it comes to ethics of my qualitative study—so I can have supporting evidence of how I define myself as the instrument of measurement, how qualified I am as a researcher-participant, how would I address the tensions that might arise, how well protected are the participants (including their confidentiality) in the study—to name a few here. We as qualitative researchers need to think through our plan of study thoroughly.—Heidi Holmes (March 3, 2006)

Research or Evaluation Questions

Preliminary identification of research or evaluation questions usually emerges from the actions described herein toward crystallizing the focus of the proposed study. Box 4.6 gives examples of transformative research and evaluation questions from published literature.

Attenborough (2007) explained the multiple sources of information she consulted before she formed her initial evaluation questions in a study of a community's response to regeneration of an old steel work area in the United Kingdom. She used "business plans, performance information, gossip, memos, minutes, reports, the Internet (for comparative data), statistics, survey findings, anything relevant that I can lay my hands on" (p. 77). She describes the results of her focusing activities:

> Within the first week, I found satisfied funders and developers, a community forum (one of two created by the authorities because the first one did not work as intended), committed and vocal community activists, disenchanted residents who had not benefited from the developments, and my employing organization perceived as a threat by two local community forums. (p. 77)

She conducted the evaluation as one major regeneration project was ending, with an intended focus on the evaluation of the next project of a similar intervention that was imminent. The evaluation questions that she generated based on this body of information included (Attenborough, 2007, p. 78):

- Why were funders and authorities proclaiming the regeneration scheme an unqualified success when the people infrastructure was falling apart, and residents were disaffected?
- What were the tasks to be carried out and the issues to be addressed in any future programmes?

Reason and Bradbury (2006b) present a five-question framework for action research that has applicability to the more broadly construed transformative research and evaluation venue. They suggest the following types of questions:

1. *Questions about emergence and enduring consequence:* What are the consequences associated with the current course of action in the community? What is the potential or realization of a sustainable change in the community?

BOX 4.6. Examples of Transformative Research and Evaluation Questions

1. How does an urban area move from recognizing the legacy of past industrial contamination to creating new economic opportunities that not only avoid further environmental degradation but also blend in economic approaches, markets, and resources brought by immigrants? (Silka, 2002)

2. What barriers confront deaf and hard-of-hearing people in their access to the justice system, and how can those barriers be overcome? (Mertens, 2000)

3. How can technology be used to improve the school experience and outcomes of deaf and hard-of-hearing students? (Johnson & Mertens, 2006). What is the role of deaf community involvement in the technology project? What strategies can be used to increase the diversity of the teaching pool for deaf and hard-of-hearing students?

4. How can indigenous beliefs and methodologies be used as a basis for effective programs to address the prevention and treatment of HIV/AIDS in Botswana? (Chilisa, 2005)

5. How can science and math research-based educational practices and curricula be localized to reflect the cultural complexity of the Puerto Rican community? (Mertens & Hopson, 2006)

6. In a co-constructed* school-to-career intervention for ninth-grade students in a predominately African American urban school setting, how are student knowledge, attitudes, and practices affected as students make the transition from middle to high school? What are the students' perceptions of the materials used, what kinds of new and relevant learning are students engaged in, and how do students report how they would use this learning as they move on to high school? (Butty et al., 2004)

7. Using a feminist and antiracist framework, how can schools that serve primarily poor, working-class youths of varying racial and ethnic backgrounds provide a safe space for critically examining how girls can prevent or delay the onset of sexual activity, build self-esteem, and increase self-sufficiency through participation in an abstinence-based, gender-specific prevention education program? (Weis & Fine, 2004)

8. How can culturally relevant and research-proven practices be used to enhance instruction in beneficial ways for African American and other students of color to facilitate literacy acquisition and development? (King, 2005)

9. What is the impact of the cut flower export industry on women's income and employment and on the division of domestic tasks between husband and wife in one region in Ecuador? (Bamberger et al., 2006, p. 105)

10. What is the impact of micro-credit on women's savings, household consumption and investment, and fertility behavior in Bangladesh? (Bamberger et al., 2006, p. 105)

(continued)

BOX 4.6. *(continued)*

11. What kind of intervention addressing domestic violence in Native American communities will reflect indigenous traditions and beliefs? (Yazzie, 2000)

12. How should schools be structured and content developed and delivered to offer equitable outcomes for aboriginal peoples in Canada? (Battiste, 2000b)

*"Co-construction is defined as evaluators' collaborating and forming genuine partnerships with key urban school stakeholder groups (educators, school administrators, students, families, and communities and Talent Development [TD] project designers and implementers) in order to conceptualize, implement, and evaluate school reform efforts in a manner that is responsive to the school's context. Co-construction, by necessity, involves a redistribution of power, assuming a kind of equality among different stakeholders. It also seeks to democratize power dynamics between evaluators and project stakeholders" (Thomas, 2004, p. 9).

2. *Questions about outcomes and practice:* What are the outcomes of the research or evaluation? Do they work? What are the processes of inquiry? Are they authentic/life enhancing? What dimensions of an extended epistemology are emphasized in the inquiry, and are these appropriate?

3. *Questions about multiple ways of knowing:* What are the validity claims for different forms of knowing and the relationship between different ways of knowing?

4. *Questions about relational practice:* What is the quality of interactions that has been developed in the inquiry and the political forms that have been developed to sustain the inquiry? How have the values of democracy been actualized in practice? What is the relationship between initiators and participants? What are the implications for infrastructure and political structures?

5. *Questions about significance:* What is worthwhile? What values have been actualized in the inquiry? To what extent have we created an inquiry process that is truly worthy of human aspirations?

The Transformative Approach in Formulating Questions

Clewell and Campbell (2002) propose a transformative research agenda that is based in feminist theory to address issues related to disparities between men and women and dominant and minority racial/ethnic groups. They recommend research that investigates:

1. The provision of quality-advanced mathematics and lab-based science courses taught by knowledgeable teachers for African American, Hispanic, and American Indian girls and boys.

2. Interventions at a precollege level that focus on generating interest in science by hands-on activities, role models through mentoring and internships, and career field trips.

3. Implications of using one's own problem-solving strategies versus "following the rules" and adults' responses to boys and girls who do develop their own strategies.

4. Workplace conditions that contribute to a feeling of comfort and support for both males and females in science and engineering.

When the concept of unearned privilege is consciously addressed in research and evaluation, the question might be: How do sexism, racism, able-bodiedism, audism, and classism serve to create barriers for women, indigenous peoples, people of color, people with disabilities, or people who are deaf?

Summary

✓ Traditional sources of information about knowledge of social issues and community needs, such as funding priorities and literature reviews, are useful for transformative research and evaluation, especially if looked at with a critical eye and an acknowledgment is made of their limitations in terms of those whose voices are given privilege through these pathways.

✓ Additional sources of information that can provide access to voices that are often excluded from traditional pathways include web-based resources, grey literature, and the lived experiences of community members.

✓ Group and individual strategies, such as focus groups and indigenous gatherings, provide strategies to bring the voices of those pushed to the margins into the conversation about the focus of the inquiry.

✓ Examples of research and evaluation questions that are framed within a transformative context take into account the community voices, as well as contextual factors such as power, privilege, discrimination, and oppression, are essential components of framing the inquiry.

MOVING ON TO CHAPTER 5...

A model of transformative research and evaluation is presented that provides a graphic depiction of community involvement, points of decision making in the research and evaluation process, and recommendations for overall methodological approaches for transformative work.

 Multiple sources of information are available to engage researchers and evaluators and community members in establishing the focus and questions for the inquiry. Going beyond traditional sources such as published literature allows for the emergence of important community-based facets of knowledge.

Note

1. Grey literature is defined as "information produced on all levels of government, academics, business and industry in electronic and print formats not controlled by commercial publishing *i.e. where publishing is not the primary activity of the producing body*" (Luxembourg, 1997; expanded in New York, 2004; see *www.greynet.org/pages/1/index.htm*. Retrieved March 2, 2006. The Grey Literature Network Service was founded in 1993. The goal of GreyNet is to facilitate dialogue, research, and communication between persons and organizations in the field of grey literature. GreyNet further seeks to identify and distribute information on and about grey literature in networked environments. Its main activities include the International Conference Series on Grey Literature, the creation and maintenance of web-based resources, a moderated listserv, a combined distribution list, and *The Grey Journal* (TGJ). December 4, 2005.
2. Both focus groups and concept mapping are discussed in detail in Chapter 8.

CHAPTER 5

A Transformative Research and Evaluation Model

Methodologically, the transformative paradigm leads us to reframe not only the understanding of our worldviews, but also to understand that subsequent methodological decisions need to be reframed as well. A researcher or evaluator may work in a setting that permits an ongoing relationship with the participants and thus could choose a cyclical approach to the inquiry. Or, researchers and evaluators may be constrained by realities of time and money such that they are limited to a shorter-term project. Within either approach, researchers and evaluators can use quantitative, qualitative, or mixed methods. However, there would be an interactive link between the researcher/evaluator and participants in determining the focus of the inquiry, methods would be adjusted to accommodate cultural complexity, power issues would be addressed explicitly, and issues of discrimination and oppression would be recognized. The researcher/evaluator would also work consciously to energize the strengths that exist in the culturally rich community.

IN THIS CHAPTER . . .

▼ A transformative model for research and evaluation is presented that illustrates the importance of community involvement, use of a cyclical strategy where possible, and options for choices of approaches and methods.

▼ Possibilities of descriptive, causal, comparative, correlational, and interventionist approaches are presented within the context of the transformative paradigm.

The transformative paradigm's methodological assumption holds that decisions about methods are made in partnership with the researcher/evaluator and members of the community in which the inquiry takes place. The degree and nature of involvement will vary depending on the context of the inquiry. The type of involvement can range from consultation with representatives from the impacted community to full involvement with the power of decision making about all aspects of the research or evaluation resting with the community. When the transformative research or evaluation accords full power to the community, the approach resembles that described by Reason and Bradbury (2006b) and Kemmis (2006) in *participatory action research* (PAR), as well as Maori research based on the principles of "by Maori, for Maori, with Maori" (Smith, 2005). The transformative paradigm, with its broad scope that encompasses research and evaluation done for the purposes of social justice and human rights, embraces such approaches whether or not PAR or indigenous methodologies are used.[1]

Transformative approaches vary along several dimensions in terms of the type and level of community involvement, the nature and length of involvement with the community, the type of research or evaluation (descriptive—needs sensing or process inquiry; or development and/or testing of interventions), and the type of data collected (quantitative, qualitative). The researcher/evaluator might guide the identification of community needs and present options for approaches that community members can consider and adapt to their own needs for information; or the researcher/ evaluator may take on a partnership role by listening to community members regarding their thoughts about methodology; or the community itself may take the leadership role in partnership with the researcher/evaluator, with community members holding the reins of power as to how the inquiry is conducted. As is clear from the preceding narrative, the transformative paradigm provides opportunities for the emergence of many models of research and evaluation. Figure 5.1 provides a graphic representation of one transformative model for research and evaluation.

Figure 5.1 depicts the nonlinear nature of the flow of decisions in planning and conducting transformative research and evaluation from a methodological perspective. The type of research or evaluation needed is determined through an interactive relationship with community members and researchers/evaluators. Broad types of transformative research and evaluation are discussed in this chapter: descriptive, causal, comparative, and correlational (e.g., needs sensing, policy analysis, group comparisons on variables that are not manipulated, or as process research/evaluation), and interventionist research or evaluation (e.g., development of interventions and determination of their impact). As there is no neat line that divides these types, especially when the inquiry process is viewed in cyclical terms, it is possible (and sometimes desirable) to use more than one of these approaches concurrently in the same study or in a series of related studies.

Given the partnership context of decisions about the research and evaluation focus and methods, the transformative research and evaluation model depicted in Figure 5.1 is based on a cyclical approach whereby the researcher/evaluator has an ongoing relationship with community mem-

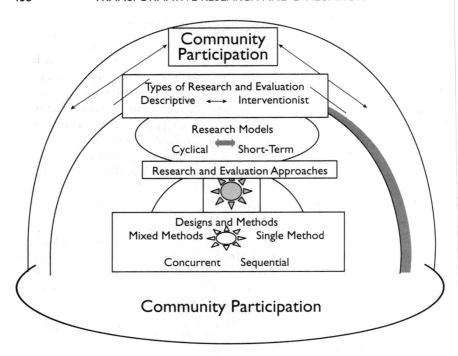

FIGURE 5.1. A transformative research and evaluation model.

bers such that the results of one cycle of inquiry feed into decision making regarding the next cycle. When real-world constraints such as time, money, or politics prohibit the use of the cyclical approach, short-term approaches can be designed in the spirit of this transformative model by engaging with community members as much as possible and providing clear recommendations for next steps in the inquiry process.

QUESTIONS FOR THOUGHT

- What are your experiences in involving communities in social action, in research or evaluation, or in some other contexts?

- What challenges did you experience or do you imagine you would experience by bringing community members into the research or evaluation process?

- What are the implications of taking a completely participatory approach, wherein the inquiry is conducted by, for, and with the community of interest, versus a partnership approach?

- How can the capacities of community members be enhanced to facilitate their involvement in the research or evaluation study?

Cyclical Models: Indigenous Peoples

Cyclical models of inquiry have been articulated by peoples who hold knowledge about ancient customs of various indigenous communities and have applied that knowledge to the research or evaluation context. For example, the Maori use group gatherings, called *hui,* for communal expression of ideas (Cram et al., 2004; Smith, 2005). The *hui* can be used for various purposes, but Maori scholars present it as a mechanism for participant involvement in the "by Maori, for Maori, with Maori" research that they advocate. Bishop (2005) describes the *hui* gatherings in this way:

> *Whakawhanaungatanga* is the process of establishing *whanau* (extended family) relationships, literally by means of identifying, through culturally appropriate means, your bodily linkage, your engagement, your connectedness, and, therefore, an unspoken but implicit commitment to other people. For example, a *mihimihu* (formal ritualized introduction) at a *hui* (Maori ceremonial gathering) involves stating your own *whakapapa* in order to establish relationships with the hosts/others/visitors. A *mihimihi* does not identify you in terms of your work, in terms of your academic rank, or title, for example. Rather a *mihimihi* is a statement of where you are from and of how you can be related and connected to these other people and the land, in both the past and the present. (p. 118)

The *hui* can serve as a venue for (1) building the capacities of indigenous researchers and evaluators to do research and evaluation (as mentioned in Chapter 3), (2) the generation of research and evaluation questions, (3) development of methodologies and protocols, (4) providing support to individuals and communities, (5) conversations about indigenous research organizations, (6) presentation and interpretation of results, and (7) plans for continued research (Smith, 2005).

African researchers and evaluators identify sources that help to build educational research and evaluation theories, models, and practices embedded in the indigenous knowledge systems, and worldviews. African communities with particular reference to Botswana have had a long history of diverse ways of processing and producing knowledge in locations such as the *kgotla* (chief's palace), shrines, and religious centers (Chilisa, 2005, p. 679). When chiefs recognize a problem in the community, they call a *pitso* (a gathering of community members) and present an agenda. The chief serves as an open-minded facilitator who listens to all voices. Botswanans work on the basis of *mmua leve oa bo a bua la gagwe,* which means, every voice must be heard. Conclusions are reached by consensus; thus knowledge is communally owned. This knowledge is then disseminated to the rest of the community through songs, plays, poems, dance, theater, and storytelling.

Student Perspective: Deaf Clubs as Communal Gatherings

Fascinating, indeed, how similar the Botswana people and Maori are with their pitso *and* hui *gathering in talking about problems and issues, respectively. Are deaf clubs the arena for gatherings like this in the deaf world?*
—*Raychelle Harris (February 8, 2006)*

Battiste (2000b) offers a model from the First Nations of Canada and many of the Native Nations in the United States based on the Medicine Wheel: "The Medicine Wheel illustrates symbolically that all things are interconnected and related, spiritual, complex, and powerful" (p. xxii). From Native American roots, Graveline (2000) suggests the medicine wheel as a metaphor for recursive research. She writes:

> I envision a fluid pattern
> Medicine Wheel as "paradigm."
>> Paradigms are beliefs that Guide "action taken in connection with disciplined inquiry," Guba says (1990, p. 17).
> Teachings of the Sacred Circle.
> Circular
>> Flowing
>>> Integrative
> Honoring Interconnectedness of All
> Balancing Mental
>> Spiritual
>>> Emotional
>>>> Physical Dimensions
> How do I get from here to there?
> Pray to the Grandmothers. (p. 364)

African Americans and Africans also provide cyclical models framed as culturally sensitive research and evaluation (Chilisa, 2005; Tillman, 2006; Hood et al., 2005). Tillman (2006) modified Kershaw's (1992) proposed Africentric emancipatory methodology and applied it to contemporary issues in the African American community. She cites the following characteristics as being a part of a culturally sensitive approach: (1) use of qualitative methods to understand the important forces in African American's lives; (2) use of those understandings to identify realities in terms of relationships; (3) identification of convergence and contradictions in realities based on understandings and "objective reality"; (4) use of a participatory approach to presenting findings and tools to empower the individuals; and (5) conduct of research that generates practical and emancipatory knowledge. Tillman emphasizes the value of maintaining ongoing and meaningful engagement with study participants.

De Jesus and Lykes (2004) present the following principles for transformative research based on their work in indigenous communities of Mexico:

- Recognizing and critically examining local, regional, and national racial dynamics, with particular focus on how racism and white privilege create and sustain oppressive structural inequalities;
- Situating oneself as "other" and questioning one's own identity politics and privilege within a praxis of solidarity with oppressed communities;
- Engaging with a more radical peace-building agenda by accompanying oppressed communities in social change efforts that seek to transform institutionalized racism and cultural and economic exploitation in order to promote a lasting peace with justice;
- Collaborating with local oppressed communities in combining creative resources and traditional indigenous practices toward action research that analyzes root causes of social oppression; and
- Actively contributing toward the co-development of community-based programs that transform structures of institutional racism and cultural and economic exploitation. (pp. 341–342)

These principles demand that researchers/evaluators adopt a role of learner within their communities, examine their own identities in the context of racism and privilege, align themselves with community groups who have a social justice agenda, examine root causes of oppression, and contribute to the co-development of interventions to further human rights. This set of principles implies the need for a cyclical approach as the researchers/evaluators and community members move through this process.

Cyclical Model: PAR

From the European roots of PAR in the 1980s comes the description of dialogue conferences (Gustavsen, 2006). In Sweden, a series of conferences were structured to allow small-group discussion of specific topics related to economic development, with a report back to a plenary session, and then a repetition of that process as members of the groups were rotated by topic. The goal was not to reach a single solution but to bring out a plurality of possibilities while building relationships that would be revisited in a sequence of conferences.

Deliberative democratic dialogue, based on Habermas's (1996, as cited in Kemmis, 2006, p. 102) theory of communicative action, is the most common format used by action researchers to work, collaborate, gather, and reflect on data. Habermas identified three features of communicative action: an orientation toward mutual understanding, a goal of achieving an unforced consensus about what to do, and the creation of a communicative space. The communicative space is created by bringing people together with a shared orientation toward mutual understanding and consensus to consider topical concerns, problems, and issues. As obvious as this might seem, creating a communicative space requires that people are brought together in meetings, in the media, in conversations with friends and colleagues, etc. Working with groups that have a prior existence, without critically examining the totality of the group, may result in the exclusion of important voices. Thus, Kemmis (2006) cites the first and central step in action research as the formation of a communicative space "which is embodied in networks of actual persons, though the group itself cannot and should not be treated as a totality (as an exclusive whole). A communicative space is constituted as issues or problems are opened up for discussion and when participants experience their interaction as fostering the democratic expression of divergent views" (p. 103).

PAR principles have been applied in a wide range of contexts, some of which have a transformative intent. Box 5.1 presents a number of examples in which researchers called for and implemented PAR in communities.

Cyclical Models: Immigrant Communities

Silka (2005) and her colleagues at the Center for Family, Work, and Community developed a research cycle model that is designed to (1) involve community members in the decision-making process, (2) provide an ongoing relationship between researchers and community members, and (3) protect individuals who might be overwhelmed by well-intentioned researchers who descend on their communities because they represent the latest "exotica" in a researcher's world. Silka developed the research cycle in conjunction with a partnership with the Hmong people in Lowell, Massachusetts, and its surrounding areas to further social justice through applied research with that community. The research cycle involves joint determination of the research question and approach, followed by data collection, analysis, and interpretation. Findings from earlier studies are used as a basis for decision making for the next round of research. Thus, community members are part of a cycle of research that addresses their needs, rather than spectators as a researcher takes data from them for purposes of knowledge creation (e.g., publication in a journal), without regard for the implications of that research for community members.

BOX 5.1. Participatory Action Research Examples

NATIVE AMERICAN INDIANS

This article presents a call for systematic change in how research and program evaluation are conducted in Indian Country. The authors do not intend to offer innovative research and evaluation methods; rather, we draw upon our collective experience, much of it based on working with individuals who have chronic illnesses and disabilities, to offer consolidated documentation for requiring that research and program evaluation in Indian Country be participatory. (Caldwell et al., 2005, p. 1)

LESBIAN, GAY, BISEXUAL, AND TRANSGENDER YOUTHS

PAR is an approach to research which empowers the community to define their own questions, lead the process of investigation, and create their own solutions for change. Through this process, the community builds skills and capacity, is able to participate in decisions affecting their lives, and engages in interactions and relationship building—all of which are the defining conditions of social inclusion. In this way PAR offers a concrete methodology to build socially inclusive policy. (Amsden & VanWynsberghe, 2005, p. 359)

POVERTY

The methods used in this study were adapted from Participatory Poverty Assessments, part of a family of participatory methodologies which have had a long association with international development work (Ros & Craig, 1997). Participatory Poverty Assessments (PPA) use participatory tools to engage households who are poor in an assessment of their own living conditions. The methods are deliberately non-technical and accessible. Visual methods are used such as mapping exercises, seasonality diagrams, timelines, and ranking exercises. Focus groups and semi-structured interviews are undertaken to draw out perceptions of well-being. The purpose of drawing on the expertise of households who are poor is not just to improve understanding, but to demonstrate the micro-effects of macro-policy (Booth, 1998). An additional purpose is to enable local people to analyse their own situation and develop the confidence to make decisions and take action to improve their circumstances. (Collins, 2005, p. 13)

The cyclical approach to researching for transformative purposes is illustrated in Silka's (2002) research on models of interdisciplinary environmental work with refugee and immigrant groups underway at the University of Massachusetts at Lowell. These models incorporate cultural traditions, environmental outreach, and economic development. Three multilevel partnership projects in which the university is involved—the Southeast Asian Environmental Justice Partnership, the Urban Aquaculture Initiative, and the Immigrant Communities Clean Production Initiative—are focused on understanding the promise and challenges that lie ahead in terms of developing community–university partnerships. The use of organized community conversations as a means to focusing the research and evaluation studies is discussed in Chapter 4.

Student Perspective: Silka's Research Cycle Model

I enjoyed the research cycle model . . . [and] the questions we should always ask about our research. The most critical area is the conflict of research purpose between the researchers and the research participants—the purpose for both are quite different: One may just want to graduate with a doctoral degree, the other wants to solve a problem in his or her community. I believe a research project can be closely aligned to everyone's purpose so everyone comes out of it satisfied. One missing aspect of this, I believe, is money. Money controls research time, design, people, etc. And who controls the money, actually controls the research.—Raychelle Harris (February 8, 2006)

I agree that time is a huge factor when doing research. We all are pressed for time. Do grants and financial assistance put burdens on researchers—to complete their research within the deadline? I experienced being stressed for a time when I did the pilot study last year [that had to be completed within the time constraints of one semester]. I could understand that I might not have done a very thorough job of my pilot study, but with the time in the way, I did the best I could. Do the researchers feel the same?—Heidi Holmes (February 8, 2006)

The issues of money, purpose, time, and control are issues that cannot be ignored. Bamberger et al. (2006) wrestled with these issues when these factors constrained a long-term cyclical approach to research and evaluation, as discussed in the next section.

Short-Term Research and Evaluation

As was mentioned previously, researchers and evaluators who work in international development or are awarded a contract with specifically defined methodologies often find themselves working under severe time constraints (from the donor agency or other funding source) that preclude the use of a longitudinal, cyclical approach.[2] Bamberger et al. (2006) address ways to incorporate the views of groups who are difficult to reach or relatively invisible (e.g., sex workers, drug or alcohol users, illegal residents, absent fathers, migrant workers, persons with HIV/AIDS, ethnic minorities, or the homeless) and how to capture data on sensitive topics (e.g., domestic violence, contraceptive use, teen gangs) while working under such constraints. The transformative spirit can still be manifest in the way the contact is made with communities in culturally appropriate ways, providing access to findings for all stakeholders, and making clear recommendations for possible future actions with regard to programs, policies, and the need for additional research or evaluation.

QUESTIONS FOR THOUGHT

- What are the implications of using a cyclical approach to research and evaluation as compared to a short-term approach?
- What are your thoughts regarding appropriate strategies when time, money, or political constraints do not allow for an ongoing cycle of research?
- What would you do if the community did not want to sustain their involvement with you as a researcher or evaluator?

Types of Transformative Research and Evaluation

Transformative research and evaluation can be descriptive, causal-comparative, correlational, or interventionist. Descriptive inquiries are conducted to get an overview of the current status, to determine needs, to document the process of a program or intervention, and/or to inform decisions about interventions. Causal-comparative approaches allow for the comparison of groups based on characteristics that the researcher or evaluator cannot manipulate (e.g., gender, race). Correlational approaches consider characteristics in terms of strength and direction of relationship (e.g., number of hours of participation in an educational experience and amount of learning that occurs). Interventionist research and evaluation examine the development and impact of a program or treatment in relation to a desired outcome.

Transformative Descriptive Research and Evaluation

Inquiries conducted to provide a snapshot in time for a community comprise descriptive research or evaluation. Heron and Reason (2006) reject the dichotomy that research purposes can be either informative (descriptive) or transformative. If the goal of descriptive research and evaluation is to provide a picture of current conditions, then that exercise in itself can be the impetus for transformational change. Thus, it is possible to start with a descriptive intent that evolves into a transformative agenda.

In some circumstances, descriptive research and evaluation can be put to the purpose of needs sensing. Various approaches can be used in a descriptive study, some of which are described in more detail in Chapter 8. One of the most common purposes of descriptive transformative research and evaluation is the collection of needs assessment data before an intervention has been implemented or when a potential revision of a program may be planned. This descriptive study of a community can be accomplished via a literature review, examination of artifacts and documents, interviews with key informants, a survey of members, or through mechanisms of group participation, some of which are rooted in ancient community traditions. The use of literature reviews and other means of focusing the research or evaluation are described in Chapter 4. In this chapter examples are provided of the use of focus groups and surveys as needs sensing instruments to be used as a basis for the design of an intervention; more specific strategies for developing and implementing focus groups and surveys as a data-collection tool appear in Chapter 7. Examples of other group participation approaches rooted in community practice appear in this chapter.

Descriptive Research and Evaluation as a Basis for an Intervention: Critique of a Needs Assessment in Africa

Chilisa (2005) critiqued a needs assessment survey that was conducted using standardized procedures with a printed form that contained closed-ended questions, written in English, and using terminology based on Western scientific language about HIV/AIDS prevention and transmission in Botswana. Tensions arose when evaluators chose to ignore the assumptions of the transformative paradigm that accurate reflection of stakeholders' understandings need to be conveyed in ways that facilitate involvement of the participant community, with recognition of and responsiveness to appropriate dimensions of diversity.

Chilisa makes four critical points:

1. In Botswana, important dimensions of diversity include the multi-ethnic nature of the population, with most of the people speaking one of 25 ethnic languages.
2. The highest rate of HIV/AIDS infection occurs in the most vulnerable populations in Botswana—that is, those living in poverty with the least amount of privilege and education.
3. The highest mortality rates were found among industrial class workers (women and girls especially) who earn the lowest wages and have the lowest education in comparison to the more economically privileged classes.
4. The meaning of HIV/AIDS (revealed in focus groups conducted by Chilisa and her African colleagues) differs from First World definitions. Botswana people have three meanings for what Westerners call HIV/AIDS that vary depending on the age at which one is infected and the mode of transmission.

Thus the needs assessment data did not accurately reflect the indigenous realities of HIV/AIDS in Botswana, nor were they responsive to the cultural complexity of the stakeholders. Nevertheless, the data were used as a basis for a prevention program that reflected a view of the Africans as a homogeneous mass for whom context-specific differences such as occupation, education, literacy levels, language, and social class were deemed irrelevant. Designing a prevention program based on the needs assessment data, these researchers made the assumption that everyone was middle class and could therefore read English. An educational campaign was developed that used billboards with text such as: "Don't be stupid, condomize" and "Are you careless, ignorant, and stupid?" Chilisa (2005) concluded: "The lack of representation of appropriate stakeholders in the determination of communication strategies resulted in messages that were offensive, degrading, and written from the perspective of a superior who casts the recipients of the message as ignorant" (p. 673). The consequence of this ill-conceived research was to delay progress in combating HIV/AIDS for the most vulnerable populations.

Chilisa (2005) recommends that the point of reference for legitimating research results should be the accumulated body of knowledge that is created by the people impacted by the program. It is incumbent upon the

researcher to interact with all stakeholder groups, including the less powerful stakeholders, to determine the local meanings attached to experiences.
She recommends that researchers work from an ethics protocol that insists
that the local language is used throughout the design of the project, the
development and implementation of the intervention, and in the presentation of the findings—especially when the less powerful stakeholders are not
familiar with English. In addition, theories, models, and practices should
be embedded in the indigenous knowledge systems and worldviews. The
diverse ways of processing and producing knowledge in Botswana involve
the proverbs, folklore, songs, and myths of that society. As Chilisa (2005)
notes, the consequences of ignoring the multiple realities, especially those
realities as they are perceived by the less powerful, is death. This example
from Botswana illustrates the importance of cultural competence in evaluation work in order to accurately reflect the needs of stakeholders in culturally complex communities.

Descriptive Research and Evaluation as a Basis for an Intervention: Needs Sensing in the Transformative Spirit

Firme (2006) describes a needs sensing study that led to an intervention
in the *favelas* (slums) of Brazil. The main purpose of the initiative was to
improve the quality of the residents' lives. The evaluation team placed high
priority on the community members' ability to identify their own needs.
Firme conducted a situation analysis to determine the demographics of the
community, as well as specific information about the needs of different
segments of the community. The results of the situation analysis were used
as the basis for designing a program called "Betting on the Future." Community members identified the following priorities: the need for attention
to children, ages 0–3, in the form of a day care center and courses for community mothers; the need for the development of a digital inclusion project
that was educational for children and adolescents and improved adults'
access to the computers and the Internet; and provision of a cultural sports
and leisure activities center for people of all ages.

The American Judicature Society (AJS) is an advocacy organization
that focuses on ethical practice within the United States judiciary. The society was approached by deaf lawyers who served primarily deaf clients with
regard to inequities in their clients' experiences in court. In response, AJS
obtained funding from the W. K. Kellogg Foundation to conduct a study
of deaf and hard-of-hearing peoples' experiences in court and the implications for professional development of judges. I conducted a transformative
evaluation of the project that began with the establishment of an advisory

board with broad representation from the deaf, hard-of-hearing, and judicial communities (Mertens, 2000). The advisory board included judges, attorneys, judicial educators, court interpreters, and police officers who were hearing, hard-of-hearing, or deaf and used a variety of communication modes and assistive listening devices, including lip reading, speaking, cochlear implants, hearing aids, and American Sign Language (ASL). Based on the recommendations of the advisory board, focus groups were held that represented different dimensions of diversity within the deaf and hard-of-hearing communities served by the courts. These included:

- Highly educated deaf professionals who used ASL
- Deaf people with less education and more communication challenges, such as deaf–blind, deaf without knowledge of ASL (i.e., dependent on gestures and limited use of signs)
- Hard-of-hearing people who used assistive listening devices
- Mexican Sign Language users

For each of these groups, a different support system was needed to facilitate communication. For example, deaf–blind individuals needed interpreters who could sign into their hands so that they could feel the signs and respond to the focus group's comments and the moderator's questions. Deaf individuals with limited language had an interpreter who was deaf himself and who acted out the comments of the group members and the moderator's questions using gestures, pantomimes, and some signs. In addition, deaf and hearing moderators ran the group and an ASL interpreter provided translation from spoken English to sign, and vice versa, as needed. Real-time captions in English were provided on television screens visible to all group members.

The results of the focus groups were used in a number of ways throughout the lifetime of the project. To begin with, the results formed the basis for the development of training materials for judges and deaf people and their advocates that was provided at different locations throughout the United States. Members of the focus groups were invited to appear in a video that was part of the training program, titled Silent Justice, that depicted challenges and strategies for improving access for deaf and hard-of-hearing people in the court system. Deaf and hard-of-hearing people were also invited to attend the training programs both as presenters and as participants. Each court system was asked to send a judge, a deaf or hard-of-hearing person, and any other court personnel thought to benefit from the training. The training ended with a session in which representatives from specific court systems developed a plan to make their courts more accessible for deaf and hard-of-hearing people. The evaluation concluded with visits from the evaluator to selected sites to determine what progress had been made in implementing the plans.

Descriptive Research and Evaluation: Short Term

When time constraints prevent a cyclical approach to needs sensing, Bamberger et al. (2006) recommend the use of rapid ethnographic methods. Beebe (2001) describes rapid assessment process (RAP; a type of rapid ethnography) as a process that takes between 4 days and 6 weeks and can be used when results are needed in a very short time frame. RAP uses strategies similar to those of the ethnographer; however, it is most commonly a team-based inquiry and uses multiple data sources and collection strategies, as well as iterative data analysis.

Causal-Comparative and Correlational Approaches

Causal-comparative and correlational approaches are commonly used when researchers and evaluators are not able to implement a treatment or program or have an interest in some inherent characteristic of individuals and another variable, such as income level, educational success, etc. Relational approaches investigate either the strength and direction of the relationship between or among variables, or group differences based on an extant characteristic (e.g., gender, hearing status, type of disability). Causal-comparative approaches are based on group differences (e.g., male/female; hearing/deaf; African American/Latino). Surveys are frequently used to gather data about such variables. When the data from surveys are treated as continuous data that are analyzed in terms of their strength and direction of relationships, they fit into the correlational category. However, when the data are used to test for group differences, they fit into the causal-comparative category.

Irwin (2005) used a longitudinal, causal-comparative survey design to address possible solutions to the troubles in Northern Ireland that have burdened that country with civil unrest for centuries. Irwin provides an example in which adversarial political parties constitute the key dimension of diversity; thus the causal-comparative independent variable was political party membership. He wrestled with the representation of stakeholders in the politically charged atmosphere of Northern Ireland in his use of public opinion polls. His preliminary work suggested that innovations that might lead to peace in that region were supported by a majority of the people;

however, they were being blocked by religious and political elites who were benefiting from maintaining social divisions and the status quo. Irwin contacted recently elected politicians from 10 different political parties and asked them to nominate a member of their team to work with him and his colleagues to write questions and run polls on any matters of concern to them. Thus, parties from across the political spectrum, representing loyalist and republican paramilitary groups, mainstream democratic parties, and cross-community parties, all agreed on the questions to be asked, the methods to be used, and the timing and mode of publication. The specific options on the survey constituted the dependent variables. The group conducted nine different polls, progressively identifying more specifically the choices for government that would be acceptable to the majority of the people. A basis for peace was found as the two groups moved from their ideal extremes to a workable middle solution.

Transformative Intervention Approaches

Intervention approaches can be used either to develop an intervention or to measure the quality and impact of an intervention (or both). The intervention may be defined by the funding agency, or it may emerge based on community needs (see Box 5.2 for examples of prescribed and emergent descriptions of interventions).

Transformative researchers/evaluators have a role to play in the development of interventions compatible with the values and traditions of a community. Battiste (2000b) emphasizes the need for theory-based educational interventions that are congruent with the culture of the community:

> What is apparent to Aboriginal peoples is the need for a serious and far-reaching examination of the assumptions inherent in modern educational theory. How these assumptions create the moral and intellectual foundations of modern society and culture has to be studied and written about by Aboriginal people to allow space for Aboriginal consciousness, language, and identity to flourish without ethnocentric or racist interpretation. The current educational shortcomings may or may not be in the curriculum, or in finance, or in testing, or in community involvement, but no one will ever know this—nor the changes necessary for improvement—without a deeper philosophical analysis of modern thought and educational practice. (p. 197)

Guzman (2003) notes that studies of interventions conducted in a transformative manner may require adjustments during the course of the investigation. Interactions between individuals and group dynamics may

BOX 5.2. Independent and Dependent Variables: Prescribed or Emergent

PRESCRIBED: SCIENTIFICALLY BASED RESEARCH

As part of *Good Start, Grow Smart,* the ultimate goal of the Early Reading First program is to improve the school readiness of our nation's young children, especially those from low-income families, by providing support for early childhood education programs serving preschool-age children so that the programs may become preschool centers of educational excellence. Many of America's young children face daunting challenges as they enter kindergarten lacking the essential reading readiness skills necessary to succeed. Through improvements in instruction and the classroom environment that are grounded in scientifically based reading research, Early Reading First helps children develop the oral language skills, phonological awareness, print awareness, and alphabet knowledge that will prepare them for later school success. Early Reading First offers an exciting opportunity to ensure that children are provided with high-quality preschool education.

From U.S. Department of Education, Office of Elementary and Secondary Education, Early Reading First Program (2006a; *www.ed.gov/programs/earlyreading/2006-359a.doc*).

*   *   *

EMERGENT: INDEPENDENT VARIABLE IN WKKF YOUTH AND EDUCATION INITIATIVE

Middle Start began as a comprehensive middle-grades improvement initiative in Michigan in 1994. Although formal funding ends in 2005, partnerships formed and lessons learned continue to spread across the United States. The Academy for Educational Development (AED) supports the Michigan Middle Start Partnership, and its National Middle Start Center acts as a clearinghouse for schools, universities, and nonprofits seeking information and resources.

Middle Start turns middle schools into learning communities by helping middle-grades educators establish working teams and access student-focused instructional methods. "This is not a cookie-cutter approach to school improvement," says Patrick Montesano, director of the Middle Start National Center at AED. But it is an adaptive tool that many schools are plying to reverse the slide in middle school student progress. "The middle grades are the time with the last-best chance to grab these kids, to help them succeed in school before it's too late," Montesano says.

Middle Start connects teachers within a school, schools in a district, and middle schools nationwide. It ends the isolation of individual teachers trying to turn students around and draws whole schools into a growing "web of support." Before Middle Start,

(continued)

lead to a better understanding of the intervention. The intervention itself may be changed by the context or by the participants, resulting in variable effects of the intervention. She writes:

> This suggests that change is not so easily assessed or engineered, but rather that it is a nonlinear process that involves the introduction of new information, and the constant reassessment of the meaning of that information in relation to the culture being examined. This interaction complicates how we create evaluation plans and how we interpret the findings of our work. As culturally competent evaluators, we must be ready to constantly reassess our evaluation plans in order to account for the never-ending changes in ecological contexts. This may mean that evaluation plans will continually change as a process of the evaluation. (p. 174)

Data-collection methods may need to be modified to capture the effects of the interventions. And, the evaluators need to be conscious of the implications of such dynamic and responsive changes in the inferences about program impact. As can be seen in the examples presented here, the researcher/ evaluator role ranges from asking questions that solicit deeper critical thinking on the part of the program developers, to working beside the program developers in a shared role.

Examples of Intervention Development

Africans and HIV/AIDS

Chilisa and Preece (2005) provide examples of how stories, poems, and songs are used in African communities to collect, analyze, deposit, retrieve, and disseminate information. They recommend the use of community stories as a basis to understand how communities have defined their problems and match solutions to the communities' perceptions. In the HIV/AIDS study that Chilisa (2005) critiqued, she poses the question: How can researchers use the communities' stories on the meaning of HIV/AIDS to conduct community-centered research? The researcher would work through a dialogue with the communities to start the research from their frame of reference.

Native Americans and Education

Native Americans provide models for the development of interventions in education and psychology. Battiste (2000b) writes:

> Little classroom research has been done on the effects of teaching students about their culture, history, and languages, as well as about oppression, racism, and differences in worldviews, but consciousness raising classes and courses at the elementary and junior high school levels, and at the college and university levels, have brought to the surface new hopes and dreams and have raised the aspirations and educational successes of Aboriginal students. Our people are slowly coming to understand that poverty and oppression are not their fault and are not the result of their faulty language, consciousness, or culture. They have begun to understand that poverty and oppression are tools created by modern society to maintain the status quo and to foster and legitimize racism and class divisions. As band [First Nations] schools offer courses in Aboriginal language and thought, and as economic opportunities are made available to Aboriginal peoples on reserves through education, racism and its residual effects in the non-Native community and family are being exposed. (p. 206)

If an educational intervention is designed to improve learning for Native Americans, it needs to reflect the culture of the aboriginal peoples. Researchers and evaluators can work with program developers and encourage responsiveness by raising such questions as: What do teaching and learning look like in a traditional aboriginal setting? Little Bear (2000) provides the following answer: For the most part, education and socialization are achieved through praise, reward, recognition, and renewal ceremonies and by example, actual experience, and storytelling. Children are greatly valued and are considered gifts from the creator. From the moment of birth, children are the objects of love and kindness from a large circle of relatives and friends. They are strictly trained but in a "sea" of love and kindness. As they grow, children are given praise and recognition for their achievements both by the extended family and by the group as a whole. Group recognition manifests itself in public ceremonies performed for a child, giveaways in a child's honor, and songs created and sung in a child's honor. Children are seldom physically punished, but they are sternly lectured about the implications of wrongful and unacceptable behavior.

Teaching through actual experience is done by relatives: for example, aunts teaching girls and uncles teaching boys. One relative usually takes a young child under his or her wing, assuming responsibility for teaching the child all he or she knows about the culture and survival. This person makes ongoing progress reports to the group, friends, relatives, and parents, resulting in praise and recognition for the child. There are many people involved in the education and socialization of a child. Anyone can participate in the education of a child because education is a collective responsibility.

Storytelling is a very important part of the educational process. It is through stories that customs and values are taught and shared. In most aboriginal societies, there are hundreds of stories of spirits, creation, customs, and values.

Native Americans and Mental Health Services

Duran and Duran (2000) assert that most of the attempts to provide mental health services to Native American people have ended in failure because they do not provide relevant forms of treatment to ethnic populations. Sociohistorical factors have had a devastating effect on the dynamics of Native American families. In order to be successful, interventions that address family violence for Native American peoples need to reflect awareness of the devastating effects of such policies as the boarding school policy in the late 1800s, which led to the systematic destruction of the Native American family system. Duran and Duran (2000) explain:

> Skepticism concerning the applicability of a purely psychological model to represent problems of family violence for Native American peoples do not mean denying the need for or the contribution of psychology in the prevention or treatment of behavioral problems. Rather, our purpose is to look deeper into the multidimensional nature of mental health for fresh perspectives and empowering interventions instead of privileging a universal scientific discourse over the voice of the subjects. A richer perspective is vital in the work of mental health professionals involved in reeducation and resocialization into appropriate family behaviors. (p. 97)

Yazzie (2000) provides an example of an approach to the provision of services, rooted in their cultural traditions, for the problem of domestic violence in Native American communities. He contrasts the peacemaking model with the Western process of responding to domestic violence by reporting a crime, possibly issuing a restraining order or an arrest, requiring courtroom appearances, and in some cases, enforcing punishment and jail time. However, this Western intervention does not address the offender's attitude or teach him or her the appropriate way to behave. Navajo methods of justice address these salient areas: They help people take a look at themselves and examine their own conduct; they foster communication of feelings; they involve everyone who is affected by the harm; and they teach proper behavior (p. 44). Yazzie (2000) describes the Navajo peacemaking tradition as a vehicle for addressing issues of domestic violence in a way that is constructive and harmonious with Native American ways of knowing:

> Peacemaking is a "walk-in" service in which a woman can request a traditional peacemaking session at a local court. The court then sends the case to a peacemaker, who invites everyone involved to attend, including the woman and her relatives, the man and his relatives, neighbours, and even social services workers. The session opens with a prayer said by the peacemaker or a respected family member. Prayer is important because peacemaking is actually a healing ceremony, and prayer gets people to commit to the peacemaking process. Now, the people who are gathered start "talking out" their problem. (p. 44)

Both husband and wife are able to express their reasons for their concerns and behaviors. False excuses such as "If my wife had dinner on the table when I got home, I would not beat her" or "I was drunk" are addressed by the peacemaker and members of the extended family who are present. The abuser is reminded of the Navajo wedding ceremony, in which the relationship between man and woman is one of reciprocity between equals. Group members discuss what should be done, including dealing with alcohol and drug abuse and possibly making use of Western treatment programs. Duran (1990) states that evaluations of such a model in mental health services for Native Americans indicate positive results.

African Americans and Education

The Talent Development (TD) Model of School Reform provides an example of a cyclical evaluation conducted from a transformative stance with specific attention to dimensions of race/ethnicity. Designed to enhance the educational experiences of students in urban schools, the majority of whom are from racial/ethnic minority groups (Boykin, 2000), this model was developed by the Center for Research on Education of Students Placed at Risk (CRESPAR), a collaborative effort between Howard University and Johns Hopkins University, as an alternative to educational reform approaches that ignore contextual and cultural issues. With an overtly transformative agenda, the evaluation of Talent Development interventions incorporates both scientific methodological and political-activist criteria (Thomas, 2004). The transformative evaluation was designed to provide information to enlighten and empower those who have been oppressed by, or marginalized in, school systems. A key element in the quality of the evaluation is the engagement of stakeholders who may have had negative or even traumatic occurrences with the school system in their youth. Evaluators demonstrate respect for the stakeholders, who have traditionally had less powerful roles in discussions of urban school reform, and create opportunities for their voices to be heard. The evaluators facilitate authentic engagement of all concerned by holding multiple meetings with the field implementers and key stakeholder groups, with the intention of obtaining genuine buy-in by these groups. To the extent possible, stakeholder suggestions are incorporated into the Talent Development activities and the evaluation.

The intervention in a TD school is an evolving entity that is developed through a co-constructive process involving the evaluators, school staff, parents, and students (Thomas, 2004). Thomas describes this process as a challenge to the conventional role of an evaluator, such that the boundary between evaluator and program designer is blurred. TD evaluators can be involved in the decision making about interventions because they have in-depth knowledge of the setting and participants, and they share the responsibility of program development, implementation, and evaluation with the program designers and implementers.

The TD evaluators also place a premium on cultural competence in the context of the urban school. To that end, they seek evaluators of color or from underrepresented groups. When this is not possible, evaluators are required to obtain a fundamental understanding of the cultural norms and experiences of the stakeholders by means of building relationships with key informants, interpreters, or friends critical to the evaluation. TD evaluators are encouraged to engage in ongoing self-reflection and to immerse themselves in the life stream of the urban school through informal discussions, attendance at meetings and school functions such as fundraisers or parent information nights. These are strategies that increase stakeholders' access to the evaluators and program implementers, with the goal being improved school performance for those who are placed at risk.

A specific application of the TD model of evaluation is described by LaPoint and Jackson (2004) in the Family School Community Partnership Program (FSCPP). Student success in high school was the desired outcome. The program staff and community members worked with the evaluator to design interventions based on the following principles: positive parenting, communication, volunteerism, at-home learning, collective decision making, and collaboration with the community.

Theory-Driven Evaluation and Logic Models

Theory-Driven Evaluation (TDE) involves an examination of the mechanisms that mediate the process and outcomes of a program or evaluand (i.e., program, policy, service, or other setting that is evaluated). It combines the use of scientific and stakeholder theory to make visible the inner workings of a program and how those workings are related to the desired outcomes (Donaldson, 2001). Logic models are tools used in some TDEs to depict the logical expectations in outcomes, given the context, resources, and interventions that are implemented with a specific group of participants (Bledsoe, 2001). Logic models provide a graphic picture as an answer to the question: "How do you expect to achieve the desired outcome?" They can involve rather simple specifications of the context, resources, activities, participants/stakeholders, outcomes, and more far-reaching impacts. Figure 5.2 is an example of a logic model for a training program.

Logic models are sometimes criticized as too simple and too linear, as not recognizing the full complexity of the context, not lending themselves to emerging designs, as possibly constraining the types of data collected, and as missing important unintended outcomes (Bledsoe, 2005). Be that as it may, a logic model can be a useful way to get a picture of what a program is intended to do and why the stakeholders believe it will, or will not, achieve the desired goals. Bledsoe notes that the development of a logic model (in a TDE) may elicit stakeholders' theories (stakeholders who might otherwise be ignored, such as those from communities of color) about what the program is intended to do and what is needed to accomplish the desired outcomes. It can also be used to surface links that are needed for the program to function, such as cultural influences, and it allows the benefit of looking at other programs and literatures to encourage a broader scope in planning and evaluating a program.

A TDE that uses a logic model usually involves a number of steps. For example, Bledsoe and Graham (2005) used a TDE approach to study an urban literacy program, where their procedures included the development of a logic model, formulation of evaluation questions, use of stakeholder program theory, and testing of appropriate evaluation questions. Bledsoe and Graham noted the usefulness of the process in terms of bringing to the surface interrelationships between dominant and minority groups, as well as relations between historically underserved African American and Latino communities. They needed to deal with the competition between

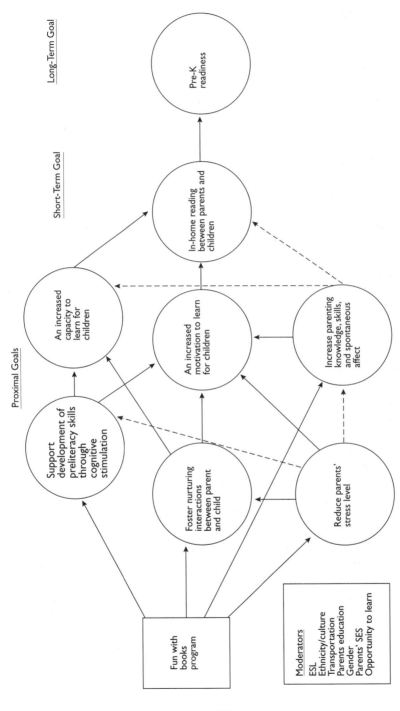

Long-Term Goal

Short-Term Goal

Proximal Goals

Pre-K
readiness

In-home reading
between parents and
children

An increased
capacity to
learn for
children

An increased
motivation to learn
for children

Increase parenting
knowledge, skills,
and spontaneous
affect

Support
development of
preliteracy skills
through
cognitive
stimulation

Foster nurturing
interactions
between parent
and child

Reduce parents'
stress level

Fun with
books
program

Moderators

ESL
Ethnicity/culture
Transportation
Parents education
Gender
Parents' SES
Opportunity to learn

FIGURE 5.2. Logic model of urban family literacy model. From Bledsoe and Graham (2005, p. 191). Copyright 2005 by Sage Publications, Inc. Reprinted by permission.

159

members of different minority groups in terms of access to valued community resources such as education.

Bledsoe and Graham (2005) made use of previous research that linked in-home reading with the development of preliteracy skills, thus enhancing school readiness. Program administrators also articulated their theory on the development of pre-literacy skills as identifying cognitive stimulation, reduced parental stress, and increased nurturing interactions as variables that influence in-home reading. They also added moderating variables to the logical framework such as English as a Second Language (which in this case meant Spanish and Polish languages in addition to English), culture, and accessibility to the weekly activities.

Brazil and the Favelas

The procedures for developing interventions and evaluation strategies in the Brazilian favelas (slum areas) emphasized social justice, capacity building, and transformation. In addition, the evaluation process had to be subtle, approaching the right people at the right time, making sure no harm was done either to the evaluation team or the community. Because these communities are severely affected by violence, mainly caused by drug trafficking, great risks were involved in the giving and collecting of information. The evaluation team emphasized the inclusion of all communities affected by the decisions. "In this context, the role of the evaluator was a proactive one in the sense of intervening to change the elements that favor social justice" (Firme, 2006, p. 5).

Theory-Driven Evaluation and Critical Systems Analysis

In Bawden's (2006) historical review of systems analysis and proposal for the integration of systems analysis with program evaluation, he describes the current state of critical systems thinking as embracing

> the idea of systems of intervention that involves stakeholder critiques of, and actions to remedy, both the social conditions in which different categories of stakeholders find themselves embedded and the boundary and value judgments that are being made, ostensibly on their behalf, by social planners or other interventionists. The focus of improvements under these circumstances results from communicative actions that deliberately confront coercive and otherwise power-limiting constraints. (p. 36)

Bawden (2006) notes that critical systems thinking is compatible with Stufflebeam's (2001) social agenda/advocacy category of evaluation approaches, in which program evaluation is used to empower the disenfranchised. However, he points to the need to extend the social justice/advocacy approach to incorporate approaches that allow judgment to be made about the merit and value of worldview transformations that are at the heart of critical systems thinking. He describes a "sea change" in the international development community that Sen (1999) refers to as *development as freedom.* From this rights-based perspective, Sen (as cited in Bawden, 2006) insists, the success of any society is to be evaluated by the extent to which the citizens within that society *are capable of living the lives that they have reason to value,* and this in turn highlights the primary significance of evaluative consciousness and active appreciation of *merit* and *worth* as central aspects of the development process (p. 38).

Bawden (2006) provides an example of critical systems thinking and evaluation in the context of a horticultural project in India. The project progressed from a focus on strengths, weaknesses, opportunities, and challenges in horticulture systems, to a focus on the "transformation of worldviews from productionism to a broader systemic perspective across broad constituencies of stakeholders of a number of various horticultural food systems. The central assumption is that such a transformation is a function of the intellectual and moral development of those stakeholders, which thus becomes the aim of the initiative and the focus of the evaluation" (p. 38).

Box 5.3 summarizes the various indicators of success in the dialogical, participative, reflective, and democratic process of critical systemic evaluation. Although this list contains challenging indicators of success, critical systemic evaluators need to meet them in order to demonstrate sensitivity to the different ways of knowing and valuing among the stakeholders. These indicators need to be interpreted so that they can be understood in the everyday language of the community.

The epistemic status of individuals is reflected in their particular worldviews. Attenborough (2007) sees critical systems thinking as a means to make explicit the relationships between systems concepts and action research concepts.

QUESTIONS FOR THOUGHT

- Having read through the many examples of transformative research and evaluation studies presented in this chapter, how would you characterize those elements that make the work transformative?
- Find examples of other studies and critique them in terms of the elements of a transformative study.

BOX 5.3. Critical Systemic Evaluation Indicators

1. Stakeholders should be able to express (and evaluate) how they come to appreciate themselves as a learning collective or subsystem of the developing system in which they are embedded, and which is itself embedded, in turn, in higher-order environmental suprasystems with both biophysical and sociocultural dimensions that present challenges as well as opportunities for further development and sustainable contexts.

2. Stakeholders should also be able to express (and evaluate) their appreciation of the systemic nature of their own learning subsystem with respect to three dimensions of learning or cognitive processing:

   a. They can process everyday matters in their search to improve circumstances that seem problematic to them in the "real world" (cognition).

   b. They can process the way by which they process those matters in seeking to improve the way they go about processing (metacognition).

   c. They can process the way that they frame the way they go about their processing and process of processing, in seeking to identify the worldviews that shape their thinking as a prelude to transforming them if they prove to be constraints to the other two levels of processing (epistemic cognition).

3. Stakeholders should be able to express (and evaluate) the systemic nature of the learning process that is relevant at each of these three levels—that is, the manner by which the different learning activities (e.g., divergence and convergence) and learning modes (e.g., empirical and ethical) interact with and inform each other.

Adapted from Bawden (2006, p. 41).

Summary

✓ A model of transformative research and evaluation was presented in this chapter that prioritizes community involvement, mixed methods, and a cyclical approach to research and evaluation, such that findings of one inquiry feed into subsequent decisions for studies and/or community action.

✓ Examples of cyclical models from indigenous peoples, participatory action researchers, and immigrant communities illustrate applications of the transformative model.

✓ Short-term research and evaluation projects may be necessary due to time, money, or other constraints. In such circumstances, efforts can be made to include the community in such a way that recommendations for further actions are possible.

✓ Descriptive approaches to research and evaluation provide a snapshot in time and can be used to assess community needs. Such information can be used as a basis for the development of culturally appropriate interventions.

✓ Causal-comparative and correlational approaches can be used when group differences that are not manipulable (e.g., gender, race/ethnicity, political parties) are important to ascertain. As is the case with descriptive studies, the findings of causal-comparative or correlational studies can be used as a basis for intervention development.

✓ Intervention research and evaluation involve the development and implementation of an intervention based on community needs. Logic models are one way of making the underlying connections between activities and desired outcomes explicit.

MOVING ON TO CHAPTER 6 . . .

Mixed-methods approaches to research and evaluation, such as experimental designs, surveys, and case studies, are examined as they are applied in the transformative context.

 If we have a prism in the window, we see different patterns of color in different parts of the room when it is early or late in the day. If we revisit the room periodically during the day throughout the seasons, we may see a pleasant surprise.

Notes

1. It should be noted that not all PAR is conducted with a social justice agenda. Kemmis (2006) identifies three forms of PAR: (1) the technical form that is aimed at increasing or decreasing a specific outcome, such as behavioral disruptions in a classroom; (2) the practical form that aims to provide information for the purpose of decision making by practitioners (e.g., teachers writing a self-reflective journal); and (3) critical or emancipatory PAR aimed at furthering social justice agendas.

2. For example, in the United States, the No Child Left Behind legislation prescribes the use of experimental and quasi-experimental designs and randomized trials.

CHAPTER 6

Quantitative, Qualitative, and Mixed Methods

The sharp separation often seen in the literature between qualitative and quantitative methods is a spurious one. The separation is an unfortunate artifact of power relations and time constraints in graduate training; it is not a logical consequence of what graduates and scholars need to know to do their studies and do them well. In my interpretation, good social science is opposed to an either/or and stands for a both/and on the question of qualitative versus quantitative methods. Good social science is problem driven and not methodology driven in the sense that it employs those methods that for a given problematic, best help answer the research questions at hand. More often than not, a combination of qualitative and quantitative methods will do the task best. Fortunately, there seems currently to be a general relaxation in the old and unproductive separation of qualitative and quantitative methods.
—FLYVBJERG (2006, p. 242)

IN THIS CHAPTER . . .

▼ Mixed-methods designs are illustrated, followed by a discussion of quantitative and qualitative approaches that can be used in such designs. Examples of how members of partnerships can address issues of cultural diversity and power inequities in transformative research and evaluation are presented.

▼ Specific quantitative and qualitative approaches are explained and illustrated as potential components of a mixed-methods approach. Ways to strengthen research and evaluation approaches through the use of culturally appropriate mixed methods are addressed extensively.

I disagree with the part of this chapter's opening quote that says the research problem drives choice of method; I believe that choice of method involves a more complex set of decisions that is driven by the researchers' or evaluators' basic paradigmatic beliefs. However, I do agree with the part of the opening quote that says it is time to move beyond the either–or stance in terms of methods to the both–and stance. Quantitative, qualitative, and mixed methods can be used in transformative research and evaluation (Mertens, 2003, 2007). These methods include traditional quantitative approaches such as experimental, quasi-experimental, causal-comparative, correlational, survey, and single-case designs, as well as traditional qualitative approaches such as group processes (e.g., focus groups or some indigenous methods), case studies, ethnographic research, phenomenological research, and PAR.[1] Gender analysis is a mixed-methods approach that provides a framework for transformative research and evaluation that has potential for transfer to other groups that experience discrimination. Mixed methods are most likely to be the approach of choice because of the need to integrate community perspectives into the inquiry process, thus necessitating collection of qualitative data during the research or evaluation process.

The advantages of using mixed-methods designs are illustrated in the Exemplary Schools Study that is part of the TD initiative (Towns & Serpell, 2004). The evaluators reported that quantitative survey responses from principals indicated that vandalism by students was not a problem. Confirming this data, the evaluation team's observations of the buildings found them to be clean and attractive. Their interview data with principals, however, revealed ongoing problems with vandalism propagated by outsiders over the weekends. In additional observations, the evaluation team noticed that school staff, students, and parents were perpetually cleaning walls and picking up garbage left from a weekend of vandalism. Hence, the evaluators concluded that the principals had reported no problem with vandalism by students because the vandalism was perpetrated by outsiders. In addition, they (Towns & Serpell, 2004) stated: "What our quantitative data could never convey was the enormous sense of shared ownership that students had for the school environment. This was a theme that was revealed in each of the student focus group interviews. Students expressed that keeping the school building and grounds clean was far from a burden; it was an activity in which they took great pride" (p. 54).

Mixed- and Multiple-Methods Approaches

Conducting mixed-methods research and evaluation studies is kind of like the "Which came first, the chicken or the egg?" question. *Mixed methods* require both quantitative and qualitative approaches. *Multiple methods* means that the researcher or evaluator uses more than one method, but the choice of methods reflects either quantitative or qualitative approaches, but not both. The linear nature of the printed text makes it extremely challenging to describe mixed-methods designs other than by explaining either quantitative or qualitative designs one after the other and then combining them. To address this challenge, various approaches that include mixed and multiple methods are described within the context of transformative research and evaluation studies, along with examples of specific designs rooted in quantitative or qualitative methods that could be used as components in a mixed-methods study.

Concurrent and Sequential Mixed-Methods Designs

Creswell and Plano Clark (2007) offer the following considerations in developing a mixed-methods design:

- Compatibility: Match the purpose, research focus, questions, and design.
- Timing: Determine the temporal relationship between the quantitative and qualitative data collection.
- Weight: Establish priority or emphasis of the qualitative and quantitative research in the study.
- Mixing: Determine when quantitative and qualitative data will be mixed in the process of research.

Based on these considerations, a rationale related to the purpose of the study needs to be developed as to why a mixed-methods design is being used. Also, a decision needs to be made whether to use a concurrent design in which the quantitative and qualitative methods occur simultaneously, or a sequential design in which one method precedes the other. Depending on circumstances, the researcher/evaluator may decide to give either equal weight to both methods, or greater weight to either the quantitative or qualitative part of the study. Mixing of methods can occur at the design stage or later in the process, such as at the analytic stage. Figure 6.1 provides examples of various mixed-methods designs.

Concurrent mixed-methods designs entail the use of quantitative and qualitative methods at the same time during a study. The TD study of exemplary schools referred to at the beginning of this chapter, exemplifies a concurrent mixed-methods design because the quantitative and qualitative data were collected in close temporal proximity to each other (Towns & Serpell, 2004). Firme (2006) also used a concurrent mixed-methods design

Concurrent Design

Sequential Design: Quantitative Followed by Qualitative

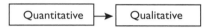

Sequential Design: Qualitative Followed by Quantitative

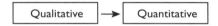

FIGURE 6.1. Mixed-methods designs.

for her evaluation of the Brazilian favela (slum areas in Brazil) project. She collected data from three kinds of checklists and interviews with beneficiaries, partners, and members of the community. Her team also collected data from unobtrusive measures, such as waiting in lines for computer access at the community center, and focus groups that were held with representatives of all program participants. The evaluators provided continuous feedback to the community throughout the process of the evaluation.

Sequential mixed-methods designs involve using either a quantitative method followed by a qualitative method, or the reverse. The Fine et al. (2004) study in California schools is an example of a sequential mixed-methods design. In May 2000, a group of advocacy organizations filed a class-action lawsuit against the state of California, alleging that poor and working-class youths were denied access to education because they attended schools that were in disrepair; staffed by undercredentialed teachers, with inadequate instructional materials and high teacher turnover. Mixed and multiple methods were used in this research, including random digit dialing surveys to generate a sample of current students and graduates of high school programs in Southern California to gather data about the students' experiences as part of the class-action suit. Here is the description of the approach:

A multimethod research design was undertaken: Surveys were completed anonymously by 86 middle and high school focus group members, prior to their involvement in the focus group discussion; 11 focus groups were facilitated with 101 youth attending plaintiff schools in the San Francisco, Oakland, and Los Angeles areas, as well as a group (of peers) in Watsonville; and 11 telephone interviews were held with graduates of California schools that fall with the plaintiff class. (Fine et al., 2004, p. 56)

A settlement was reached and approved by the court in March 2005 that requires that all students have instructional materials and that their schools are clean and safe. The settlement also provides strategies to increase the quality of teaching. Schools will be held accountable for accomplishing these goals and will be given $1 billion to do so.

Greene (2008) argues for the inclusion of another important dimension in the consideration of mixed-methods designs, that is, the degree and timing of integration of the various methods and the data that result. She describes "component designs" as those in which the different methods are independently implemented throughout the study, with linkages occurring only at the end after all the data have been analyzed. Such an approach might have the power to support conclusions if a convergence of findings emerges from different methods. If the results do not support each other, then this offers an opportunity for thought that Thomas Cook (1985) labeled an "empirical puzzle" (as cited in Greene, 2008, p. 23). The second design Greene describes is the integrated mixed-methods approach in which the mixing of methods occurs throughout the study, creating opportunities for "conversations" across methods as ways of generating additional insights regarding the phenomena under study as well as the methods that are being used.

Mixed-methods research and evaluation are growth areas in social science research. Witness the *Handbook of Mixed Methods in Social and Behavioral Research* (Tashakkori & Teddlie, 2003), the *Journal of Mixed Methods Research*, the annual International Mixed Methods Conference in Cambridge, United Kingdom, and an increasing number of texts that address mixed-methods approaches (e.g., Creswell & Plano Clark, 2007; Greene, 2008; Mertens & McLaughlin, 2004). As Greene points out, the use of mixed methods is a generative area for researchers and evaluators: "The process of developing a thoughtful and appropriate mixed-methods design is less a process of following a formula or set of prescriptive guidelines and more an artful crafting of the kind of mix that will fulfill the intended purposes for mixing within the practical resources and contexts at hand" (p. 129).

A cyclical model of research and evaluation is compatible with either concurrent or sequential, or component or integrated designs. Short-term studies can also use mixed methods, usually concurrently. However, if a single method is dictated by the funding agency, then researchers and evaluators can provide guidance as to next steps to encourage a cyclical approach, albeit with less certainty that follow-through will occur. This also means that the descriptive and interventionist research and evaluation approaches can be found in a study that begins with descriptive work to identify the issues and interventionist work to implement potential solutions.

Mixed Methods: What Is Being Mixed?

Bryman (2004) conducted a literature review of research designs that used mixed-methods research. He noted that experimental and quasi-experimental designs were the least represented in the journals surveyed (3%). The most common design was a cross-sectional one for the collection of both qualitative and quantitative data (63% of all articles). Of these, 42% used a survey instrument and personal qualitative interviewing. Another 19% used case studies, either with one case or multiple cases. This next section provides a description of the case study approach and then considers case studies from different theoretical perspectives.

Case Studies

Case studies are multifaceted strategies used to explore a bounded system and can involve collection of both quantitative and qualitative data (see Box 6.1). This section lays out steps in the conduct of transformative case studies. The first step, identifying the boundaries of the case, involves selecting the place and people and the potential intervention, as well as the time period for the case study. Decisions about place, people, and all aspects of the study are decided as a part of group process, including the level of participation in terms of researcher/evaluator and community members. The research or evaluation questions and purpose can be developed as a part of this process in conjunction with members of the community. Next, data-collection methods and decisions about instruments need to be made. Typically, case studies include interviews/surveys, observations, and document review, and if in an educational setting, can include an assessment of learning. The specifics of data collection using these strategies are presented in Chapter 8, data analysis strategies are in Chapter 9, and reporting options are in Chapter 10. The conduct of a transformative study is

BOX 6.1. Case Study: Classrooms as Learning Portals

INVITATION

How can I teach my deaf students math skills that go beyond drill and practice? How can I teach in a way that helps students learn higher-order critical thinking and problem-solving skills? These are questions that many teachers of deaf students ask themselves. Team leaders from the Join Together grant have developed strategies that represent promising practices to improve deaf students' learning in content subjects through the use of technology. You are invited to be part of a team of educators that is conducting case studies as a means to collecting data to support the use of these as evidence-based practices in deaf education.

BOUNDING THE SYSTEM

1. *Decide on the intervention/strategy.* Go to the *www.deafed.net* website. Notice that there are recommended practices such as teaching *step-by-step strategies* for problem solving in mathematics that extend beyond drill and practice to math and science processes that require *higher-order critical thinking* and problem-solving skills.

Related Technologies

- ❐ Math Pad—demonstrates step by step, one problem at a time, how to complete math problems.
- ❐ Math tutorial websites—*www.webmath.com*
- ❐ A Math Dictionary for Kids (website)

Video mini-studies explain projects or lessons that require higher-order critical thinking and problem-solving skills. In addition, there are bulletin boards for all the grant objectives (content competence, teacher diversity, faculty competence in technology, technology infrastructure, and multistate collaboration). Choose one or more of the strategies that you want to try in your classroom.

2. *Decide on a level of participation from the following options:*

❐ Level 1: Faculty and collaborating faculty. Faculty collaborates with another faculty, from another deaf education program, who is incorporating the same Recommended Practice(s).

❐ Level 2: Faculty, collaborating faculty, and Master Teacher. Instructor collaborates with another faculty member and also incorporates into instructional activities, in some way, a Master Teacher. Such collaboration may include, but is not limited to, (1) a presentation (either face-to-face or via technology) to the class on how the Master Teacher actu-

(continued)

BOX 6.1. *(continued)*

ally uses the selected Recommended Practice(s); (2) a demonstration of a lesson where the Recommended Practice is used, to preservice teachers either in the Master Teacher's classroom or via technology (e.g., video conferencing or videotape); or (3) another option developed by the instructor and the Master Teacher.

❐ Level 3: Unit option: Faculty, Master Teacher, and student teacher. Faculty and Master Teacher agree upon one or more Recommended Practices appropriate for the target students and appropriate to the selected Content Standard ("target students" are real students to whom the lessons will be "pitched"). Faculty and Master Teacher develop a unit of instruction to teach the selected Content Standard. The unit plan is to (1) provide a description of the class, (2) include at least one of the Recommended Practices (understand that some of the practices have a stronger research base than others), and (3) must include appropriate technology uses as identified on *www.deafed.net* and in the Recommended Practices list. The unit plan must be comprehensive and include as much practical information for teachers as possible. An excellent example of a comprehensive unit can be found by going to *www.deafed.net/publisheddocs/titanic%2012.doc*. Faculty, Master Teacher, and student teacher develop assessment rubric(s) that can be used with the target students.

PURPOSE AND QUESTIONS

Establish a purpose for doing the case study. For example, find out how effectively the strategy enhances higher-level thinking and problem solving in mathematics. Add research questions that relate to the purpose:

What forms of technology did I use and how did these support the math methods course curriculum?

How did the learner(s) respond to the use of this strategy?

In what ways did this integration of instructional technology and content impact on student learning?

Who will be involved? Decide who the participants will be and who else needs to be involved in the process (a collaborating faculty member, classroom teacher, Master Teacher, students, parents, administrators, aides?). Decide how they will be involved and what their role will be (learner, critical friend, advisor, another pair of eyes?). The post-report, which includes an evaluation of the process, varies depending upon the choice of participation level. It can include (1) a comparison between present instruction and the instruction enhanced with the Master Teacher's collaboration; (2) sample comments from students that led the faculty to believe that the students understood the material sufficiently to use the practice; and (3) a sample lesson plan developed by preservice teachers that incorporates the Recommended Practice(s).

rarely as straightforward as the listed steps imply, as seen in the following example.

Opfer (2006) conducted an evaluation of a charter school initiative in a southern state with a history of racial segregation that placed social justice issues in the foreground. At the beginning of the evaluation Opfer was concerned that state officials were "unwilling to publicly acknowledge that parents could, and had, set up charter schools with the expressed intention of segregating their (White) children from children of other races" (p. 271). The case study questions were developed by state officials and proved to be problematic in terms of making recommendations related to inequities. Sample questions included:

1. How did charter schools compare with traditional public schools in the state with regard to student achievement and stakeholder satisfaction?
2. How was the charter school concept being implemented in the state?
3. What implementation issues were arising in charter schools and what were the impetuses for these issues? (p. 275)

Opfer (2006) used several sources of data for the case study: discussion groups with parents and teachers; site visits and observations at 14 charter schools selected to represent regional variations, school levels, and school types; interviews with principals and teachers; and documents related to curricula, academic offerings, communications with parents, student demographics and achievement, and charter school annual reports to the state. She reported on the discrepancy between the demographics in one county in which 92% of charter school students were white, whereas 71% of the students countywide were black. In addition, she provided qualitative data from parent interviews that illustrated their racist attitudes and a desire to have their children educated in a segregated setting. The state department of education officials who had commissioned the study asked her to remove that finding. Their public reason for this request was that the evaluation should focus on overall patterns in the charter schools, not on one particular school. They privately shared their concerns with the evaluator that the charter school was in a district with a powerful member of the state's education committee and that it would be problematic if the finding was included in the report. Opfer then analyzed racial representation in charter schools across the state. Statewide, 12 of the 28 charter schools' demographic data revealed a 20% difference between the district's demographics in terms of race and that of the schools; 10 of the 12 had at least 20% more white students and 2 had 20% more minority students. She rewrote the report to indicate this pattern as a social justice concern. The state department officials subsequently ended communications with Opfer, removed that section from the report, and withdrew the contract they had offered her to do a follow-up evaluation of the charter schools.

Opfer (2006) offers an analysis of the lack of action by the state in terms of an inconsistency between individual beliefs (inequity by state officials) and the political culture (in this case, a belief in individual parental choice and that parental choice is working based on higher achievement levels). In addition, school officials felt that presenting charter schools as a source of social justice concerns would threaten the advances that they had made in increasing overall funding for education in the state.

Opfer's work is transformative in a number of ways. First, she examines inequities in access to school resources on the basis of race and reports egregious inequities in one charter school. Second, she provides evidence of a pattern of inequities in the charter schools. Third, when her work is made to "disappear" in the educational bureaucracy, she completes and publishes a thoughtful analysis of the reasons that her findings were removed from the report and the inaction of the state department officials with regard to this issue in terms of racism and political power.

Myths and Counterarguments about Case Studies

Case studies have often been criticized because it is not possible to establish causation, and the "results" are not generalizable. Yet, their use in transformative research and evaluation is critical because they allow for the type of relationships to develop that are needed for systematic collection of data for the purpose of social transformation. Because of the importance of case study methods in transformative work, the issues related to critique and defense are discussed in this section.

Flyvbjerg (2006) provides critics' arguments and his own counterarguments related to the issue of generalizability of case study research and evaluation. He presents the argument and its counterargument as follows:

Argument: "The view that one cannot generalize on the basis of a single case is usually considered to be devastating to the case study as a scientific method" (p. 224).

Counterargument: "One can often generalize on the basis of a single case, and the case study may be central to scientific development via generalization as supplement or alternative to other methods. But formal generalization is overvalued as a source of scientific development, whereas 'the force of example' is underestimated" (p. 228).

Ruddin (2006) extends this argument in asserting that it is false to think that a case study cannot grant unswerving information about the broader class. Rather, the strength of a case study is that it captures "reality" in greater detail and thus allows for both the analysis of a greater number of variables and for generalization from the concrete, practical, and context-dependent knowledge created in the investigation. He further explains: "We avoid the problem of trying to generalize inductively from single cases by not confusing case inference with statistical inference. Case study reasoning would be seen as a strong form of hypothetico-deductive theorizing, not as a weak form of statistical inference" (p. 800).

Stake (2005) places the burden of generalizability on the writer (presumably the researcher/evaluator or a team of writers) and the reader. The writer reports a case using "thick description" (Geertz, 1973), meaning with sufficient details about the context, actors, operations, behaviors, vitality, and trauma that a reader can understand that case. Stake weighs the cost of trying to compare the specific case to other cases against the gain in presenting the uniqueness of a particular case. He sees formally designed comparisons as competing with learning from a specific case. Readers will make comparisons based on their previous knowledge and experience with similar or different cases. It is then incumbent upon readers to make reasonable generalizations once they understand the specifics of the researcher's or evaluator's presentation of the case.

Flyvbjerg (2006) also addressed the misunderstanding about case study research that this method is useful for generating hypothesis in the early, pilot stage of a research program, whereas hypothesis testing and theory building are best carried out by other methods later in the process (p. 234). He contends that case studies are useful for both generating and testing hypotheses, among other uses. Because of their focus on an in-depth approach, case studies may well be better suited to test hypotheses and build theories than other approaches.

Morse (2006) contends that qualitative researchers can address research problems that quantitative researchers do not see as researchable, thus laying the groundwork for valuing qualitative inquiry as a necessary and essential research method that makes a contribution in this evidence-based research world. She places her arguments within a medical context related to attaining health. She states: "Nurses know that attaining health is a *behavior*, a lifestyle, an attitude, not solely the success of drug therapy" (p. 417). Hence, qualitative methods hold potential for reducing morbidity and mortality and making the provision of health care more humanistic.

Case studies have also been criticized because they are viewed by some as allowing more room for the researcher's or evaluator's bias to impact the findings than other methods, and are thus less rigorous than are quantitative, hypothetico-deductive methods. Flyvbjerg (2006) contends that such an accusation is based on a lack of understanding of what is involved in case studies. Also, the question of subjectivism and bias applies to all methods, not just to the case study and other qualitative methods. For example, bias can be present in the researcher's or evaluator's choice of categories and variables in a quantitative investigation. The probability of bias being present in any type of research or evaluation is a product of the choices made throughout the process and the breadth and depth of the member checking to ensure that the work is culturally competent. The theoretical frameworks discussed in Chapters 1 and 2 provide additional examples of how case studies can be conducted in a transformative spirit. The next sections explore critical race, feminist, and indigenous theoretical frameworks within the context of transformative case studies.

CRT and Case Studies

Madison (2005) states that CRT leads us away from understanding race as a biological component to thinking about the power dynamics that hold race in place. What are the ideologies, images, and institutions that perpetuate racism? The CRT framework provides a "more radical discussion of social and political power, [and] we see how race is formed and embedded by class and economic stratifications. . . . Critical race theory analyzes the complex machinations of racialization in the various ways it is created, sanctioned, and employed, but it also illuminates the various ways race is an effect of our imagination and how racial symbols and representations determine our understanding and attitudes about race in the first place" (pp. 72–73).

CRT calls for a reexamination of the concept of race by recognizing that it is not a fixed term; rather it is fraught with social meaning and is influenced by political pressures. Parker and Lynn (2002) make the argument that case study methodology is appropriate as a means to capture the CRT narratives and stories that challenge preconceived notions of race and support the development of legal narratives of racial discrimination. The "thick descriptions" and interviews can be used to illuminate both institutional and covert racism. The researcher or evaluator can use interviews to construct narratives that can be used in legal cases to document racial bias in officials or discriminatory policies and practices.

As an example of the integration of case study methods and CRT, Parker and Lynn (2002) cite the civil rights case in which Navajos in Utah sued the school district for discriminatory educational policy practices such as tracking, operating virtually dual school systems based on race, and not providing bilingual services (*Myers v. the Board of Education of San Juan County*, 1995; Villenas, Deyhle, & Parker, 1999). The case study approach allowed for the use of expert witness testimony and personal narratives to be used in establishing the school district's intent to discriminate. Deyhle (in Villenas et al., 1999) used the term *social justice validity* to describe a type of research validity that is "grounded in social justice and commitment on tribal nation terms and long-term involvement in challenging White supremacy over tribal nation affairs" (p. 11).

Feminist Theory and Case Studies

Watts (2006) used a feminist theoretical framework in her case study of barriers that women face in the highly male-dominated profession of civil engineering in one large consulting firm in the United Kingdom. Watts explained that her use of a feminist theoretical base included explicitly addressing her own characteristics and experiences in the context of the study; examining power relations between herself and participants; allowing the participants' voices to be heard; providing reciprocity to the women who participated in the data collection; and using the findings to improve the lives of women. However, Watts also reported that the use of the term *feminism* created a negative reaction from the participants; therefore, she chose not to reveal her theoretical framework during the study. She used a multiple-methods approach that included semistructured interviews with 31 women and 14 months of fieldwork involving observation and unstructured interviews. Watts describes her ethical dilemmas as she proceeded with data collection; however, she felt that obtaining data on the barriers women experience in this profession outweighed concerns about concealing the theoretical framework of the study.

For example, the women described incidents at building sites where men made disparaging and sexually suggestive remarks. The women indicated that these comments were unwelcome and made them uncomfortable, but they tended to dismiss them as circumstantial and isolated—as a normal part of the workday. Using a feminist theoretical framework, Watts identified the power relations in this patriarchal system that are associated with discriminatory practices against women. Instead of overtly challenging men who engaged in sexual harassment, the women learned to refuse to give the expected reaction. Watts sees this as a small, incremental strategy that fails to address the wider gender-based power imbalance. She shared her report with management and participants, indicating that the problem is systemic and requires systemic change. The responsibility for addressing this issue should not rest on the shoulders of individual women.

Indigenous (Postcolonial) Theories and Transformation

Indigenous (postcolonial) theories play two roles in framing research and evaluation studies: They both study the oppression of the dominant social structure and they support a positive and proactive stance for what indigenous people view as appropriate outcomes of the research or evaluation (Clarke & McCreanor, 2006). Clarke and McCreanor's indigenous Maori research study examined the dominant culture's response to sudden infant death syndrome in the Maori community, as well as the conflict between the dominant culture and the Maori culture when an infant dies. The dominant culture seeks to assign blame and does so by removing the child's body so that medical tests can be conducted. The Maori parent wants to keep the baby close until appropriate support mechanisms in terms of community members can be put in place. The forceful removal of the infant's body greatly complicates the grieving process for Maori family members, who believe that the dead body should not be left alone. Clarke and McCreanor also noted supportive strategies that appeared to lessen the negative impact, such as the presence of Maori community members who acted as liaisons between the grieving family and the police and coroners. They conclude that an indigenous Maori theoretical framework leads to a challenge of the investigative processes following the sudden death of an infant in that the dominant society's postmortem protocols lead to more harm in the grieving family than would occur if an indigenous investigative strategy were used.

Ethnography

Ethnography is a commonly used qualitative method of describing and analyzing the practices and beliefs of cultures and communities (Patton, 2002). It is possible to combine ethnography with other approaches in a mixed-methods study or to conduct a case study using ethnographic methods. A mixed-methods approach combining ethnography and surveys was proposed by Bamberger et al. (2006); teams of evaluators conducted a survey of households in a primarily poor and minority community to determine reasons for use or nonuse of rural health centers. Their mixed-methods design followed these steps:

- Conduct rapid ethnographic studies in a small number of communities to identify some of the issues and question formats that would be most appropriate for the survey.
- Select a sample of households for the surveys and a subsample for ethnographic studies of families and health services.
- Compare information from the survey and the ethnography for key variables (e.g., use of health services).
- Prepare separate quantitative and qualitative reports and have the teams meet to discuss the areas of agreement and disagreement.
- Conduct follow-up fieldwork to check on inconsistencies and possibly prepare additional cases to illustrate key points.

Mienczakowski and Morgan (2006) used an ethnographic approach in their action research studies of schizophrenia, drug and alcohol abuse and detoxification, recovery from sexual assault, and other health-related topics. They described a two-phase process, starting with intensive ethnographic data collection through an informant-led process, during which the informants decided the purpose of the inquiry and joined into the data collection. Data were collected by means of participant observation as well as by interviews conducted by the medical staff, student nurses, and other team members. They returned the data to the informants for additional comment, guided by a specific question: "What do you want to tell an audience of medical health workers, health service providers, care-givers or young people about the experience of schizophrenia or alcoholism or sexual assault or cosmetic surgery or acquired brain injury or cancer or unemployment or suicide or whatever the subject of the research is?" (p. 177). From their responses, the researchers compiled a list of themes, which informants were asked to validate. These themes were then used as a basis for the development of a script using the voices of the stakeholders in the form of an ethno-drama.

Mienczakowski and Morgan's (2006) approach was transformative on a number of dimensions. First, they framed their study in relation to the lives of the most marginalized—people with schizophrenia, alcohol and drug users. Their informants helped develop the research focus and participated as co-researchers in the data collection. The meaning of the data collected was vetted through the informant group. Recommendations for specific transformative action were made based on the input of the participants. Further details about this approach for the creation of recommendations for dissemination of results are included in Chapter 10.

Critical Ethnography

Just as with case studies, the theoretical framework that is brought to the ethnographic study can enhance the transformative potential of the work. Critical ethnography begins with an ethical responsibility to address processes of unfairness or injustice within a particular lived domain (Madison, 2005). The term *ethical responsibility* refers to a compelling sense of duty and commitment based on moral principles of human freedom and wellbeing, and hence a compassion for the suffering of living beings. The critical ethnographer contributes to transformative knowledge and discourses of social justice. Critical ethnography depends on theory as a way to illuminate a social phenomenon—whether it is Marxist, queer, postcolonial theory (as discussed below) or feminist, critical race, or another commensurate theoretical framework.

Marxist Theory

Marx focused on how the economic system influenced social structure and interactions. Systems such as capitalism and the accumulation of wealth, trade rules, and the machinery of production, distribution, consumption, and reproduction work to support the rich at the expense of the poor. Hence, this theoretical framework focuses on class divisions among groups of people in terms of their access to economic resources (Madison, 2005, p. 52). Marx argued that economic conditions determine our reality.

Queer Theory

Understanding the sexual politics that surround the personal and public domains in which each person must navigate is elaborated in the articulation of queer theory (Madison, 2005). Queer theory challenges conventional categories of sexuality and gender. Plummer (2005) asserts that there is no specific method that is associated with queer theory, however, he does describe text analysis, ethnographies, and case studies as being amenable to the application of queer theory. Queer theory ethnographies focus on specific sexual worlds and challenge assumptions about conventional understandings of such groups as gay, lesbian, bisexual, transsexual, and transgendered people. Another preferred strategy for investigations rooted in queer theory is textual analysis of, for example, films, literature, television, opera, and musicals. Mass media representations of sexuality are critically analyzed in terms of their portrayals of sexuality, with specific focus on homosexuality and homophobia.

Postcolonial Theory

Postcolonial theory argues that in countries with a colonial past—whether it is the Americas, Asia, or Africa—postcolonialism entails

> "all the culture affected by the imperial process from the moment of colonization to the present" (Ashcroft, Griffiths & Tiffin, 1998, p. 2). Therefore, when the critical ethnographer enters into a country with a colonial past, they [*sic*] also enter into a postcolonial present, with all the symbolic and material remnants passed down from the history of colonialism. Because postcolonial theory asserts that the aftermath of the colonial past exceeds the historical moment or transition from colonials to independence, we examine how the colonial epoch—for better and for worse—profoundly affected education, language, geographic borders, religion, governmental structures, and cultural values that are carried forth to the present and will continue to be carried forth in the future. (Madison, 2005, p. 47)

The purview of this examination includes remnants that continue in the present setting, such as settlement and dislocation, economic and material stratification, strategies of local resistance, as well as issues of representation, identity, belonging, and expressive traditions.

Madison (2005) lists the following elements in the research design for a critical ethnography:

- A statement of your research problem or questions.

- A description of your data-collection methods, including interviewing, journaling, and coding processes, and how these will be accomplished with the researcher as a co-performer in the field or participant observer.

- An explanation of your ethical methods and how the welfare of the participants will be put first by protecting their rights, interests, privacy, sensibility, and offering reports at key stages to them, including the final report.

- A description of the participants in terms of population, geographic location, norms and rules, significant historical and cultural context, and expectations for key informants.

- A time frame for entering the field, collecting the data, departing from the field, coding and analysis and completion of the written report, and/or public performance.

- Use of a critical theoretical framework in the design, implementation, and dissemination of the study.

Phenomenology

Husserl's (1970) phenomenological philosophy provides a basis for research and evaluation that is sometimes described as phenomenological inquiry. However, phenomenology encompasses multiple perspectives; it is not a "single unified philosophy or standpoint" (Moran, 2000, as cited in Madison, 2005, p. 57). Types include transcendental phenomenology, existential phenomenology, hermeneutical phenomenology, and phenomenology that emphasizes Marxist theory, feminism, and semiotics. The basic premise of phenomenology is that the perceiver determines meaning, and therefore it is human perception, not external influences or objects in the material world, that is at the core of the analysis. This approach emphasizes the importance of understanding participants' narratives from their own points of view by focusing on how subjectivity is formed and expressed.

Gubrium and Holstein (2002) discuss a phenomenological foundation for research that is designed to link the apprehension of meaning to social action while taking into account cultural, historical, and institutional concerns. Their description of phenomenologically based interpretive practice is commensurate with the transformative paradigm. Schutz's (1970) work aligns Husserl's philosophical stance with ethnomethodology as a research strategy that attempts to identify how individuals experience the world. People who share understandings about phenomenon in the world will see the world in similar ways. The researchers' responsibility is to suspend their own understandings of commonly accepted phenomenon in a search for the understandings that are constructed by members of the community.

Jimerson and Oware (2006) describe ethnomethodology in simplistic terms as "conduct explains codes," where codes are accounts of how people explain their behavior (conduct). Ethnomethodologists study the telling of codes. Jimerson and Oware used ethnomethodology to study how black male basketball players explain their conduct by telling the "code of the streets" (a term taken from Anderson, 1999). In terms of data collection, the authors interacted with their fellow players during pick-up basketball games that were captured on videotape over a 7-month period by Jimerson's uncle. Using ethnomethodology, they found that the code of the street centers on respect, and that respect is associated with defusing danger, "handling women," and dealing with each other. For example, the men talked about ways to avoid public danger, especially when encroaching unintentionally upon gang territory. The code was revealed by explaining how a companion had made a mistake and how they had taken control of the situation, thus engendering respect from their friends. The men used the code to explain their behavior in a setting where mutual understandings existed. Given the high death rate among black men, sharing the code has implications for their survival.

Participatory Action Research

Fals Borda (2006) describes the historical development of PAR as the recognition of an empathic attitude toward others, called *vivencia* (meaning, life experience), which is "necessary for the achievement of progress and democracy, a complex of attitudes and values that would give meaning to our praxis in the field. From this time on, PAR had to be seen not only as a research methodology but also as a philosophy of life that would convert its practitioners into 'thinking feeling persons' " (Fals Borda, 2006, p. 31). "If applied in earnest, this participatory philosophy could produce personal behavioural changes as well as deep social/collective transformations and political movements" (p. 30).

PAR seeks to empower community members to define their own research questions as well as lead the inquiry process and create their own solutions for change (Amsden & VanWynsberghe, 2005). The intent is to build community members' research capacity so that they can participate in the decisions that affect their lives through engaging in interactions and relationship building with each other and the researchers. PAR provides a concrete methodology for creating socially inclusive policy. (See Box 6.2 for an example of PAR.)

PAR methods include an iterative group-based process that involves the use of visualization methods to broaden the inclusiveness of the process, enabling people to represent their knowledge using their own catego-

---

BOX 6.2. Participatory Poverty Assessments

Participatory poverty assessments (PPAs) use participatory tools to engage householders who are poor in an assessment of their own living conditions. The methodology is deliberately nontechnical and accessible. Visual methods are used, such as mapping exercises, seasonality diagrams, timelines, and ranking exercises. Focus groups and semistructured interviews are conducted to draw out perceptions of well-being. The purpose of drawing on the expertise of householders who are poor is not just to improve understanding but to demonstrate the micro-effects of macro-policy (Booth, 1998). An additional purpose is to enable local people to analyze their own situation and develop the confidence to make decisions and take action to improve their circumstances (Collins, 2005, p. 13).

ries and concepts, and an explicit concern with the quality of interaction, including a stress on personal values, attitudes, and behaviors (Heron & Reason, 2006). The general format of PAR includes these elements:

1. The group decides on the focus and questions for the research.
2. Researchers and participants observe, engage in action, observe and record.
3. Researchers and participants immerse themselves in action and elaborate and deepen their understandings.
4. Group members reassemble and share their knowledge, using this iteration as an opportunity to revise their plans for the next cycle of research.
5. This cycle might be repeated between 6 and 10 times depending on the complexity of the research context.

Heron and Reason (2006) suggest that groups composed of 6–12 members are the most effective.

Greenwood and Levine (2007) note that action research (AR) is not limited to group meetings and qualitative methods. They indicate that the key characteristics of transformative action research are action, research, and participation. Action research is viewed as a research strategy that "generates knowledge claims for the express purpose of taking action to promote social analysis and democratic social change" (p. 5). The nature of the desired social change is an increased ability of involved community members to control their own destinies in a more just environment. They reject the separation of applied and basic research within the context of AR, noting, for example, that knowing how much heavy metal is in the ground water can serve as a basis for transformative action research. Greenwood and Levine (2007) summarize: "Surveys, statistical analyses, interviews, focus groups, ethnographies, and life histories are all acceptable, if the reason for deploying them has been agreed upon by the AR collaborators and if they are used in a way that does not oppress the participants" (p. 6).

Appreciative Inquiry

Appreciative inquiry (AI; as noted in Chapter 1) is based on the theoretical framework of positive psychology (Seligman, 2006). AI has excellent potential to be applied for transformative purposes because it focuses on the strengths, rather than deficits, in a community. Ludema et al. (2006)

take the position that action research has generally failed to bring about social transformation because it has focused on a problem-oriented view of the world. Such a critical stance serves to contain conversation, silence marginal voices, fragment relationships, erode community, create social hierarchy, and contribute to cultural enfeeblement—thereby allowing scientific vocabularies of deficit to establish the very conditions they seek to eliminate. As people in organizations inquire into their weaknesses and deficiencies, they gain an expert knowledge of what is "wrong" with their organization, and they may even become proficient problem solvers, but they do not strengthen their collective capacity to imagine and to build better futures. Ludema et al. recommend that action research be paired with AI to counteract these blocking factors and to foster the ability to work toward constructive change that relies on the capability of a group or organization to see and produce alternative realities through language (p. 157).

The methods associated with AI include four phases, with a cycling back at the end of the fourth phase, based on the assumption that organizations want to move forward and that people will contribute to that process if they feel their views and skills are valued (Ludema et al., 2006).

- The *first phase is topic selection*. Groups are encouraged to pick a topic that highlights their ideals and achievements. Researchers can stimulate discussion with questions such as: "What do you really want from this process? When you explore your boldest hopes and highest aspirations, what is it that you ultimately want?" (Ludema et al., 2006, p. 159).

- The *second is the discovery phase*, during which participants search for factors that give life to the organization. What is best about this organization? In this particular setting or context, what makes organizing possible? "What gives life to our organization and allows it to function at its best? What are the possibilities, latent or expressed, that provide opportunities for even better, more effective and value-congruent forms of organizing?" (Ludema et al., 2006, p. 161).

- The *third phase is to dream about what could be*. By focusing on positive ways of seeing the organization, individuals are encouraged to share creative and constructive ideas that paint a picture of their organization at its best. The length of time for each phase is dependent on the complexity of the research focus and the size of the organization. It is possible that the dream phase will not occur until the second year of an inquiry. The dream phase can be accomplished by organizing a series of retreats at which participants can recount their peak experiences as they envision their ideal organization in a safe environment.

- The *fourth phase is to design the future through dialogue.* The participants discuss ways to reach their dreams. It is important at this phase that everyone is included and supported in the conversation.

- At the end of the fourth phase, there is a cycling back, referred to as *destiny,* which includes the extension of invitations to an ever-growing group of people to engage in conversations about how the future can be constructed through action. Action is undertaken and reviewed and revised. *AI then cycles* again through the process as the organization comes to learn more about what it means to function at its best.

Morsillo and Fisher (2007) provide an excellent example of combining AI and action research in their work with a diverse group of disadvantaged secondary school aboriginal youths in Australia who expressed alienation from their neighborhoods and a likely disengagement from school. Morsillo and Fisher adapted the AI process into four steps by first asking the students to appreciate the best of what is going on in their lives by having them play a game in which they identified things about which they felt passionate (e.g., sports, adventure, music, dance). The second step, dreaming or envisioning what could be, was accomplished by having the students create visions for positive community improvement and engage in transformative discussions. The third step, design, was accomplished when the students created community projects that included cycles of planning, acting, and reflecting. For example, they designed and implemented projects such as a drug-free underage dance party, a cultural festival for immigrants, and an aboriginal public garden. The fourth step, destiny (or sustaining what will be), was taken when the students engaged in narratives of enhanced community connectedness. The researchers' results indicated that the students felt they did have the strengths needed to carry out the projects, they appreciated having someone believe in them enough to really listen to them and let them design and implement their projects, and, in the end, they expressed greater connection to the community than they had felt in the beginning of the study. The students cycled back to various activities, such as submitting a grant proposal to fund the development of the aboriginal garden and the youth theater project.

Experimental and Quasi-Experimental Designs

Although not the only way to test the impact of an intervention, experimental and quasi-experimental designs are relevant approaches in many such situations. As Mark and Gamble (2009) write, there is nothing inherently evil about wanting to know if an intervention is effective or if it is more effective than another intervention. In fact, establishing that an intervention is effective may have stronger ethical claims than depending on perceptions of effectiveness. Hence, use of such designs in transformative studies is not prohibited, but the transformative paradigm leads to an awareness of particular issues that might not be considered under other paradigmatic frameworks.

In experimental or quasi-experimental studies, an intervention (e.g., new teaching practice, prevention program for HIV/AIDS, nutritional supplements, free contraceptives) is called an *independent variable*. The *dependent variable* is that aspect of the participants that the researcher or evaluator hypothesizes will change as a result of being exposed to the intervention (e.g., knowledge, skills, attitudes, income, health). If the researcher or evaluator has the power to randomly assign groups to receive an intervention or to be placed in a control group (i.e., to receive no treatment or to receive an alternative treatment or placebo), then an experimental design can be used. If two or more groups are to be compared, one of which is to receive the intervention, and if the researcher/evaluator cannot, for logistical and/or ethical reasons, randomly assign participants to groups, then a quasi-experimental design can be used. Theoretically, an experimental design allows for the control of more threats to internal validity in the research than does the quasi-experimental design. However, the qualifying clause, *if the researcher/evaluator cannot for logistical and/or ethical reasons randomly select or assign participants* is an important "if."

The Helsinki agreement (Okie, 2000) states that participants in the control group should not receive "no treatment." Rather, they should receive the most appropriate treatment, given current knowledge of interventions, that is possible for that particular context. This principle or standard holds true for both experimental and quasi-experimental designs, and it addresses, in part, concerns around the issue of withholding treatments—whether the intervention involves drugs with the potential to save lives, housing programs, or educational programs. Decisions about the withholding of treatments should be made in consultation with community members. An additional criterion that enters into design decisions is the researcher's basic belief system with regard to control over the implementation of an intervention and consideration of the community's voice.

A simplistic experimental design might look like this:

$$R \quad X_1 \quad O_1$$
$$R \quad X_2 \quad O_1$$

where the R means that participants were randomly assigned to groups to receive either the experimental treatment or the placebo/alternate treatment; X is indicative of a treatment (independent variable), which in the simple design shown above, would mean that there are two levels of the independent variable (the experimental treatment and an alternative treatment); and O means the outcome or observation (dependent variable). The two rows indicate two different groups who are being studied in this experiment. Both groups will receive the same measurement instrument at the end (the dependent variable). If it is possible to give a pretest to the two groups, then the design would look like this:

$$R \quad O_1 \quad X_1 \quad O_2$$
$$R \quad O_1 \quad X_2 \quad O_2$$

Experimental designs are said to protect the internal validity of the study by controlling for extraneous variables that might influence the dependent variable, such as age, gender, intelligence level, or socioeconomic level. By randomly assigning participants to groups, theoretically, the background characteristics of the participants should balance out and not have a systematic effect on the outcome (as might happen if participants in one group were older or more intelligent than those in another group—a threat to validity known as *differential selection*).

Bamberger et al. (2006) suggest that experimental designs involving random assignment can be used when there are insufficient resources to provide a particular intervention to everyone. Then the intervention can be assigned at random by the use of a lottery to see who is in the experimental group and who is in the control group. Examples in international development include the random assignment of training programs for teachers or the use of special textbooks or technology-based resources (e.g., educational TV). Carvello and White (2004) describe the use of randomized lotteries to assign people to treatments when more poor communities request a service than can be met by available resources. A lottery is held to see which communities will receive a service such as clean water, improved sanitation, or a new health center. Although ethical concerns still arise with the denial of treatment, some researchers and evaluators justify this approach on the principle that demand outstrips supply, and the communities will have another opportunity to apply for the service in future years.

Quasi-experimental designs are similar to experimental designs except that the participants are not randomly selected or assigned to groups (see Box 6.3). Thus, concerns *do* arise with regard to differential selection.

BOX 6.3. Quasi-Experimental Design: Interviews and Multivariate Analysis

The World Bank conducted a mixed-methods evaluation of a development project in Ecuador. The evaluators were interested in assessing the impact of the cut-flower export industry on women's income and employment and the division of labor between husband and wife. They wanted to create groups of participants who participated in the cut-flower industry and groups of those who did not; however, it was not possible to randomly assign people to these two conditions. Therefore, they used a nonequivalent control group design by comparing two sets of families: those who participated in the cut-flower business and those who lived 100 miles away in another valley without access to this business. The methodology included the use of interviews and sophisticated multivariate analysis of variance. The dependent variables included women's employment and earnings and the number of hours spent by husband and wife in domestic chores. They also collected data on family size and the educational level of both spouses. The multivariate analysis of variance allowed for the control of these background characteristics before testing the effects of the independent variable on the dependent variables. Statistically significant differences were found between the two groups on each of the dependent variables: The women who worked in the cut-flower industry made more money and had a more equitable distribution of chores than those who lived 100 miles away (without access to this business). Newman (2001) noted the limitations associated with this design in that preexisting differences between the two groups might have accounted for the results.

Although this validity threat cannot be completely overcome, researchers and evaluators can collect additional background information about the different groups and use that to support equality of two or more groups.

A quasi-experimental design might look like this:

$$
\begin{array}{cc}
X_1 & O_1 \\
\hline
X_2 & O_1
\end{array}
$$

Here the X's refer to the independent and placebo or alternate treatment and the O's refer to the dependent variables. Note that there is no R preceding each line, indicating that the groups were accepted intact rather than being randomly assigned. In addition, the line separating group one and group two is another indication that the two groups were not randomly assigned to conditions. Sometimes the comparison group is selected because it is matched in some ways with the experimental group; however, it does not receive the independent variable as a treatment. This is called a nonequivalent control group design.

If it is possible to do a pretest on the treatment and control/alternate treatment groups, then the design might look like this:

$$O_1 \qquad X_1 \qquad O_2$$
$$\overline{}$$
$$O_1 \qquad X_2 \qquad O_2$$

The Talent Development model discussed in earlier chapters used a quasi-experimental design to determine the effects of the interventions in math and reading (Balfanz, Legters, & Jordan, 2004). The researchers had students from three neighborhoods in Baltimore use the instructional program and compared them to students from three matched control schools. All six schools were drawn from the same neighborhoods and had similar demographics. Their academic histories were similar in that all had experienced a long history of low attendance rates, low achievement, and low graduation rates.

Robert Moses, a civil rights activist, developed the Algebra Project, an intervention designed to address the right of low-income African American children to learn the higher mathematics that serve a gatekeeping function for opportunities in science and technology (Lee, 2004). Moses assessed the strengths in the students' homes and the community and developed a method of teaching algebra that reflected their experiences and strengths mapped onto the rational number system. For example, students took rides on public transportation (with which they were very familiar) and created math problems from their observations of mathematical concepts involved in train and bus travel (e.g., distance, time, money). They described these concepts first in their home language, then they learned to translate these problems into a pictorial representation, and finally into a formal algorithmic representation. Currently, the Algebra Project is implemented across the nation and serves over 40,000 students.

Quasi-experimental designs using matched control groups indicate that the students who participated in the Algebra Project achieve significantly higher scores on standard tests of algebra concepts and enroll and succeed in more advanced mathematics courses (Moses & Cobb, 2001; Moses, Kamii, Swap, & Howard, 1989; West & Davis, 2005). Interestingly, Davis, Greeno, and West (2000) received a National Science Foundation grant to study, using ethnographic techniques, the causal factors that underlie the success of the Algebra Project.

Preexperimental designs are also used; that is, an intervention is applied to one group and a measure of the intended dependent variable is obtained either twice (before and after the intervention) or once (only after the intervention). Of course, this type of design is fraught with difficulties when trying to make a causal claim because of the many possible intervening variables. However, a transformative researcher or evaluator might argue that if the changes from pre- to posttesting are vetted through the community, and there is a sense that this program is working for the betterment of their interests, then the traditional criteria used to determine validity may not be as important.

As noted by Bamberger et al. (2006), focusing exclusively on dependent measures either in a pre–post or post-only design yields information on changes in the dependent variable but does not provide insights into how the intervention was implemented, the quality of the implementation, how the intervention could be improved during the project, questions concerning who had access to the intervention and who did not, and other contextual variables that would explain success or failure. Transformative work would support the addition of process evaluation strategies that are quantitative or qualitative as a mixed-methods design to answer these information needs.

Ethical Issues

Impact evaluations that rely on collecting data from control groups are sometimes unethical because they exclude people from program benefits. Some argue that this criticism applies only when resources are available for serving everyone as soon as the program starts (Savedoff, Levine, & Birdsall, 2006, p. 23). When funds are limited or programs need to be expanded in phases, it might be impossible to provide services to all potential beneficiaries at any time. Savedoff et al. contend that choosing who initially participates by lottery is no less ethical (and perhaps even more so) than many other approaches. Some programs are allocated by lottery when they are oversubscribed (e.g., school choice in the United States or voucher programs in Colombia) or for transparency and fairness (e.g., random rotation of local government seats to be set aside for women in the Indian elections). Furthermore, whenever there is reasonable doubt of a program's efficacy or concerns with unforeseen negative effects, ethics demands that the impact be monitored and evaluated. For example, in Mexico opponents of a conditional cash transfer program in the mid-1990s argued that giving funds to poor mothers might increase their vulnerability to domestic abuse. A well-designed impact evaluation was able to put those serious concerns to rest. Many well-intentioned social programs are like promising medical treatments—we cannot really know if they do more good than harm until they are tested. Finally, starting with a properly evaluated pilot program can greatly increase the number of eventual program beneficiaries, because the evidence of success will provide support for continuing and expanding an effective program.

Mark and Gamble (2009) suggest five considerations when contemplating the use of experimental or quasi-experimental designs. First, the importance of the potential findings needs to be established in terms of improving society. Second, there needs to be real uncertainty about the best course of action. Third, it should be likely that an experiment would provide better information than alternative approaches. Fourth, it should be plausible that the study results will be used to inform discussion about changing the policy, program, or practice in question. Fifth, the experiment should respect participants' rights, for example, by not being coercive and not leaving participants worse off than if they had not been in the experiment. All of these considerations are complex and potentially may conflict with one another. Hence, the use of these approaches, like any transformative work, is a thinking person's game.

Mark and Gamble (2009) suggest several strategies that can be used when contemplating these approaches, such as the use of power analysis to determine the minimum number of people needed in a study as a way to limit the number of people placed at risk. Stop rules can be established so that if unusually positive results are found early in the study, these can be shared with others sooner rather than later. Or if the converse is true, if unusually negative results are associated with a treatment, the experiment can be stopped early. In addition, designs can be developed that enable the disaggregation of data by different types of subgroups that might be hypothesized to have differential experiences with the interventions.

Survey Design and Correlational and Causal-Comparative Studies

Generally survey designs are descriptive, cross-sectional, or longitudinal. Descriptive surveys give a snapshot in time of the variables being studied. Cross-sectional surveys illustrate how different sectors of a sample respond to the survey items (e.g., third graders vs. sixth graders) about a specific topic (e.g., attitudes toward school). Longitudinal surveys follow a cohort through a prolonged period of time; for example, surveying a group of third-grade students, waiting 3 years, then surveying them again in sixth grade. The advantage of a cross-sectional survey is that researchers and evaluators can obtain information about both younger and older respondents at the same time. However, by waiting 3 years, the survey data can be obtained from the same group at each age. The disadvantage of the latter strategy is that researchers and evaluators have to wait 3 years to find out how students' attitudes toward school change from third to sixth grade.

Survey data can be used as descriptive data, as a basis for group comparisons, or as an indicator of the relative strength and direction of two variables. In the former case, the example given above, comparing third- and sixth-grade students, would be a causal-comparative approach. If researchers and evaluators instead used the number of years in school as a predictor variable with regard to attitudes toward school, they would then have a correlational study. Transformative research and evaluation that use surveys are conducted under similar conditions as those described for the other approaches discussed in this chapter.

Survey as Intervention

Irwin's (2005) longitudinal causal-comparative survey to address possible solutions to the troubles in Northern Ireland that have burdened that country with civil unrest for centuries is an example of a transformative approach. In this study, adversarial political parties constitute the key dimension of diversity; thus the causal-comparative independent variable was political party membership. Irwin wrestled with the representation of stakeholders in the politically charged atmosphere of Northern Ireland in his use of public opinion polls. His preliminary work suggested that innovations that might lead to peace in that region were supported by a majority of the people; however, they were being blocked by religious and political elites who were benefiting from maintaining social divisions and the status quo. Irwin contacted recently elected politicians from 10 different political parties and asked them to nominate a member of their team to work with him and his colleagues to write questions and run polls on any matters of concern to them. Thus, parties from across the political spectrum, representing loyalist and republican paramilitary groups, mainstream democratic parties, and cross-community parties, all agreed on the questions to be asked, the methods to be used, and the timing and mode of publication. The specific options on the survey constituted the dependent variables. The group conducted nine different polls, progressively identifying more specifically the choices for government that would be acceptable to the majority of the people. A basis for peace was found as the groups moved from their ideal extremes to a workable middle solution.

Irwin experienced several challenges. Early in the process, the British and Irish governments were opposed to the use of an independent needs-sensing activity. Not only did they not want to participate in the writing of any of the questions, design of the study, or funding of the effort, they objected to Irwin's presence in the building where he met with the politicians. However, the stakeholders overruled the government officials and went forward with the process, making public the results of each poll. The results of the ninth poll indicated that a majority of the electorate would say *yes* to a referendum that would bring peace through a power-sharing agreement between the British and Irish governments. By insisting on the representation of long-time adversaries in the planning and implementation of the polling, Irwin was able to contribute significantly to the Belfast Agreement that was passed by the people. The building of a political consensus, while time consuming and difficult, was necessary to reach an agreement that could help to build peace in the world.

Irwin notes a number of critical areas of conflict that exist in the world, some of which are decades and even centuries old for example, Greek and Turkish Cypriots, Israelis and Palestinians, Serbs and Albanians in the former Yugoslav Republic of Macedonia, and the English, Americans, and Iraqis. In order for public polling to be successful as a means of contributing to world change, researchers or evaluators must identify the appropriate dimensions of diversity that need to be represented at the table. This might include both moderate and extremist groups, as well as liberal and conservative politicians, grass-roots community organizations, and religious groups. If the appropriate stakeholders are not identified or not involved in a meaningful way, then the results of the survey have much less potential to be linked to the desired social action. This topic is further explored in the discussion of the relevant dimensions of diversity within the research or evaluation context in Chapter 7.

Gender Analysis: A Mixed-Methods Approach with Potential Transfer to Other Groups That Experience Discrimination

Gender analysis frameworks are methodologies that make use of observation techniques such as participant observation (a variety of participatory rural appraisal techniques) or more formal surveys that provide quantitative data (March et al., 1999). Used to assess inequalities in women's and men's social roles, these frameworks are rooted in the international development community but have applicability in a broader context. March et al. (1999) explain:

> Gender analysis: Such an analysis explores and highlights the relationships of women and men in society, and the inequalities in those relationships, by asking: Who does what? Who has what? Who decides? How? Who gains? Who loses? When we pose these questions, we also ask: Which men? Which women? Gender analysis breaks down the divide between the private sphere (involving personal relationships) and the public sphere (which deals with relationships in wider society). It looks at how power relations within the household interrelate with those at the international, state, market, and community level. (p. 18)

Gender analysis frameworks can be problematic depending on the political and cultural contexts in which they are applied. Key terms used in gender frameworks may be difficult to translate or may be interpreted as insensitive to the indigenous culture or personal lives of the participants. Even the term *feminist* may not be acceptable to some constituencies because of the political baggage that it carries (Whitmore et al., 2006). As Watts (2006) found in her work with civil engineers, and Mertens (Whitmore et al., 2006) found in her work in Africa with an international donor organization, the word *feminist* was not a comfortable fit, although the participants acknowledged the usefulness of feminist theory in understanding inequities based on gender. In the African context, the term *feminist* was associated with the concerns of white women, lesbians, and women who were hostile toward men, and as such, was not a term the participants were willing to acknowledge as a basis for their work with women in Africa. Specific examples of gender analysis frameworks are presented in Chapter 8 on data collection.

Rigor in the Process of Research and Evaluation

Lincoln and Guba (1985) developed criteria for evaluating qualitative research. These criteria can be adapted for use with transformative research and evaluation studies, whether quantitative, qualitative, or mixed methods are used. Researchers and evaluators strive to achieve internal validity or credibility; that is, if an intervention is used, are any changes in the outcomes of interest adequately proven to be due to the intervention? What additional contextual variables contribute to the outcomes? If a study is descriptive, how congruent are the results with the reality as perceived by the participants? Lincoln and Guba suggest specific strategies to enhance the trustworthiness/internal validity of research, including:

- *Prolonged and substantial engagement and persistent observations.* Did researchers or evaluators stay long enough to reach a state of saturation, such that salient issues could be identified accurately? This needed saturation level involves not only the length of the study but also the time on site and the number of times and circumstances that were observed. In addition, issues of insider–outsider need to be considered, and the process of building relations and trust. For example, Nichols and Keltner (2005) conducted a study of Native Americans in whose community they were well-known. They attended tribal meetings, pow-wows, naming ceremonies, honoring ceremonies, traditional ceremonies, and family gatherings.

- *Peer debriefing.* Did the researcher/evaluator talk over the study as it was in progress with a "disinterested" third party? What criteria were used to choose the peer debriefer? What role did the peer debriefer play? The criteria of having a disinterested party as a peer debriefer is not set in stone, however. Many researchers and evaluators work in teams and use frequent discussions to reveal aspects of the study that might remain under the surface without such an effort.

- *Progressive subjectivity.* To what extent did the researcher/evaluator engage in self-reflection throughout the study? How was this accomplished? Did he or she make note of initial hypotheses and feelings and revisit them throughout the study? Did he or she include data from the reflective exercises in the report of the findings?

- *Member checks.* How did the researcher/evaluator check the believability of the results with the participants from various constituencies? What contribution did these member checks make to the study? How were member comments integrated into the results? For example, Nichols and Keltner (2005) shared their findings formally and informally with the informants, family associates, and advisory board members at various times during the study. The community members confirmed or refuted the findings at these meetings.

Lincoln and Guba (1985) proposed a second category, transferability, as a parallel to external validity. *External validity* means that the sample is statistically representative of the population, and hence, theoretically, the results of research and evaluation studies can be generalized from the sample to the population. *Transferability* refers to the ability of the researcher/ evaluator to present the findings to readers so that they can assess the transferability of the results of one study to another situation. As mentioned previously in this chapter in the discussion of case studies, the report writer needs to provide sufficient detail ("thick description") so that the reader can make a judgment as to the transferability of the information from the specific case investigated to the reader's own circumstances. For example, if a study is conducted in one residential school for deaf students, the reader needs a sufficient description of the particular school to be able to make a judgment about its relevance in another school setting.

Lincoln and Guba (1985) also identified dependability as the corollary to reliability. *Reliability* refers to a measurement's ability to yield similar results from one time to the next, without intervention. If the research or evaluation study is conducted in circumstances undergoing change, then *dependability* would mean that such changes are being tracked and documented. Lincoln and Guba called this process a *dependability audit.* Yin (2003) recommends tracking changes by maintaining a detailed protocol that notes each step in the inquiry process.

Confirmability is the third major category of rigor and parallels the concept of objectivity. *Objectivity* refers to the degree to which researchers and evaluators need to make judgments about the meaning of results and the extent to which those judgments might bias the results. Because judgment is required in all types of research and evaluation regarding what data to collect, how to collect it, and how to interpret it, Lincoln and Guba (1985) suggest the use of a *confirmability audit,* which allows for a tracking process to cover the study from the collection of raw data to the identified outcomes. Data excerpted from field notes or interviews can be used to support the themes that are reported, thus supporting that these results are not the product of the researcher's or evaluator's imagination or bias.

The final category of rigor is *authenticity,* which means that researchers and evaluators present a fair and balanced view of the research, and that community members are able to use the information for the furtherance of social justice and human rights. Although the criteria associated with authenticity appear in Chapter 1, they are listed again here as specific criteria for assessing rigor in transformative work (the first three criteria are elaborated in Kirkhart, 2005; others are found in Mertens, 2005; and Lincoln & Guba, 2000).

- Experiential: How is the experience of the people involved in the research/evaluation changed as a result of their participation?

- Consequential: What are the consequences of the inquiry in terms of furthering social justice and human rights?

- Interpersonal: How have the relationships among researchers/evaluators and participants changed?

- Ontological: How has the nature of reality been modified to contribute to social justice goals?

- Catalytic: What actions resulted from, or are potentially possible as a result of, the study?
- Critical reflexivity: How do the researchers/evaluators and participants understand themselves differently?
- Reciprocity: What has the research/evaluation contributed to the community?

QUESTIONS FOR THOUGHT

- Locate research and/or evaluation studies in your area of interest. Critically analyze them on the basis of the criteria for rigor that are presented in this chapter. How do the researchers/evaluators manifest transformative principles in their work?

- *An overarching transformative question to guide reflection on the quality of the work:* What evidence is there that the researcher/evaluator and community members developed the design to be responsive to the practical and cultural needs of specific subgroups—on the basis of such dimensions as disability, culture, language, reading levels, gender, class, race/ethnicity, and other contextually dependent dimensions of diversity—toward the pursuit of social justice?

- Discuss possible methods to be used in a research or evaluation study with members of the community in which you wish to work. What are the various reactions that you receive when you describe different methods?

Summary

✓ Concurrent or sequential mixed- and multiple-methods designs are recommended in transformative research and evaluation.

✓ The methods that are mixed are borrowed from scholarly literature that describe quantitative and qualitative approaches, such as case studies, ethnography, phenomenological studies, participatory action research, appreciative inquiry, experimental and quasi-experimental designs, survey research, and gender analysis.

✓ Theoretical frameworks that are compatible with the transformative paradigm are discussed for the various methods, such as feminist, CRT, indigenous, postcolonial, Marxist, and queer theories.

✓ Specific conditions apply to the use and combination of these approaches in transformative research and evaluation studies, based on the researchers'/evaluators' assumptions. Specifically, the goals of human rights and social justice are placed in the foreground, resulting in methodological decisions rooted in culturally respectful, reciprocal relationships between researchers and community members that advance the stated goals.

✓ Criteria for rigor apply in transformative research and evaluation in terms of the extent to which the researcher/evaluator and community members developed the design to respond to the practical and cultural needs of specific subgroups on the basis of such dimensions as disability, culture, language, reading levels, gender, class, race/ethnicity, and other contextually dependent dimensions of diversity.

MOVING ON TO CHAPTER 7 . . .

Chapter 7 examines the process of identifying the dimensions of diversity that are relevant in particular contexts, presents strategies for sampling or selecting people to be involved in the inquiry and determining the levels of their involvement, and describes supportive mechanisms with which to increase the probability of authentic involvement and the role of ethical review boards from institutional and community-based perspectives.

How many ways can we look at the same thing? If we try to count the rainbows or measure the light waves, do we get the same information as when we stand in awe at the miracle of a rainbow?

Note

1. PAR was presented as a model in the previous chapter. In this chapter PAR is presented from a more specific methodological perspective. The topic of discourse analysis, a qualitative approach, is treated in the chapter on data analysis (Chapter 9).

CHAPTER 7

Participants

Identification, Sampling, Consent, and Reciprocity

Individuals whose sexual orientation or gender identity does not conform
to societal norms are ostracized and even victimized. As a result,
LGBTQ[1] youths remain more vulnerable to suicide and other mental
health issues (Elze, 2002; Roberts, Grindel, Patsdaughter, Reardon, &
Tarmina, 2004), to victimization in school (Elze, 2003; GLSEN, 2006),
lower academic achievement, and lower college attendance (GLSEN,
2006) than their non-LGBTQ peers. In addition, both LGBTQ youths
and adults receive strong negative social and political messages about
their sexual orientation, with some being encouraged or even forced to
undergo "conversion" therapies designed to "set them straight."
—DODD (2009, p. 476)

IN THIS CHAPTER . . .

▼ Sampling is reframed with a transformative eye, with specific focus on

   ▼ The myth of homogeneity

   ▼ Understanding the contextually relevant dimensions of diversity

   ▼ Theoretically important characteristics (e.g., trust)

   ▼ Impact of labels (e.g., at risk vs. resilient)

▼ Culturally appropriate strategies are discussed to enable researchers and
evaluators to overcome barriers to inclusion and to issue an authentic
invitation to people in the community to engage in the inquiry process. This
discussion includes examples of the types of support that have been found to
be important for a variety of communities.

▼ The roles and functions of ethical review boards are examined.

▼ The issue of reciprocity is discussed in terms of avoiding the use of coercion
or taking advantage of others, as well as providing appropriate compensation
for participation.

Using the transformative paradigm, sampling is reframed to (1) reveal the dangers of the myth of homogeneity, (2) understand those dimensions of diversity that are important in a specific context in order to avoid causing additional damage to populations by using labels that can be demeaning and self-defeating, and (3) recognize the strategies needed to remove barriers to participation in research or evaluation studies. The myth of homogeneity is evidenced when generic labels are used to describe a culturally complex group of people, without recognition of that complexity. For example, gender provides one example of a dimension of diversity that is generally thought to be unproblematic when the two options—male and female—are offered for self-identification. Although the use of these two options may be sufficient in some venues, the opening quotation of this chapter illustrates how a transformative lens can reveal consequences associated with operating from the dominant culture's perspective that gender is a bidimensional characteristic.

Social Justice: Dimensions of Diversity and Cultural Competence

- Gertrude Stein: Rose is a rose is a rose . . . (1913)
- But, is an African an African an African? (Chilisa, 2005)
- Is a person with a disability a person with a disability a person with a disability? (Mertens & McLaughlin, 2004)

Saying "Rose is a rose is a rose" is a comment on an individual whom Stein characterizes by the use of the rose as metaphor. However, Stein's admiration for her friend Rose is sometimes mistranslated as "a rose is a rose is a rose." I doubt that a gardener who cultivates roses could be found who would agree with that statement. As a researcher or evaluator, the absurdity of saying an "African is an African is an African" should be equally obvious. Yet, much research and evaluation are conducted that do not incorporate the complexities of African values and experiences. The implications of such research and evaluation in terms of social justice and human rights are far more serious than simply misquoting Gertrude Stein.

Because the transformative paradigm is rooted in issues of diversity, privilege, and power, recognizing the intersection of relevant dimensions of diversity is a central focus. Researchers and evaluators raise questions to program personnel and participants to consider the relevant dimensions of diversity, especially with regard to traditionally underserved groups—

whether based on race/ethnicity, gender, socioeconomic class, religion, disability status, age, sexual orientation, political party, or other characteristics associated with less privilege—and ways to structure program activities and measure appropriate outcomes, based on those dimensions. For example, if the central focus of a program is race and ethnicity, what other dimensions need to be considered? Gender, disability, SES, reading level, or home language other than English? Length of time with HIV/AIDS infection, role in the family, access to medications, presence of supportive community? Participation in various political parties that have a history of adversarial relationships?

Cultural competence is a necessary disposition when working within the transformative paradigm in order to uncover and respond to the relevant dimensions of diversity. Some semblance of cultural competence is required to identify those dimensions that are important to the specific context. Who needs to be included? How should they be included? How can they be invited in a way that they feel truly welcome and able to represent their own concerns accurately? What kinds of support are necessary to provide an appropriate venue for people with less privilege to share their experiences with the goal to improve teaching and learning? Or health care? Or participation in governance? Or reduction of poverty? What is the meaning of interacting in a culturally competent way with people from diverse backgrounds?

How can relevant dimensions of diversity be identified and integrated into programs designed to serve populations characterized by a diversity that is unfairly used to limit their life opportunities? Understanding the critical dimensions of diversity that require representation in order for transformative research or evaluation to contribute to social change is dependent on the realization that relevant characteristics are context dependent. Important questions include:

What are the dimensions of diversity that are important in this study?

Who is on the program team?

Who is on the research or evaluation team?

How reflective are team members of the targeted community?

How can stakeholders be identified and invited to participate in a truly welcoming manner?

What support is needed?

What sampling issues need to be addressed?

To what extent do underrepresented groups (disaggregated) have input into decisions about what and how issues will be addressed and how the impact of the interventions will be measured?

How is resource distribution affecting the ability of stakeholders to benefit from the innovations?

Who cannot participate and why?

How can power differences be safely acknowledged and accommodated?

Gender

Kadour (2005; as cited in Kosciw, Byard, Fischer, & Joslin, 2007) provides additional evidence of the consequences of omitting a broader range of options when gender is defined as male–female in research about youths. For example, the Centers for Disease Control published a special issue of *Morbidity and Mortality Weekly Report* that focused on suicide, and, despite considerable consensus about the potential for gay youths to be at risk for suicide, there was no mention of sexual orientation. As Kadour points out "data are a cornerstone of any public health system, and the lack of data on sexual minorities correlates with the failure of public health to address this group's needs" (p. 31). When studies fail to ask participants about their sexual orientation or their gender identity, they are eliminating the opportunity for the particular needs of those individuals to be identified. Studies on intimate partner violence, school bullying, or cardiovascular disease that omit sexual orientation and gender identity can be used to justify programming for those issues in general, but not to justify the need for programs specifically for LGBTQ individuals.

Dealing appropriately with this population requires clarity about such terms as *sex, sex identity, gender,* and *gender identity.* Referring to the ontological assumption of the transformative paradigm leads us to query the historical, cultural, and biological bases for defining these concepts. Mertens et al. (2008) note that the World Health Organization (2007) recognizes sex as a biologically based category and gender as a psychological feature associated with biological states. The American Psychological Association (2008b) extends this understanding of gender by describing it as a psychological phenomenon referring to learned sex-related behaviors and attitudes. Diamond (2000) describes gender identity as one's sense of maleness or femaleness, including awareness and acceptance of biological sex. I and my colleagues (Mertens et al., 2008) continue to explore the meaning associated with this set of complex concepts:

Although sexual identity is fluid and created by individuals, communities and socio-historical events (Frable, 1997), sex itself is usually tied to observable genitalia yielding two primary (male and female) and one blended (intersex) categories. Gender, then, refers to an individual's internal awareness and experience of gender and includes the five accepted categories of heterosexual, homosexual, bisexual, transgendered, and asexual. Ultimately, there are eleven sexual identities which take the categories of sex and combines them with concepts of gender: heterosexual male, heterosexual female, bisexual female, bisexual male, lesbian woman, gay man, pre- or postoperational MTF (male to female) or FTM (female to male) transsexual, and asexual. These eleven identities represent a useful set of descriptive categories for investigating how gender differences can impact meaning-making and lived experiences (West & Zimmerman, 1985). Ontologically, a transformative paradigm would lead the researcher to question the potential of discriminating against some realities by imposing the normative heterosexuality inherent in limiting gender queries in the form of M and F. (p. 85)

Race/Ethnicity

In the United States, race and ethnicity are commonly viewed as salient dimensions of diversity that require focused attention. The U.S. Census (2001) categories for race and ethnicity provide another example of issues that arise in sampling based on what is gained and what is lost by reducing sampling to generic categories. The minimal categories for race in the U.S. Census in 2001 included seven categories:

- White
- African American
- American Indian and Alaska Native
- Asian
- Native Hawaiian and Other Pacific Islander
- Some other race
- Two or more races

There are also two minimum categories for ethnicity: Hispanic or Latino and Not Hispanic or Latino. Hispanics and Latinos may be of any race. Although data such as those yielded by the U.S. Census are useful for broad generalizations, they also obscure important differences in the population of the United States.

Race has been considered in terms of a biological phenomenon as well as from the social constructionist perspective (Kendall, 2006). Science has been unable to produce sufficient supportive evidence that race is a biological phenomenon, hence, the interest in understanding how we create the meanings we give to race and ethnicity. The social construct of race has developed on the premise that some people have greater inherent worth than other people. To be specific, society has held the belief that, and operated as if, white people are superior to people of color.[2]

The American Psychology Association's *Guidelines on Multicultural Education, Training, Research, Practice, and Organizational Change for Psychologists* (2002) focus primarily on four racial/ethnic groups because of the unique salience of race/ethnicity for diversity-related issues in the United States. They developed guidelines for research (and evaluation) for inquiries conducted with Asian American/Pacific Islander populations, persons of African descent, Hispanics, and American Indians. The American Psychological Association used race/ethnicity as the organizing framework; however, they also recognized the need to consider other dimensions of diversity. This need is acknowledged in the following guiding principle:

> Recognition of the ways in which the intersection of racial and ethnic group membership with other dimensions of identity (e.g., gender, age, sexual orientation, disability, religion/spiritual orientation, educational attainment/experiences, and socioeconomic status) enhances the understanding and treatment of all people. (p. 19)

As noted previously, the Talent Development Model of School Reform provides an example of an evaluation conducted from a transformative stance with specific attention to dimensions of race/ethnicity because it is designed to enhance the educational experiences of students in urban schools, the majority of whom are from racial/ethnic minority groups (Boykin, 2000).

The Promoting Reflective Inquiry in Mathematics Education (PRIME) project provides another example of the importance of stakeholder involvement in a project focused on Native American students (Saylor, Apaza, & Austin, 2005). Disaggregated results from multiple measures confirmed the gap between Native Americans and non-Native Americans in terms of achievement in mathematics. Whereas 70% of white students in the school system achieved proficiency at grade level, only 40% of Native American students did so. In addition, the proficiency rate for Native Americans was reported to be inflated because well over half of the Native Americans entering high school dropped out before graduation.

Course-taking patterns revealed that Native Americans were nearly absent in upper-level math courses: of the 140 Native Americans who started as an elementary grade-level cohort, 15 succeeded in algebra in 2003–2004 and only 3 passed the advanced placement (AP) calculus course. The evaluators scheduled frequent meetings with project directors to review their findings. The evaluators felt frustrated because the tribal representatives did not come to the meetings to discuss the evaluation findings, even with repeated invitations.

A transformative lens focused on this evaluation that revealed differential experiences in math in a comparison of white and Native American students elicits such questions as the following:

What is the importance of involving members of the Native American community in the early stages of this project?

How can members of the Native American community be involved?

Who in the Native American community needs to be involved?

What are the political ramifications of demonstrating the gap in achievement and access to advanced math and science courses between white and Native American students?

How can evidence of an achievement gap be obtained and be viewed as information of value to the Native American community, rather than as a negative reflection on their community?

How can the evaluator encourage program developers to identify those contextual variables that exert a causal influence in determining learning?

Once the gaps have been identified, how can the interventions be structured so that they are responsive to the context in which the people live?

How can evaluators encourage program staff to be responsive to the multiple dimensions of diversity?

LaFrance (2004) provides many insights into the conduct of culturally competent evaluation in Indian country, starting with the recognition of the need to follow traditional lines of authority in contacting members of a tribal nation.

Caldwell et al. (2005) identify two fundamental considerations that are important when research is conducted with American Indians and Alaska Natives (AI/AN): tribal sovereignty and diversity. Both groups are sovereign political entities with their own form of governance, culture, and history. It is a mistake to view AI/ANs as a single minority population. There are over 560 native nations and tribal entities in the United States, each with its own culture and political issues. In Alaska there are at least four different cultural groups: Eskimos, Aleuts and Alutiq, Athabascan Indians, and Northwest Coastal Indians.

Nichols and Keltner (2005) provide additional insights into the diversity of AI communities by noting that according to the 2000 census, there are 4.1 million Native Americans in the United States. Many of the tribes are very small (having less than 1,000 members) and are dispersed in urban areas and rural communities. "Some tribes have no land base at all, some AI families move on and off the reservation land and others have been in the same location for generations. There are 278 reservations, the largest being the Navajo. An estimated 200 indigenous languages still survive, the majority of which can be spoken by only a few elders" (Utter, 1993; as cited in Nichols & Keltner, 2005, p. 31).

Diversity in the Latino Community: Challenges and Resilience

The Latino population in the United States is very diverse in regard to ethnicity, age, geography, mobility, and legal status (Cardoza Clayson et al., 2002). Cardoza Clayson et al. note that assets and deficits coexist in this group:

> For example, the lives of California's migrant farm workers are shaped by historical racism, current anti-migrant sentiment, and the globalization of capital across the U.S.–Mexico border. While many families have strong ties, spiritual connections and cohesive cultural practices, they may also suffer from the effects of poverty, violence, and chemical dependency. In some California new migrant communities, neighborhood in and out migration reaches 50% per year. Yet, existing within these mobile neighborhoods are structures, sometimes invisible to outsiders, spoken, unspoken, formal and informal rules, and culture and gender-specific imperatives. We argue that to conduct evaluations within these communities a substantive understanding of the particular community context must be achieved. (p. 36)

Immigrant Communities

Lee (2004) provided insights into variations in immigrant communities that have an impact on their willingness to, and comfort level with, participating in research and evaluation studies. She examined concepts of civic participation in four different immigrant groups: the Chinese, South East Asian, Indian, and Caribbean communities. She reported that historical contexts played a major role in the willingness of individuals in those communities to engage in research and evaluation studies. More concern was expressed about revealing any personal information by those who came from countries in which expression of opinions had been severely repressed.

In addition, if the oppressor's language was English, it was easier for immigrants who had "benefited" linguistically from colonial schooling to feel comfortable engaging in civic activities in the United States. All the groups showed differences in their concepts of civic participation that were related to issues of comfort in the majority society and historical models of civic participation in their home countries.

Third/Developing World

Varadharajan (2000) notes that scholars of color have resisted the homogenization implied in the term *Third World* in Western discourse by calling for an acknowledgment of the fundamental differences among and within Third World nations:

> They have argued, simultaneously, that Third World cultures must be granted an existence independent of their erstwhile colonizers. They believe that the identity of these cultures should be formed in the process of contending with their own imperatives rather than in the process of reacting to colonial ones. Postcolonial critics are challenging Western critical frameworks on the grounds that they alienate members of Third World cultures from their own realities, induce slavish conformity on the part of postcolonial intellectuals (who should know better than to collaborate with their masters), and remain deaf to "Native" responses to the Western critical reception of texts as well as to the texts themselves. (p. 144)

African and Botswana Diversity

Chilisa (2005) argues that First World researchers commit the "sameness error" of viewing "Africa and its inhabitants . . . as one mass exhibiting the same characteristics and same behavior, irrespective of geographical boundaries, diverse languages, ethnicity and particular institutional practices" (Teunis, 2001, as cited in Chilisa, 2005, p. 671). In official government publications about Botswana's health conditions, the Annual Sentinel Surveillance Reports, partial information about HIV/AIDS is given by blocking local views of the epidemic and its modes of transmission, and by ignoring context and basic demographic variables such as occupation, education, and social class. Based on the assumption that the vulnerable groups are middle class and can read English (both assumptions being false), interventions are developed that consist of information, education, and communication materials in English that are context and culturally insensitive.

Donors fund research and evaluations of HIV/AIDS as well as teachers, schools, and universities. However, these priorities are mythical. Chilisa,

Bennell, and Hyde (2001) reveal significant poverty dimensions associated with HIV/AIDS, with the less privileged, the less educated, and the poorly paid women and girls experiencing high mortality rates. The industrial-class workers of the University of Botswana, for example, who earn the lowest wages and have the lowest education in comparison with other cash-income groups, had the highest mortality rates. Primary school teachers also had high mortality rates in comparison with secondary teachers and university lecturers who earned higher wages and higher level of education.

Botswana is the third largest natural diamond producer in the world and has one of the highest gross domestic product (GDP) per capita on the continent. However, marked inequities are evident in the distribution of wealth and its accompanying privileges. For example, 50% of the people live below the poverty line, and women form the majority of the poorest. With a population of about 1.7 million people, it is a multiethnic nation, with inhabitants speaking more than 25 languages. In the early 1990s, Botswanans had an average life expectancy of 65 years; however, with the onset of the HIV/AIDS epidemic, that number has fallen to 45 years. It is projected that 22% of the population will be infected by 2010.

Chilisa's (2005) description of the way in which she addresses diversity in the African context is exemplified in this citation, in which she explains the dimensions of diversity that are important to recognize with regard to social structures, as well as perspectives of community versus individuality. She writes:

> The production of knowledge was facilitated by indigenous researchers/ intellectuals that included chiefs, poets, social critics, diviners and story tellers guided by the community's values and ways of perceiving reality. Most African communities with particular reference to Bantu people of southern Africa, for instance, view human existence in relation to the existence of others. Among views of "being," for instance, is the conception that "*ntuh, nthu ne banwe*" (a person is because of others) or "I am because we are." This is in direct contrast to Western views that emphasize individualism: "I think therefore I am." Most African worldviews emphasize belongingness, connectedness, community participation and people centeredness. (p. 679)

Diversity among the Maori

The Maori place high value on sharing stories about their origins (*whakapapa*). Carter (2004, as cited in Cram et al., 2004) says:

> Some people aren't going to choose to fully participate. So *iwi* (regional tribe) membership will continue to be diverse and complex because of the changes

that have occurred and continue to occur in Maori society. I think research-ers need to be aware of this dynamic nature of *whakapapa* (identifying your roots), because it's not just about going to a little bounded group and they're all going to be the same, and all going to have the same ideas. So people need to be aware of the way *whakapapa* is dynamic and the way that it challenges traditional notions of what makes up a Maori group, in particular what makes up an *iwi*, *hapu* (local tribe), or *whanau* (family) group and that, of course, is made up now of very complex and diverse relationships. (p. 160)

Student Perspective: Diversity—Race and Deafness

What about diversity in the Maori community? Are they all the same? From a deaf perspective, to what extent do Maori values/culture overlap with the deaf community? There is a sharing of anger, frustration, discrimination, and oppression. Some reject this description of the deaf person's experience. I see different types of cultural values, what about studying deaf people? Should we come up with different cultural values within the deaf culture, such as hard of hearing, cochlear implants, oral, little hard of hearing, deaf of deaf, deaf of hearing, etc.? There is no one approach to the group of deaf people like the Maori approach. How's it work with Maori? Are they all the same?—Heidi Holmes (February 5, 2006)

Disability

People with disabilities comprise the largest minority group in the United States. Because prevalence figures are dependent on the definition of dis-ability and judgments made about who should be labeled with having a particular disability, it is difficult to precisely identify the number of people with disabilities. Males are significantly overrepresented in special educa-tion, as are culturally and linguistically diverse students. This overiden-tification can be linked to unfair, unreliable, and invalid assessment and diagnostic practice and/or to a lack of cultural competence on the part of school personnel. Underidentification of girls is linked to a lower prob-ability that they exhibit behavioral problems in conjunction with learning challenges. Hence, they must experience more significant deficits than do boys in order to gain access to special education services (Mertens, Wilson, & Mounty, 2007).

Intersections of Disability, Race, and Gender

Important research and evaluation implications arise when we consider the intersection of race/ethnicity, gender, and disability in a context of social change. Seelman (1999) reported that there is great diversity within the

20% of the U.S. population with disabilities. For example, women have higher rates of severe disabilities than men (9.7% vs. 7.7%), whereas men have slightly higher rates of nonsevere disabilities. Considering both sex and race, black women have the highest rate of severe disability (14.3%), followed by black men (12.6%). Rates of severe disability for men and women who are Native American, Eskimo, or Aleut are nearly as high, and Native Americans have the highest rates of nonsevere disability. Researchers and evaluators who are aware of the diversity within the disability community can use this information to avoid errors based on assumptions of homogeneity, and they can increase the potential for their work to address marginalized populations by including appropriate subgroups.

Rousso and Wehmeyer (2001) examined the intersection of gender and disability in their book *Double Jeopardy*. They conclude that disparities on such indicators as educational- and employment-related outcomes support the idea that girls and women with disabilities are in a state of double jeopardy. The combination of stereotypes about women and stereotypes about people with disabilities leads to double discrimination that is reflected in the home, school, workplace, and the larger society.

However, not all indicators support the position that males with disabilities are favored over females. The U.S. Department of Education (2004) reported that males, especially those from minority ethnic and racial groups, are diagnosed as having disabilities in much greater numbers by a ratio of about two males for every one female. According to the Civil Rights Project at Harvard University, black children constitute 17% of the total school enrollment of those labeled mentally retarded, and they show only marginal improvement over a 30-year period (Losen & Orfield, 2002). During this same period, disproportionality in the areas of emotional disturbance and specific learning disabilities grew significantly for black students. Furthermore, between 1987 and 2001, there was a fourfold increase in the proportion of students from homes where the first language was not English (i.e., primarily Spanish-speaking families) identified with a disability (U.S. Department of Education, 2002). Researchers and evaluators need to be aware of these complexities because people with disabilities are likely present in almost all stakeholder groups (Gill, 1999; Mertens et al., 2007). Awareness of issues related to differential access and outcomes at the intersection of race, disability, and gender is particularly relevant for evaluators whose work relates to the "No Child Left Behind" agenda.

Meadow-Orlans et al. (2003) provide an example of working within a culturally complex community where the primary focus was the hearing status of children. They used a mixed-methods design to evaluate satisfaction regarding services offered to parents of deaf and hard-of-hearing children. A national survey of parents of young deaf and hard-of-hearing children revealed different levels of satisfaction with services when the data were disaggregated by race/ethnicity, parental hearing status, child's hearing level (deaf or hard of hearing), presence of additional disabilities beyond deafness, and parent's choice of communication mode for his or her child. In order to gain a more thorough understanding of the reasons for differences in reported levels of satisfaction based on these dimensions of diversity, the national survey was followed by individual interviews with the specific goal of determining the supportive and challenging factors associated with each group's experiences.

As the individual interviews proceeded, it became clear that racial/ethnic minority parents were not appearing in adequate numbers in the follow-up data collection. The investigators conferred with the leaders of programs that served parents and children primarily from racial and ethnic minority groups. They recommended the use of focus groups held at the school site with the invitation issued by the school staff who normally worked with the parents, and the provision of food, transportation, and child care. Under these circumstances, it was possible to gain insights from the less represented stakeholders with regard to program satisfaction.

The need for accommodations to authentically include people with different communication choices was critical to obtaining accurate data. Parents who were deaf were interviewed through the use of an on-site interpreter who voiced for the parents' signs and signed what the interviewer said to the parents. By being culturally aware and responsive to the demands of this complex community, the research team was able to identify sources of both support and challenge that were common across groups, as well as those that were unique to specific groups. Information of this type is important for programs that serve diverse clients, as well as for the parents themselves.

More elaborate accommodations may be necessary depending on the context and the dimensions of diversity that are salient in that context. For example, in a study of court access for deaf and hard-of-hearing people across the United States, Mertens (2000) worked with an advisory board to identify the dimensions of diversity that would be important and to devise ways to accommodate the communication needs of the individuals who were invited to focus groups to share their experiences in the courts. The advisory board recognized the complexity in the deaf community in terms of communication modes. Thus, the needs of individuals who were well educated and sophisticated in the use of American Sign Language were accommodated by deaf and hearing co-moderators, along with an interpreter who signed for the hearing moderator and voiced for the signing participants. In addition, individuals (court reporters) skilled in real-time captioning produced text of the verbal comments, which appeared on television screens visible to the group members. When deaf people who were less well educated and had secondary disabilities were invited to share their experiences, additional accommodations were necessary. As mentioned previously, a deaf–blind participant required an interpreter who signed into her hands so that she could participate in the discussion. One individual did not use ASL as a language, but rather communicated using some signs and gestures. For this individual, the evaluators provided a deaf interpreter who could watch the signs of others and "act out" the communications occurring in the group. Users of Mexican Sign Language required the use of a Mexican Sign Language interpreter, who then translated the participants comments into ASL, and those were translated by a third interpreter who voiced in English.

Student Perspective: Diversity and Deafness

Speaking of horizontal marginalization, I see that within the deaf community—the subgroups of the main group (the oralists, the cochlear implanted, the hard of hearing, etc.). They could be marginalized from the "mainstream" society and further marginalized by their own people.—Heidi Holmes (February 8, 2006)

QUESTIONS FOR THOUGHT

- How would you determine the dimensions of diversity that are relevant in your particular context?
- How could you use mixed methods to enhance your understanding of cultural diversity in your research/evaluation?
- What is the importance of understanding the meaning of the concept of cultural competence in the context in which you work?
- How can improved understandings of the community be linked to social justice?

Student Perspective: Power and Language

In some school systems, those who are deaf are usually accompanied with the label communication disordered because many deaf are in speech therapy. In the school system's view, since we can't speak clearly, we have a communication disorder. That is a strange label since there are other ways to communicate with other human beings. We could write on a paper, gesture, or use some other communication system. The hearing administrators who run the school system have a very limited view of communication. I guess it is only fair to label the hearing manually disordered since they cannot sign clearly.—Matt Laucka (September 2004)

Those in power have the advantage of choosing the labels or categories into which those with less power are placed. For example, Cardoza Clayson et al. (2002) describe the origins of *Latino* as a political term used to designate a heterogeneous Caribbean and Latin American population sharing a historical background and cultural perspectives. In actuality, Latinos come from various countries (e.g., Mexico, El Salvador, Guatemala), and have unique cultures that have been formed though their geographical and historical locations. In each country there are also multiple levels of development, wealth, and racial mixtures. People who are labeled *Latino* may also build part of their identity on the basis of their representation in the media, ability to migrate, exposure to other cultures, access to technology, and their transnational networks. Patterns of settlement and migration are important for understanding and working with Latino communities.

Madison (1992) critically examined the use of the label *at risk* that was used in programs to serve youths from poverty areas in one state. Based on interviews with various stakeholder groups, she ascertained that *at risk* carried meanings such as parents who don't care about their kids and kids with a high probability of failure. Both staff and youths expressed similar interpretations of the term. Her findings provide evidence of the potentially powerful deleterious effect of particular labels. In the Talent Development Project (Thomas, 2004), the evaluators deliberately chose to use the term *placed at risk* to indicate that the tenuous circumstances in which the youths found themselves resulted from inadequate societal response, rather than parent or youth failures.

Rationale for Sampling Strategies

Before choosing a sample, thought should be given to the population of interest, the relevant dimensions of diversity in the population, implications of how those dimensions are defined and labeled, supports and accommodations needed for appropriate inclusion of sample members, and recruitment and reciprocity strategies. Sampling strategies can be probability-based, purposeful, or convenient, depending on the purpose of the research or evaluation and access to the people who will participate in the study. The following section discusses decision points in terms of sampling strategies, transformative ethics, and ethics associated with institutional review boards.

Flyvbjerg (2006) discussed options for sampling in the context of conducting a case study that are applicable more generally to those considered when selecting a sample for a research or evaluation study. He identifies two basic strategies: random selection (probability-based) and theoretical selection. A third strategy is also commonly used: convenience sampling, meaning that the researchers/evaluators collect data from anyone who can be accessed conveniently. Random selection strategies are more commonly used in quantitative methods; however, they need not be restricted to that type of approach. Theoretical strategies are more commonly associated with qualitative approaches, but they can also be used in quantitative studies. The techniques of random selection and the use of average cases are used when researchers/evaluators want to see a representative sample, not overpowered by extreme elements in the population. However, Flyvbjerg argues that the extreme case could allow insight into deeper causes behind a problem and its consequences.

To accomplish random selection, a list of individuals who are members of the target population is needed, from which individuals from that population are randomly selected to participate in the study. If there is a comparison group, then the individuals are divided randomly into intervention and comparison groups (called *random assignment*). Random selection from a population means that every person has an equal chance of being selected. In its simplest form, it can be accomplished by putting all the names in a hat and drawing out names one by one. More sophisticated means use computer-based selection programs. (See Box 7.1 for an explanation of various strategies for probability-based sampling.) Proponents of random selection argue that use of such a strategy eliminates sources of variance that could obscure program effects. However, programs often are designed to serve a specific group of people; for example, women who have been abused, deaf people in courts. Hence, it may not be possible to get a full list of all the people that the program is designed to serve. It may also not be possible, for logistical or ethical reasons, to randomly select people to receive services or not.

Purposeful or theoretical sampling strategies are also included in Box 7.1. As mentioned previously, these sampling strategies are based on the researcher's or evaluator's conscious decision to obtain data from individuals based on a rationale that they are the best sources of such information. People or cases may be chosen because they exemplify certain theoretically important characteristics or because their life experiences reflect critical cultural or historical positioning in regard to the phenomena under study.

BOX 7.1. Random Sampling and Theoretical Sampling

RANDOM SAMPLING STRATEGIES

Simple random selection	If the population is known and a list of accessible members of the population is available, then the researcher can randomly select individuals by drawing names out of a hat, using a table of random numbers, or using a computer-based procedure. The goal of random selection is to obtain a sample that is representative of the population.
Stratified random selection	If the conditions for random selection prevail and there are subgroups in the population that might not be adequately represented using simple random sampling, then the sample can be stratified (divided) into subgroups first, and then randomly sampled within groups.
Cluster sampling	If the population can be depicted by a map (e.g., a neighborhood), then the researcher can randomly sample specific locations (e.g., blocks) and then sample all the people in that block.
Systematic sampling	If the population list is in no particular order, then the researcher can systematically select every fifth (or tenth or nth) name, depending on the size of the population and sample desired.

THEORETICAL SAMPLING STRATEGIES

Average cases	To obtain individuals who represent "average" on the dimensions of interest.
Extreme/ deviant cases	To obtain information about unusual cases—especially those that are especially good/problematic, best/worst, richest/poorest, or other dimensions that are relevant to the phenomenon under study.
Maximum variation cases	To obtain information from individuals who exhibit significant differences on important dimensions of diversity.
Critical cases	To obtain information that permits logical deductions of the type (e.g., If this is [not] valid for this case, then it applies to all [no] cases.).
Snowball sampling	To obtain information when you do not have a full list of people or the intended participants are difficult to find, start with someone who you do know and ask him or her to recommend others who either agree or disagree or might be able to present confirming or divergent points of view.

In some populations, it is less likely that their names will be publicly available on lists; for example, those engaged in illegal activities or those who are members of invisible minorities. Examples of a variety of purposeful or theoretical approaches follow.

Example of Theoretical Sampling: Native Americans

Nichols and Keltner (2005) used a theoretical sampling strategy in an ethnographic study of the traditional values, beliefs, and cultural responses of family adjustment to disabilities in two American Indian communities. They sought individuals in the community who were dealing with the family challenge of adjusting to children with disabilities because they believed that such informants could provide rich and meaningful data. Their initial criteria for selection included having a child with a disability, having a child without a disability, being a tribal leader, being an elder in the community, and being a service provider who worked with AI children with disabilities in the community. They asked an advisory board to nominate potential participants. This method resulted in a diverse and representative group that included 26 AI families with children with disabilities, 36 AI families with children who did not have disabilities, 20 service providers, 15 tribal leaders, and 23 AI elders.

Inclusion and Illusions

Flyvbjerg (2006) recommends use of the critical case as having strategic importance in relation to a general problem. As an example he used a study of the effect of organic solvents on the brain. Rather than selecting a random sample of businesses that use organic solvents, he selected a business that had met all the safety regulations for cleanliness and air quality. He reasoned that if a higher rate of brain damage was found in such an exemplary critical case, it would be found in other businesses with less stellar records as well. Use of the critical case strategy is dependent on prior experience with the phenomenon under study, as there are no universal principles to guide such a selection. It is a process of thinking through what is the most likely or least likely case that would allow the researcher or evaluator to either confirm or refute hypotheses.

Kumar and Saidah (2005) provide an example of critical case sampling in their studies following the tsunami relief efforts in Southern India. They identified two individuals, both of whom had disabilities. The first, Kannan, was a 21-year-old man who was the proprietor of a public telephone office (i.e., he had a telephone that local people without telephones could use to make a call). He was born with a congenital physical disability and survived polio in childhood. In the tsunami, the office was completely destroyed. He received relief services and his business was thriving in short order. The second, Durga Devi, was also a survivor of childhood polio. At the time of the tsunami, she did not have a job, although she lived just 200 yards from Kannan's telephone business. She lost everything in the tsunami. She has not received any relief aid. She says: "The tsunami almost took my life, almost killed me. My new life after the tsunami, some days, I think will be the thing that finally kills me." What is the difference between these two individuals that makes them critical cases? Kannan had an address and Durga did not. Without an address, Durga could not support her application for relief.

Snowball Sampling

Schalet, Hunt, and Joe-Laidler (2003) conducted a study of ethnic gangs in San Francisco Bay Area over a 4-year period. They conducted over 600 interviews with gang members; 61 of the interviews were with female members. They used the snowball sampling approach, asking respondents who were gang members to recommend others. They then conducted a second study for an additional 4 years, using the same strategy. This time, they had 39 female gang members. They found this strategy to be useful because they could not get a list of gang members, females are less frequently members of gangs than males, and they needed entry into the community from trusted sources.

Illusion of Inclusion: Tensions in Transformative Participatory Research

Gaventa and Cornwall (2006) recognize the myth of homogeneity in their writings about PAR. They indicate that researchers need to be wary of knowledge that is viewed as valid because it was constructed by the community or the people, rather than by researchers. However, the presentation of knowledge as valid because it emerged from consensus may be disguising important differences in the targeted community. This point brings to mind Reason and Bradbury's (2006a) question about the data reflecting a plurality of voices in the community. What is the assurance that community-based knowledge is not a reflection of the dominant discourse (see Chilisa's concerns described in Chapter 3 about being co-opted into the dominant discourse at the risk of ignoring her knowledge base as an indigenous Botswanan)? As Reason and Bradbury note:

Little attention is generally given to the positionality of those who participate and what this might mean in terms of the versions they present. Great care must be taken not to replace one set of dominant voices with another—all in the name of participation (p. 76).

The dangers of using participatory processes in ways that gloss over differences among those who participate, or to mirror dominant knowledge in the name of challenging it, are not without consequence. To the extent that participatory processes appear to have taken place, and that the relatively powerless have had the opportunity to voice their grievances and priorities in what is portrayed as an otherwise open system, then existing power relations may simply be reinforced without leading to substantive change in the policies or structures that perpetuate the problems being addressed. In this sense, participation without a change in power relations may simply reinforce the status quo, adding to the mobilization of bias the claim to have a more "democratic" face. The illusion of inclusion means not only that what emerges is treated as if it represents what "the people" really want, but also that it gains a moral authority that becomes hard to challenge or question (Reason & Bradbury, 2006a, p. 77).

Recruitment of Participants

Participants can be recruited by a variety of means. Access and context variations determine which approach will be successful. If a community is physically gathered in a defined space, it may be possible to hold a meeting and explain the purposes of the research or evaluation study and recruit volunteers at that time. If members of the community are likely to be physically present in a space but asynchronously, it may be possible to post an invitation to participate on a bulletin board or elevator wall. If the community is spread out across a larger area, mailings or electronic communications via listservs or e-mail may reach the appropriate persons.

Researchers and evaluators report volunteering at various agencies or centers in order to get to know the community in a way that also allows them to give a useful service to the members. Collins (2005) began recruitment of participants in a poverty assessment project by volunteering at a food co-op. She also met with the executive director and co-op workers to get permission to present the intended research to the co-op members. The co-op leaders decided that participation in the research project could count for the monthly work requirements for the members. The researcher invited participation at a regular monthly meeting of the co-op members. Collins describes that meeting as follows: "The researcher introduced the project by explaining that the intent of the research was to have people speak for themselves rather than someone else speaking for them. Examples were given of some of the topics that might be discussed and several questions were answered" (p. 13). The members voted to allow the study to proceed, but individuals were to decide for themselves if they wanted to participate. At the end of the meeting, only the few women who signed up participated over the length of the study.

The researcher gained insights into the members' reticence to be involved in the research through conversations with co-op members as she carried out her volunteer shifts and by discussions with the small group of research participants. The members did not feel comfortable revealing information about themselves because there was an atmosphere of distrust that had been created several years ago when funding cuts led to the establishment of a fraud line so recipients could report on each other. This mistrust and reluctance to participate in research signal yet another cautionary note with regard to the myth of homogeneity. Collins (2005) notes that gender, age, and ethnicity are not the only dimensions of diversity that need to be acknowledged. An assumption of solidarity and harmony in a community can also lead to additional challenges in recruiting participants and in the willingness of individuals to reveal data about themselves. The women who did participate suggested that in addition to distrust, people who came to the co-op might want to get only the food, not to socialize. They might be embarrassed that they are in the situation to need the food, or they might just want to be by themselves. Collins (2005) concludes:

> It needs to be recognized that participation by its very nature must be an invitation, not a requirement. It must meet the needs of those who are asked to participate. For most members of the co-op what had been an anticipated benefit of participation, an alternative way to meet co-op work requirements that involved informal and closer social interaction with other co-op members, was not perceived as a benefit. Participatory research has a tendency to stress the solidarity of communities and to picture community as a natural social entity (Cleaver, 2000). In reality, communities often embody "both solidarity and conflict, shifting alliances, power and social structures" (Cleaver, 2000, p. 45). It is important not to deny the presence of conflict, but to make both the forces of inclusion and exclusion part of the analysis. (p. 14)

Ethical Review Boards and Protection of Human Participants

Ethics from a Regulatory Perspective

As mentioned in previous chapters, professional associations and indigenous peoples have developed guidelines or codes of ethics. In many countries, governments and other institutions have established ethical review boards for the protection of human (and animal) participants in research and evaluation studies. In the United States, institutional review boards (IRBs) are mandated by the National Research Act, Public Law 93-348, and require that all human trials conducted by federally funded institutions have IRB approval. Many researchers and evaluators encounter challenging questions about the ethics of their planned studies within the context of their institutions' ethical review boards or human subjects committees. The U.S. federal regulations are included in Title 45 *Code of Federal Regulations* Part 46 that are accessible from university research offices, reference librarians, or the Office for Protection from Research Risk in the National Institutes of Health (NIH; located in Bethesda, Maryland). Information on IRB requirements in many locations is available on the Internet. The historical origins of IRBs in the United States can be found in the Belmont Report (National Commission for the Protection of Human Subjects of Biomedical and Behavioral Research, 1979), and the NIH website has a tutorial that addresses human subject approval processes and institutional review at *ohsr.od.nih.gov/cbt.*

In the United States, research ethics involving human participants are based on three principles that serve as justifications for the many ethical prescriptions and evaluations of human actions: respect, beneficence, and justice, as set forth in the Belmont Report (National Commission for the Protection of Human Subjects of Biomedical and Behavioral Research, 1979). *Respect* is defined as treating people from diverse backgrounds and cultures with courtesy, and vulnerable populations are singled out for additional protection. *Beneficence* includes securing the participants' well-being by doing them no harm, maximizing possible benefits, and minimizing possible harm. The principle of *justice* is meant to ensure that participants benefit from the research and that the procedures are fairly administered and thoughtfully prepared. Emanating from these principles are concepts such as confidentiality, anonymity, and informed consent (see Box 7.2 for an explanation of these terms). The following section explores exceptions to IRB approval and indigenous ethics review boards.

Exceptions to IRB Approval

U.S. IRBs need to approve all research that involves human subjects, with a few exceptions. There are no clear-cut distinctions made by IRBs with regard to the need for approval of studies that are categorized as research or evaluation. Even if you think your study might fall into one of the exempt

BOX 7.2. Confidentiality, Anonymity, and Informed Consent

CONFIDENTIALITY AND ANONYMITY

Confidentiality means that the privacy of individuals will be protected in that the data they provide will be handled and reported in such a way that it cannot be associated with them personally. *Anonymity* means that no uniquely identifying information is attached to the data, and thus, no one, not even the researcher, can trace the data back to the individual providing it.

INFORMED CONSENT

Informed consent is a process, not just a form. Information must be presented to enable persons to voluntarily decide whether or not to participate as a research subject. It is a fundamental mechanism to ensure respect for persons through provision of thoughtful consent for a voluntary act. The procedures used in obtaining informed consent should be designed to educate the subject population in terms that they can understand. . . . The written presentation of information is used to document the basis for consent and for the subjects' future reference.

From *ohrp.osophs.dhhs.gov/humansubjects/guidance/ictips.htm* and *bms.brown.edu/fogarty/consent.htm*.

categories, you should contact your institution's ethical review board because most still require an abbreviated review to establish the legitimacy of the exemption. Two exemptions follow:

1. Research that is conducted in established or commonly accepted educational settings, involving normal education practices, such as instructional strategies or classroom management techniques.
2. Research that involves the use of educational tests if unique identifiers are not attached to the test results.

Note: An interesting development occurred with regard to IRB approval for oral-history proposals for research. The Office for Human Research Protections, the federal office that oversees the use of human volunteers in research, decided that oral-history interviews generally do not fall under the government's definition of research and therefore do not need to be regulated by institutional review boards. The rationale was that the federal definition of research that involves human subjects has as its goal a systematic investigation designed to develop or contribute to generalizable knowledge. Because oral history involves the study of a particular past, rather than to identify generalizable principles, it does not fit the federal definition of research that requires human subject protection. At the time of this writing, the decision covers only researchers financed by the Department of Health and Human Services. Updates on this situation and its broader impact can be found at the websites for the Office for Human Research Protections, the American Historical Association, and the Oral History Association (Brainerd, 2003).

Indigenous Ethics Review Boards

Many indigenous communities have established 'ethical review boards on their own terms. Caldwell et al. (2005) provide an example of this type of guidance in Native American tribes:

> In general, research in Indian Country may have neither more nor fewer ethical problems and dilemmas than research conducted elsewhere. Still, issues such as cultural competence, relatively high rates of poverty, illness, and prevalent rural infrastructure deficits can exacerbate ethical problems. Making judgments about ethics and values can be challenging to researchers because of potentially conflicting roles and circumstances. For instance, the sponsor of the research may have agendas, rules, and expectations that are different from or in conflict with those of the tribe(s) participating in the study. In such circumstances, it is prudent for the researcher to seek guidance from a project advisory committee, the research sponsor, and/or legal authorities without disclosing information that would violate the identity of the research participant(s) or violate the confidentiality of participant data. (p. 10)

Although IRBs were established to protect individuals from harm, they have come under criticism for a number of reasons. Because IRBs have their origins in the medical research community, they may be biased more favorably toward, and more knowledgeable about, quantitative research and evaluation strategies (Simons, 2006). Cheek (2005) notes that ethics committees may reject a proposal that makes use of a design that is not a randomized control trial "on the basis of 'poor design'—and, thus, 'unethical research'—that will result in no benefit, or even possibly in harm, to research participants" (p. 397). Their rationale for rejecting the study is because it is unscientific and not able to be generalized. Cheek raises these key questions:

- What constitutes scientific merit and who determines this? (p. 397)
- Will the research be based on practices that treat people as the objects of research and provide them with limited opportunities to contribute to the production of knowledge, or will it be based on collaborative practices that view people as participants in the production of knowledge? (Stuart, 2001, p. 38, in Cheek, p. 399)
- What are the dangers of "quick turnaround" research? Would this . . . encourage the rise of an atheoretical set of qualitative techniques designed for expediency and framed by reductionist understandings of what qualitative research is and might do? (p. 404)

A second criticism of IRBs is that they work to protect the institution, rather than the individual (Christians, 2005; Simons, 2006). They argue that protecting the institution from litigation is the priority, rather than the protection and benefit of those who participate in the research or evaluation studies, and that such a position lacks ethical integrity.

Confidentiality: Protecting Children

Because children are viewed as a vulnerable population, legislators have implemented additional safeguards for them. Such U.S. federal legal requirements concerning confidentiality draw from the following legislation:

1. The Buckley Amendment, which prohibits access to children's school records without parental consent.
2. The Hatch Act, which prohibits asking children questions about religion, sex, or family life without parental permission.
3. The National Research Act, which requires parental permission for research on children.

There are, however, circumstances in which the IRB can choose *not* to require parental permission:

1. If the research involves only minimal risk (i.e., no greater risk than in everyday life), parental permission can be waived.
2. If the parent cannot be counted on to act in the best interests of the

child, parental permission can be waived. This circumstance usually involves parents who have been abusive or neglectful.

Confidentiality: Alternative Strategies

An additional layer of confidentiality protection may be achieved by obtaining certificates of confidentiality, which protect identifying information from subpoena for legal proceedings (Dodd, 2009). Certificates of confidentiality provide protection against "compelled disclosure of identifying information about subjects enrolled in sensitive biomedical, behavioral, clinical or other research. The protection is not limited to federally supported research" (retrieved January 21, 2008, from *www.gov/ohrp/ humansubjects/guidance/certconf.htm*). The NIH's website notes that the certificates are granted when disclosure of study information "could have adverse consequences for subjects or damage their financial standing, employability, insurability, or reputation" (retrieved January 21, 2008, from *www.grants.nih.gov/grants/policy/coc*).

For example, for LGBTQ youths who are not "out" to their parents or who live in unsupportive or even violent homes, requesting parental consent for a research study involving LGBTQ issues could pose a serious risk. According to Dodd (2009):

> In such cases a researcher may request that an independent adult advocate, who has an existing relationship with the youth through a social service agency or school, be used to establish informed consent (Elze, 2003) or that the sponsoring agency be judged *in loco parentis* and therefore provide informed consent (Martin & Meezan, 2003). . . . Disclosure of sexual orientation or gender identity may have a negative impact for the individuals involved as subjects risk job discrimination, strained or severed family relationships, and possibly even violence. (p. 482)

As a part of the confidentiality issue, participants should also be informed that researchers and evaluators are required by law to inform the appropriate authorities if they learn of any behaviors that might be injurious to the participants themselves or that cause reasonable suspicion that a child, elder, or dependent adult has been abused.

It is sometimes possible to obtain data within the context of anonymity by having someone other than the researcher/evaluator draw the sample and delete unique identifying information. Sieber (1992) also suggests the possibility of having a respondent in a mail survey return the questionnaire *and* to mail *separately* a postcard with his or her name on it. Thus, the individual would be noted as having responded, and second mailings need only be sent to those who had not yet done so. However, in many instances, this method is not feasible. In such circumstances, arrangements to respect the privacy and confidentiality of the individuals in the study can be done by coding the data obtained and keeping a separate file with the code linked to unique identifying information. The separate file can then be destroyed once the necessary data collection has been completed.

Problems with confidentiality arise especially if the community of interest is small. For example:

> Tribes often do not object to the identification of the tribe or communities in research reports. However, when research is conducted on sensitive topics, a tribe may insist that the research report not identify the tribe or communities participating in the research. Protecting the privacy of research participants and keeping their identity anonymous can pose a special challenge for small tribes and communities. As one example, if the program being evaluated is small, it can be almost impossible to maintain the anonymity of key informants. (Caldwell et al., 2005, p. 10)

Student Perspective: Small Community and Confidentiality Concerns

Gallaudet is such a small world—for deaf people and conducting research with/or on them might be redundant? or beneficial? or . . . ? Again, confidentiality raises tensions for the IRB approval of qualitative research: the collaboration, the interactivity, and democratic ethics. . . . If the reason for the IRB is to protect the institution, not the participants . . ., how do we fully protect the participants in qualitative research if we intend to collaborate with them, to interact fully with them as researcher–participant, and how do we draw our "ethics boundaries" with the participants? Like I said, I need to cover all bases with these questions in mind with justifications from other qualitative researchers.—Heidi Holmes (March 4, 2006)

Research and Evaluation Ethics and Indigenous Knowledge Systems

Chilisa (2005) provides insights into the dangers associated with transferring the Western and Northern concepts of research ethics to postcolonial settings in that this may further privilege such practices and ethics. She criticizes accepting the definition of ethics as the regulations of conduct for a given profession or group. Critical questions to ask with regard to ethical conduct in postcolonial settings include these:

- Can there be universal research and evaluation ethics?
- Can such ethics be value free and inclusive of all knowledge systems?

Chilisa (2005) explains:

> Ethical issues in research include codes of conduct that are concerned with protection of the researched from physical, mental, and/or psychological harm and where the assumption is that the researched might disclose information that might expose them to psychological and physical harm, which includes discrimination by the community or the employer. The codes of conduct to protect the researched include ensuring anonymity of the researched and confidentiality of the responses. This dimension of the ethical codes emphasizes the individual at the expense of the communities and society to which findings from the study can be generalized or extrapolated. Paradoxically, while in quantitative research one of the main aims is to generate laws and principles that govern the universe, the universe is not protected against harmful information by the sample researched. The assumption made is that research procedures which include sampling, validity and reliability in quantitative research clear the findings of any respondent and researcher biases that cannot be considered universal.
>
> While generalization of findings is clearly an essential ethical issue to consider, disrespect and psychological harm to communities, societies and nations to which research findings are generalized or extrapolated is another dimension. (p. 675)

Chilisa (2005) warns against the privilege that First World researchers have enjoyed by making use of the written word as their forum for legitimizing knowledge. She writes:

> Unfortunately, the majority of the researched, who constitute two-thirds of the world, are left out of the debate and do not therefore participate in legitimizing the very knowledge they are supposed to produce. The end result has been that ethics protocols of individual consent and notions of confidentiality have been misused to disrespect and make value judgments that are psychologically damaging to communities and nations at large. But, above all, the production of knowledge continues to work within the framework of colonizer/colonized. The colonizer still strives to provide ways of knowing and insists on others to use these paradigms. In the postcolonial era, however, it is important to move beyond knowledge construction by the Western First World as the knower. Resistance to this domination continues and it is attested, among other things, by the current African Renaissance. (p. 677)

Hence, ethical conduct needs to consider access to information for participants in a way that is responsive to the different kinds of knowing that characterize the diverse communities.

Ethical Review Boards and Informed Consent

Corbin and Morse (2003) emphasize the need for participants to fully understand what it means to participate in terms of risks and benefits, especially when there are cultural or language differences. It is the researcher's and evaluator's responsibility to make sure that participants understand their rights, including their right to withdraw from the study at any time. Researchers and evaluators need to consider not only emotional risks but also social, political, legal, and economic complications that might result from participation in the study.

The American Anthropological Association's (2004) paper on IRBs and ethnography raises the question of whether written informed consent is required to document participants' consent:

> It is often not appropriate to obtain consent through a signed form—for example, where people are illiterate or where there is a legacy of human rights abuses creating an atmosphere of fear, or where the act of signing one's name converts a friendly discussion into a hostile circumstance. In these and in other cases, IRBs should consider granting ethnographers waivers to written informed consent, and other appropriate means of obtaining informed consent should be utilized.

> The Common Rule clearly allows IRBs to authorize oral informed consent. Section 46.117(c) of the regulations permits the waiver of written consent, either if the consent document would be the only form linking the subject and the research and if the risk of harm would derive from the breach of confidentiality or if the research is of minimal risk and signing a consent document would be culturally inappropriate in that context. Section 46.116(d) authorizes the IRB to waive informed consent or approve a consent procedure that alters or eliminates some or all of the elements of informed consent if four conditions are met: (1) the research is of no more than minimal risk; (2) the change in consent procedures will not harm the respondents; (3) the research could not "practicably be carried out without the waiver or alteration"; and (4) whenever appropriate, additional information will be provided to subjects after participation.

> These regulations can be interpreted to provide alternative means of obtaining consent. Consent can be assumed in instances where the respondent is free to converse or not with the researcher or evaluator and is free to determine the level and nature of the interaction between participant and the research or evaluation team. This in no way absolves the anthropologist from

clearly informing participants about the purpose and procedures of the study, its potential risks and benefits, and plans for the use and protection of ethnographic materials gathered during the study.

There are also situations in which some community authority must approve the research or evaluation before any individual community member is asked to participate. In some communities an individual would be put at risk of community sanction if he or she agreed to participate in a project without the formal approval by community authorities. In some cultural settings, a spouse or male household-head, rather than an individual person, may be the culturally or legally appropriate agent to provide consent.

In reviewing particular cases posing complex ethical questions, an IRB that does not have an ethnographer on its panel should consult an outside expert with knowledge of ethnographic approaches and/or the particular context in which the study will take place.

Ethics Committees: Navigation

You should always contact your own institution's ethical review board to find out its policies and procedures early in your planning process. Sometimes such a review can occur in stages if you are planning to conduct pilot work or obtain funding from an external agency. In any case, you should be prepared to submit your proposal in the appropriate format to the review board well in advance of the time that you actually plan to start data collection. The committee members need time to read and discuss your proposal, and they might have questions that will require some revision of your planned procedures. Lead time, an open mind, and a cooperative attitude help. There are a number of potential points of tension in the review process. For example (Cheek, 2005, p. 397):

- If, for example, it is necessary for researchers or evaluators to state clearly, before research begins, each question that they will ask participants, this makes the emergent design of some qualitative approaches extremely problematic.

- If the ethics review board asks you to modify your proposal in a way that appears to compromise the approach you wish to take, what do you do (e.g., if someone will not sign the form, exclude them)?

Cheek (2005, p. 398) suggests the following strategies as ways to work with an institutional review board:

- Write to ethics committee; explain how you filled in the form, why you did it that way, especially with respect to not being able to provide certain details until the study is actually underway.

- Explain how the initial approach will be made to participants, and outline the general principles that will be employed regarding confidentiality and other matters.

- Suggest that, if the committee would find it useful, you are happy to talk about the study and discuss any concerns committee members might have.

- See your role as "researcher/evaluator as educator." Frame your responses in terms of the understandings of research and evaluation that the committee brings to the table . . . understandings of ethics . . . philosophical debates about the nature of knowledge and the way that it is possible to study that knowledge.

Other helpful strategies include:

- Find out as much as possible about the processes used by the committee and ask to see examples of proposals that have been accepted.

- Speak to others who have applied to the committee previously.

Power, Trust, and Reciprocity

Cheek (2005) describes the need to have a trusting relationship between researchers and participants. Although he sets his comments within a qualitative context, they have applicability in the broader transformative context:

> Qualitative approaches to research are premised on an honest and open working relationship between the researcher and the participants in the research. Inevitably, in such studies the researcher spends a great deal of time with participants getting to know aspects of their world and learning about the way they live in that world. At the center of a good working relationship in qualitative research is the development of trust. Furthermore, as qualitative researchers, we all have dealt with issues such as participants feeling threatened by the research and therefore concealing information, or participants who are eager to please us and give us the information they think we want to hear or that they think we need to know. (p. 401)

QUESTION FOR THOUGHT

Think about Watts's (2006) dilemma, which was presented in Chapter 6. She was interviewing female civil engineers who reacted negatively to the word *feminist*. She decided not to use that word in her description of the study for the participants, even though she knew she was using feminist theory as her theoretical framework. What are your thoughts about her decision set in contrast to the recommendation in this section that the researcher or evaluator establish an honest and open relationship with participants?

In addition to the strategies for building trust discussed in Chapter 3, other actions can be taken at the point of identifying potential participants. Tell participants who the funder is and the purpose of the funding. Be honest in your promises of anonymity/confidentiality. Participants may have a realistic reason to fear that they will be "punished" if they say something that offends the funder. If you cannot ensure anonymity (e.g., because of a small community), then make this clear to the participants. What will you do with the information? Who will have access to it? How will their rights to confidentiality be ensured? Inform participants if any issues arise about ownership of the data and the way it will be disseminated.

Reciprocity, as discussed previously, can consist of sharing information, writing letters, making phone calls, etc. (Corbin & Morse, 2003). There is also the responsibility to publish findings and to do justice to the participants and their culture. Researchers and evaluators may benefit in terms of reputation and funding. In the transformative spirit, both the researchers/evaluators *and* participants will benefit by societal changes that further social justice.

ETHICAL REVIEW BOARD QUESTIONS FOR THOUGHT

- Is research or evaluation done for the academic community or for participant communities? Or both? What are the ethical implications if you include participants' use of the study findings as a priority?

- What does beneficence really mean? No harm? A coupon to eat at a fast-food restaurant? Or . . . ?

- How can you ensure full and authentic informed consent of your participants?

- How can you address ethical review boards' concerns about the use of more interactive designs that may involve the collection of data in your own community?

- What are the implications of ethics from the indigenous voice perspective (see American Anthropological Association's website)?
- What is the meaning of ethics as defined from a social justice perspective?

Summary

✓ Sampling issues in the transformative paradigm highlight the dangers associated with accepted conventional wisdom in terms of dimensions of diversity, both in terms of ignoring minority positions and the complexity associated with such positions.

✓ Cultural competence is a disposition that is required to understand how to approach communities in a respectful way, to invite participation, and to support that participation.

✓ Relevant dimensions of diversity are contextually dependent. In this chapter, examples were presented that include race/ethnicity, disability, indigenous populations, women, and immigrants.

✓ Probability-based, theoretical, and convenience sampling strategies were identified, as well as the tensions that are associated with representation in samples.

✓ Ethical review boards that are established by government entities were contrasted with ethical concerns from an indigenous perspective.

✓ Issues of power, trust, and reciprocity were revisited in this chapter.

MOVING ON TO CHAPTER 8 . . .

Once the participants for a study have been identified, then it is time to make decisions about the specific data-collection methods, instruments, and strategies to be used. Critical factors include choosing data-collection strategies that are culturally appropriate, involving community members, reflecting an understanding of the community context, and reinforcing a trusting relationship between researcher/evaluator and the community. Chapter 8 includes description of such data-collection techniques as personal reflections, interviews, focus groups, gender analyses, visual data collection, surveys, and tests. Examples of these approaches are presented as they have been applied in transformative research and evaluation studies.

Some people love prisms; some people hate them. I know someone who is annoyed by the way the colors splash around the room when the prism swings in the window.

Notes

1. LGBTQ stands for lesbian, gay, bisexual, transgender, and queer. Kosciw, Byard, Fischer, and Joslin (2007) define *transgender* as a term that "loosely refers to people who do not identify with the gender roles assigned to them by society based on their biological sex. Transgender is also used as an umbrella term for all those who do not conform to 'traditional' notions of gender expression, including people who identify as transsexual, cross-dressers, or drag kings/queens" (p. 553).
2. I never knew why white people were called Caucasian. I came upon this explanation in Kendall (2006): In her essay "Why Are White People Called Caucasian?" Nell Irvin Painter identifies Johann Friedrich Blumenbach as the person who popularized the application of Caucasian to white people. An 18th-century social scientist, "Blumenbach . . . created a system of racial classification. Caucasian refers to the Caucasus Mountains, two ranges in what was then Russia and is now Chechnya, which he believed were extraordinary and produced 'the most beautiful race of men.' Blumenbach identified Caucasians as the 'primeval' race because Noah's Ark rested on Mount Ararat after the biblical flood and that mountain is part of the Caucasus range" (p. 44).

CHAPTER 8

Data-Collection Methods, Instruments, and Strategies

Transformative results are most immediately captured through personal reflections (evocative) of those with first-hand knowledge of what has occurred and, for "harder" results, through documentation of shifts in indicators (evidential) of health or life status of individuals, organizations, or communities affected. Because these results are unique to the individual, organization, or community realizing them, those most profoundly affected are best positioned to reflect on and share the implications of what has occurred. Such reflections may be captured through journals, interviews, focus groups, or other forms of self- or group expression. Concrete evidence of change, such as improvements in personal health (physical, mental and/or spiritual), organizational climate, community health statistics, and quality-of-life indicators, should follow the breakthrough events in relatively short order if the events truly were transformative.
—GROVE, KIBEL, AND HAAS (2005, p. 7)

IN THIS CHAPTER . . .

▼ Overarching issues related to decision points and planning for data collection are presented.

▼ Specific data-collection strategies are used to illustrate the transformative approach, including interviews, observations, document and artifact reviews, gender analyses, community-based data collection, visual data, surveys, and tests.

Researchers and evaluators who place their work within different paradigms approach data collection differently. For example, in the post-positivist paradigm, it is assumed that a quantitative, standardized instrument decreases the bias of the researcher/evaluator, allowing him or her to remain neutral, present the questions in exactly the same way to each person, and analyze the data into a numeric value with a determinable margin of error. In the constructivist paradigm, the researcher/evaluator would establish rapport with the people in the study through sustained contact and anticipate multiple constructions of reality in the words of the persons with the lived experience. Data-collection strategies would primarily include interviews, document and artifact review, and observation.

In the transformative paradigm, the researchers/evaluators begin with the acknowledgment that there is a power differential between themselves and the people in the study. They need to understand the community through some kind of sustained involvement such that community members would trust them enough to give accurate information to them. Together, the community and researchers/evaluators make decisions with regard to a data-collection method that is culturally appropriate, reflects a deep understanding of the cultural issues involved, builds trust to obtain valid data, makes modifications that may be necessary to collect data from various groups, and links the data collected to social action. The quotation that opens this chapter makes the point that multiple methods of data collection are recommended to provide evidence in transformative research and evaluation studies.

Data-collection techniques in the transformative paradigm often have labels similar to those used in general methodology textbooks. The difference in the transformative paradigm is in the choice, development, and implementation of the data-collection strategies so that they are grounded in the community and the furtherance of human rights. Data-collection techniques described in this chapter include personal reflections, interviews, focus groups, gender analyses, visual data collection, surveys, and tests. The examples used to illustrate transformative data collection provide insights into how these approaches are shaped for social justice purposes.

Reliability and Validity/Dependability and Credibility

The American Educational Research Association, American Psychological Association, and the National Council on Measurement in Education (1999) publish *Standards for Educational and Psychological Testing* that describe recommended practices with regard to reliability and validity when tests are used. Their recommendations are relevant in research and evaluation contexts that use many types of quantitative measures. Reliability of quantitative data is defined as a measure of stability or consistency in a measurement instrument. It can be established by administering an instrument more than once and comparing the results or by using a statistical process that indicates the degree of consistency (see Box 8.1 for

BOX 8.1. Types of Reliability

QUANTITATIVE DATA

Repeated measures:

❏ Coefficient of stability: An instrument is administered once and after a period of time is administered again. The results are compared using a statistic such as a correlation coefficient (see Chapter 9). This is sometimes called test–retest reliability.

❏ Alternate-form coefficient: Parallel forms of the same instrument are administered to the same group of people and the results are compared as in the coefficient of stability.

Internal consistency:

❏ A statistical technique such as the Kuder–Richardson formulae or Cronbach's alpha are used to compare the internal consistency of items on an instrument to see if respondents are consistent in the way they respond to the overall instrument.

Reliability with observers recording quantitative data:

❏ Interrater reliability: Consistency across observers is calculated either as a correlation or as a percentage of agreement by comparing a sample of their observations of the same setting.

❏ Intrarater reliability: Consistency within observers is calculated using a statistical technique to determine if an individual is consistent in the way he or she records his or her observations.

QUALITATIVE DATA

Dependability: The observer keeps a case study protocol that provides evidence of when and why changes in understanding emerge as the data picture becomes more complete.

examples of types of reliability). These procedures are appropriate when an instrument is used to measure a unitary characteristic and are less so when measuring a multidimensional characteristic. Item response theory can be used to determine the goodness of fit for each item on a test with the model, yielding an alpha level that indicates divergence from the model at a specified significance level.

In terms of qualitative data, Guba and Lincoln (1989) note the expectation that insights based on data will change as the picture becomes more complex. Hence, the idea of consistency is not applicable to the collection of qualitative data. However, if reliability is reframed to mean dependability, then the researcher/evaluator can offer evidence to support his or her claims of the quality of the data. Yin (2003) recommends the use of a case study protocol to track the details of data collection at each step in the process, thus providing a publicly inspectable audit trail of when and how understandings change based on the data that are available at any point in time.

Validity is a concept that is used in a variety of ways in a research or evaluation context. Earlier chapters discuss validity in terms of research and evaluation designs and approaches. Recall that Guba and Lincoln (1989) reconceptualized validity in qualitative research in terms of the credibility of a study's findings, and in Chapter 6, I argue that this reconceptualization has applicability in terms of the criteria used to judge the rigor of a study. In this chapter, the focus on validity shifts from the overall findings of a study to specifically looking at validity as a unitary concept that measures the degree to which all accumulated evidence supports the intended interpretation of data for the proposed purpose (American Educational Research Association et al., 1999; Messick, 1995). Types of evidence that can be used to establish validity include: comparing the outcomes of an instrument to a theoretical model, comparing the items to an established body of information (e.g., the curriculum that was taught in schools or professional development), and comparing scores against a known criterion (e.g., Graduate Record Exam scores against college grade-point averages) (see Box 8.2).

Validity is a controversial concept in transformative research and evaluation because of the inherent cultural baggage it carries via concepts such as personality characteristics, intelligence, and attitudes that are measured in a social science context. Guba and Lincoln's (1989) concept of credibility as the qualitative parallel to validity informs our thought about the quality of measurement and data collection in a transformative sense. The essence of credibility is the correspondence that can be demonstrated between the way community members actually perceive constructs and the way the researcher/evaluator portrays their viewpoints. The strategies

---

BOX 8.2. Validity-Related Evidence: Quantitative Data

VALIDITY AS UNITARY CONCEPT

❏ **Construct validity:** To what degree does all accumulated evidence support the intended interpretation of scores for the proposed purpose? This is inclusive of content-, criterion-, and consequential-related evidence (Messick, 1995; American Educational Research Association et al., 1999).

❏ **Content-related evidence:** Items on an instrument are compared to the content that they are purported to cover, such as school curricula or professional development materials.

❏ **Criterion-related evidence:** If an instrument is being used to measure a current behavior, then a comparison is made based on the scores on the measure and observations of current behavior (e.g., an instrument to measure depression is compared against behaviors exhibited by individuals diagnosed with depression). If an instrument is being used to predict aptitude or success in the future, then the scores are compared against the behavior that it is intended to predict when the time is appropriate for that behavior to be manifest (e.g., scores on an entrance exam and eventual performance in a program).

❏ **Consequential-related evidence:** Researchers and evaluators need to be sensitive to the consequences associated with using information from measures, especially in terms of social inequities that result in lack of access to certain segments of society to resources that impact on performance on the measures (e.g., deaf children who are diagnosed as mentally retarded because the tests are presented in printed English, rather than in their visual language).

---

for demonstrating credibility in qualitative research and evaluation studies were discussed in earlier chapters. As a review from Chapter 6, here is the list of strategies:

- Prolonged and substantial engagement
- Persistent observations
- Peer debriefing
- Progressive subjectivity
- Member checks
- Multiple data sources

Pilot tests are recommended to determine not only validity/credibility and reliability/dependability of data-collection instruments for the intended purposes, but also the appropriateness of data-collection procedures to the intended community members. The avoidance of bias is the key concept in data collection in the transformative paradigm. Although all researchers and evaluators need to be aware of the importance of avoiding bias on the basis of gender, race/ethnicity, sexual orientation, disability, religion, or other dimensions of diversity, work in the transformative spirit places these concerns front and center. Feminists identify numerous issues related to gender bias in measurement, including use of sexist language and norms based on one gender group applied to other groups (Eichler, 1991). The *Standards for Educational and Psychological Testing* (American Educational Research Association et al., 1999) contains Standard 7.2, which is a strong statement with regard to bias in testing:

> When credible research reports that differential item functioning exists across age, gender, racial/ethnic, cultural, disability, or linguistic groups in the population of test takers in the content domain measured by the test, test developers should conduct appropriate studies when feasible. Such research should seek to detect and eliminate aspects of test design, content, and format that might bias test scores for particular groups. (p. 81)

Language as a Critical Issue

Choice of language is a critical decision point for data collection in transformative research and evaluation. A first step in this process is an awareness of which languages are in use by which segments of the community. A common practice in translation is to have the text translated from the original language into the target language and then have that translated version retranslated into the original language, a process known as *back translation*. This is a useful but not entirely effective measure to take when language differences are important in the context of an inquiry. The researcher or evaluator needs to realize that translation of an instrument is not evidence of cultural competence in a community. Language is part of a full set of cultural baggage, and the researcher/evaluator needs to be cognizant of the wider cultural implications of the use of language. Guzman (2003) notes:

> While translating a measurement tool or having someone who speaks the language of the target population is a step in the direction of cultural sen-

sitivity, these two steps do not constitute cultural competency. As evalua-tors, we must realize that there is much more to how language functions in a culture, and that a mere translation of certain concepts or measures will not fully capture the experience of the participants. . . . If an evaluator is not fully aware of a particular culture and how their linguistic patterns shape the behavioral patterns of the individuals from that culture, then the evaluator cannot make logical assessments about the impact of a certain intervention. (p. 177)

Cardoza Clayson et al. (2002) provide additional insights into cultural issues around translation of data-collection instruments in their study of civic engagement in Spanish-speaking communities in the United States. They state:

> Translation is not a matter of literally translating from English into Spanish or back translation from Spanish into English. Translation without contex-tualization can lead to miscommunication, particularly when working with people from different countries of origin. Interpretation and translation are inherently tied. When the dimensions and subtleties of the word are contex-tualized, clarified and thus, interpreted, translation becomes possible. Thus, in the case of "trust" or "civic engagement" the relevance of the concepts in the countries of origin are central to translating between evaluation stake-holders. For those from the United States context (funders) civic engagement had an inherently different meaning than it did for those from the commu-nity (grantees). Thus, an early evaluation step was to interpret the meanings of these terms and then to translate them to different stakeholder groups. (p. 40)

Cardoza Clayson et al. (2002) suggest that the evaluator needs to ensure not only that translations are done accurately from a linguistic perspective, but also from a conceptual perspective. They describe this role of the evalu-ator as one of mediation to clarify concepts so that a common language of communication is established.

QUESTIONS FOR THOUGHT

- What languages do you speak/read/write/sign competently?
- What experiences have you had in other cultures?
- If you are called upon to work with a community in which a variety of languages is used, how would you proceed?

Planning Data-Collection Strategies

The general steps for planning data-collection strategies in the transformative spirit share much in common with the steps taken in other approaches. A brief overview of the steps is presented in this section, followed by details of specific data-collection strategies that illustrate transformative approaches.

1. In conjunction with community members, decide on the data-collection strategies (e.g., personal journaling, observations, interviews, surveys, visual strategies, or tests). Figure out what types of accommodations might be necessary (e.g., interpreters, visual depictions of language or concepts, a person to record responses).

2. Plan to do a pilot test with your data-collection strategies before collecting the actual data. If you are seeking approval from an ethical board in the United States, all data-collection instruments and procedures need to be submitted to the appropriate reviewing body.

3. Decide how many times you will interact with participants; this may not be definitively known at the beginning of the study, but think about how many times you expect to interact with participants and adjust as necessary.

4. Plan what you will say to participants when:
   • Making first contact to set up the data collection
   • Beginning the data collection and ensuring informed consent

5. Decide how you will record the data (e.g., self-report, audiotape, videotape, notes taking).

6. Think about aspects of data collection to consider during the process, such as questions or issues to be explored; note that these may vary for different participants (e.g., students, teachers).

7. Ensure quality of the data (e.g., fill in notes immediately after interview or observation, check tapes for clarity, send transcript to participants to review).

8. Plan how to complete the data collection (e.g., reviewing data with the participants, providing reports).

Specific Data-Collection Strategies

Data-collection strategies in the transformative paradigm are taken, in part, from the data-collection strategies commonly used in social science research and evaluation studies in general. Familiar strategies such as observation, interviews, document review, and testing can be used in a transformative study. However, as has been made clear throughout this text, the philosophical assumptions of the transformative paradigm guide the inquirer into a conscious awareness of cultural concerns and acknowledgment of power issues at this stage of the research. In addition, transformative researchers and evaluators have developed strategies based in community roots that are specific to addressing issues of social justice. Examples of these approaches are described in the following sections.

Observation

Observation is a powerful data-collection strategy that is essential to transformative work. Observations can be conducted formally or informally, but it is difficult to conceive of a researcher or evaluator conducting a study in a context in which he or she has not been "face-to-face" with the community members. Observations can be made by using a field notes approach and/or noting specific behaviors of interest. For example, I often start my observations by (1) sketching the area to set the notes in context, (2) labeling the people in the observational setting by using a code that protects their identity, (3) noting who is talking to whom, and (4) noting what is being said. The number and length of observations vary from study to study. However, such behavioral categories as *on task/off task, reading, writing, information seeking*, or *discussion* can be noted on an ongoing basis in a classroom or other contained setting.

Various roles are possible for observers, ranging from total membership in the community to being actively or peripherally involved. The choice of an observation role, as well as the schedule and venues for observations, should be made in conjunction with the community discussions that precede data collection. Patton (2002) provides an extensive list of possible areas/points to notice when observing:

- *Program setting:* What is the physical environment like? Try to be specific enough that a person who has not been physically present can "see" the venue.

- *Human and social environment:* What patterns of interaction, frequency of interactions, and directions of communication occur? What variations occur on the basis of gender, race/ethnicity, disability, or other observable dimensions of diversity? How do these variations change during the observation?

- *Program activities and behaviors:* What is happening at the beginning of the observation? In the middle? At the end? Who is present and involved? How does this involvement change during the observation? What variations are observable? How are participants reacting at different points of time?

- *Informal interactions and unplanned activities:* What is going on when no formal activities are underway? Who talks to whom about what?

- *Native language:* What is the native language in the setting? This can mean a spoken, printed, or visual language. It can also mean specific terminology and how that is specifically used in the observed setting.

- *Nonverbal communications:* What do body language and nonverbal cues suggest? How do people get the attention of one another? What physical activities are observed (e.g., fidgeting, moving around, expressions of affection)? How do people dress and space themselves?

- *Unobtrusive measures:* What physical clues are observable, such as dust on, or signs of extensive use of, materials?

- *Observing what does not happen:* Based on prior knowledge and expectations, what is *not* happening that might have been expected? For example, a particular person may be absent or uninvolved, or an activity that is scheduled does not occur.

QUESTIONS FOR THOUGHT

- Use the preceding list of observable items above and conduct an unobtrusive observation in a public area. How useful is this list for framing your observations?
- What did you see that you wanted to know more about?
- How would you proceed past this preliminary observational period if you were to continue to collect data in this setting?
- What are the limits of data collected by means of observation?

Document and Artifact Review

For document and artifact data, a wide variety of sources is available, for example, written, electronic, or hard-copy articles ranging from official documents (e.g., marriage certificates, file records) to documents prepared for personal reasons (e.g., diaries, letters). Other sources include photographs, websites, meeting minutes, project reports, curriculum plans, etc. In making decisions about documents and artifacts, it is important to keep in mind issues of power and privilege that typically result in the preservation of some groups' documents, whereas others, having been assigned less importance, were either not in a format that could be preserved (e.g., in written form), or if they were created, they were destroyed.

Documents and artifacts are valuable in that they can provide background that is not accessible from community members. They can also be used as a basis of conversation with community members to stir memories that might not rise to the surface without such a catalyst. Researchers and evaluators must be cautious in the use of extant documents and artifacts, however, because they reflect only those experiences that have been preserved, thereby eliminating the possibility of the viewpoints of those whose data are not accorded that privilege.

Personal Reflections

Personal reflections were discussed extensively in Chapter 3. The notes kept in journals can be used as data to elucidate critical hypotheses, assumptions, and points of insight that are relevant for the study. This data can also be used to document the changes in the researcher's/evaluator's emotional state as he or she moves through the process of data collection and interpretation. Autoethnography represents the study of self using an ethnographic lens, making personal reflections the major data source for that inquiry (Jones, 2005).

Interviews

Roulston, deMarrais, and Lewis (2003) note the complexity of the interviewing process as well as the many types of interviews, ranging from general qualitative interviewing, in-depth interviewing, phenomenological interviewing, focus group interviews, oral histories, and ethnographic interviews. Each type of interview is associated with different procedures, and details about these procedures can be found in many good qualitative research and evaluation books, as well as in the *Handbook of Interview*

Research: Context and Method (Gubrium & Holstein, 2002). Roulston et al. identify a number of challenges in the interviewing process, including (1) responding to unexpected participant behaviors (e.g., revelation of an emotionally volatile condition, such as when a respondent reports having just learned that her husband was having an affair), (2) dealing with the consequences of a researcher's/evaluator's own actions and subjectivities (this relates back to knowing oneself), (3) phrasing and negotiating questions (e.g., allowing the participants' comments to lead the interview process and keeping the focus on the intended topic), and (4) dealing with sensitive issues (e.g., asking about racism or sexism). One good practice to consider is to keep a reflective journal and listen to audiotapes, watch videotapes, or read transcripts of the interview with these challenges in mind (Gubrium & Holstein, 2002).

Steps in the Interview Process

Corbin and Morse (2003) describe four phases in the interview process. Despite the fact that they specifically place their process within the context of conducting unstructured interviews, the manner in which they describe the phases resonates with the transformative approach to data collection, no matter which type of interviewing is being conducted.

The Preinterview Phase. The researcher/evaluator first contacts potential interviewees to set up an appointment to discuss the study and determine their interest in participating. At the first appointment, the researcher/ evaluator:

- Explains the purpose and process of the interviewing to be sure that the participant fully understands the process.
- Explains about confidentiality or anonymity.
- Answers questions.
- Asks the participant to sign the informed consent form (although this is not always possible depending upon cultural norms; see Chapter 7 on informed consent).
- Gets permission to record the event (again, if this is possible given the cultural norms).

Participants are reminded that they can withdraw from the study at any time without penalty. The researcher/evaluator and participant engage in small talk and develop a sense of trust (or not), making this phase very important. The issue of reciprocity is salient at this stage: What will participants get from sharing their stories? What can the researcher/evaluator offer that is of value to the participants? As Corbin and Morse (2003) note, participants can gain a number of benefits from being interviewed, such as:

- Validation of their worth and the importance of their experiences
- Obtaining needed information about a possible service
- A sense of relief at unburdening themselves
- Hope that their story will help others
- Making sense out of things by talking them through

Parents of deaf and hard-of-hearing children participated in lengthy interviews in which they described the diagnosis of their child and subsequent life experiences (Meadow-Orlans et al., 2003). One mother offered the following statement toward the end of her interview: "I hope that it helps somebody else. I really hope it helps some other parent some day— that would make me feel really good" (p. viii).

The Tentative Phase. At the beginning of the interview itself, the participant is still "feeling out" the interviewer to determine his or her emotional reaction and level of trust. Often the interviewee shares more background information in this phase as he or she gains a sense of what feels comfortable to reveal to the interviewer. Verbal and nonverbal behaviors are critically important now for conveying a sincere interest in the participant's story.

Novice interviewers may try to rush this phase or impose their own controls on the participant to try to get him or her to come to the point. This imposing behavior may emerge because the novice is uncomfortable with pauses and silence and responds by interjecting additional comments and questions into the interview. Learning to interview effectively comes with practice and constructive feedback. The novice can pilot-test the interview questions and strategies and then review the transcripts to see where he or she needs to modify behaviors. Good interviewing requires patience, sensitivity, humility, and honesty.

The Immersion Phase. Participants vary in the amount and depth of the information they share. Interviewers need to communicate their acceptance of participants' styles of conveying their thoughts and feelings. If participants express their thoughts in a nonlinear way, interviewers can allow them to continue as long as they feel comfortable and make a note to return to a topic that might need further clarification. Depending on the topic of the interview, participants may become very distressed and cry or express other strong emotions. Good interviewers convey support for participants by reaching for a hand to touch, offering assurance, and then sitting silently. Interviewers might also share their own feelings of anger or sadness in a similar situation, without shifting the focus of the interview to themselves. The purpose of interviewers is to really listen and learn from their interviewees. Good interviewers will not end an interview with participants in distress. They will wait for individuals to regain composure and then inquire whether they want to take a break or end the interview and perhaps schedule another time to talk more. It may be necessary to stop or postpone discussion on a particularly painful topic or even to end the interview altogether.

The Emergence Phase. Interviewers usually bring closure to the interview by making sure that participants are in control. They might summarize and clarify issues that emerged during the interview. Depending on the nature of the interaction, interviewers and participants may continue to converse about topics that may seem irrelevant to the interview focus. Participants may ask questions of interviewers about their own experiences. At these times, it is not unusual for participants to add some insights that are relevant to the topic. The human mind is complex, and once it begins a journey of remembering, it is possible that thoughts and feelings will emerge after the "pressure" of the interview seems to be over.

Self-Care of the Interviewer

Interviewing can be quite demanding on the interviewer (Corbin & Morse, 2003). Being involved with participants in an empathetic way requires investment of a lot of energy. Although the intensity of interviews certainly varies, interviewers need to be conscious of the toll such work can take on them. In one study I conducted of a cultural exchange program for deaf students from Costa Rica and the United States, I did site visits and interviewed the students in Costa Rica, along with their families and internship placement staff. Each day, these interviews involved four languages: ASL, Costa Rican sign language, spoken English, and spoken Spanish. At the end of the day, several of the host families offered to take me out to dinner. Despite my fear of potentially insulting them by refusing, I often had to make apologies and just go to bed. Working in four languages all day exhausted me.

Cultural Factors in Interviewing

Studies that used interviews with various racial and ethnic groups provide insights into cultural factors that need consideration with this approach. For example, Guzman (2003) describes the aspect of Latino culture that views elders and scholars as deserving respect. This attitude may be evidenced in interview situations with Latinos who do not make direct eye contact or feel reticent to express their true feelings about how an intervention impacted them, whether positively or negatively. In the U.S. mainstream culture, this behavior might be interpreted as meaning the person lacked engagement with, or felt no impact from, the program. Guzman suggests that this situation might be remedied by having a member of the Latino community conduct the interview.

Nichols and Keltner (2005) provide an example in which they interviewed over 140 people in a study of Native American community perspectives of families caring for a child with disabilities. They asked the local advisory board to nominate the interviewers. They provided extensive training for the interviewers to ensure the quality of the data and the confidentiality of the participants, and the researchers visited the participating communities regularly to be sure that the data were being collected as planned. The interview guide was developed in collaboration with the local advisory boards in order to be responsive to the participants' culture in context and form. The interviewers took notes and audiotaped the interviews. Each interview consisted of 11 open-ended questions, a sample of which appears in Box 8.3. Interviewers began with general questions about family life and the hopes and worries that families with small children have in their community. They then moved on to ask about the nature of contact that participants had experienced with people with disabilities. Subsequent questions were designed to build on the community tradition of storytelling.

Community Involvement: Key to Interview/Observation

Cardoza Clayson et al. (2002) describe the importance of community involvement in their work in Hispanic communities. They combined observation and participation in the community with their desire to conduct interviews. Their attendance at a Christmas Posada was viewed as essential to the quality of the data collection, based on this example:

> At one Christmas Posada a community member said to us " . . . you see (over there) Maria, she knows everything but unless Pedro says you're ok . . . she

---

BOX 8.3. Native Americans' Perspectives on Children with Disabilities: Sample Interview Questions

One of the best ways to learn about community life is through stories that people share with each other. Do you have a story to tell that features someone with a disability? Family stories sometimes include ways siblings or cousins help each other. Tribal stories sometimes tell about people who had a disability but helped the tribe or community in some way. Could you tell us any stories about a person with a disability in your family or tribe?

All of us have heard different people talk about the good things that happen to them and talk about the bad things that happen to them. Most people live their lives in a way that is comfortable for them (doing certain things, at certain times like dancing or special ceremonies, giving a ride to a cousin who needs to go into town, or listening to elders). Sometimes Indians call this living in harmony and teach their children how to live in harmony. Can you tell me some things you know that families can do to help their children with disabilities live in harmony?

Sometimes families need help with meeting the special needs of their child with disabilities. Depending upon what the special need may be, families may try to use a variety of resources or services. Some of these resources may be within the family (grandmother's advice, uncle familiar with Indian medicines, sister who also has a child with a disability) or some of these resources are from organizations like churches or support groups, or some resources may be from the mainstream society (schools, clinics, physicians). In our community, what kind of resources do you think families use? Would you recommend them to a family you know and cared about? If you would not recommend a resource, could you tell us why not?

From Nichols and Keltner (2005, pp. 38–40).

---

isn't going to talk to you . . . people are afraid of La Migra (the Immigration and Naturalization Service-INS)." We have found that the "outsider" role severely limits the ability of evaluators to identify and understand the more invisible structures, spoken, unspoken, and formal and informal rules that govern complex community initiatives. Attending celebrations, like *Posadas*, while time intensive, is a primary method for information gathering and understanding the generalities and specifics of community functioning. (p. 38)

Community Patterns of Engagement

Smith (2000) provides insights from her experiences in the Maori community about how cultural patterns of engagement influence the collection data:

Maori research projects have employed multidisciplinary approaches to a research "problem." Maori researchers have themselves developed methods and approaches that have enabled them to do what they want to do. They have gone into the field (that is, their own territory or *rohe*) to interview subjects (sometimes their own relations or *whanaunga*) whom they have identified through various means (including their own networks). They have now filled out their questionnaires or interview schedules and head back to the office to analyze and make sense of their data. During the course of their encounter, they are often fed and hosted as special guests, they are asked questions about their family backgrounds, and they are introduced to other members of the family, who sometimes sit in on the interview and participate. Sometimes, if the subject is fluent in Maori, they switch back and forth between the two languages, or, if they think that the researchers cannot understand Maori, they try even harder to speak "good" English. If the researchers are in their home, they may see photos of family members in the lounge. Sometimes it is hard to tell that the "subject" is Maori. Sometimes they say things a researcher may feel uneasy about, sometimes they come right out and ask the researcher to do something for them, and sometimes they are cynical about and hostile to the questions being asked. When the researcher leaves, it is with the silent understanding that they will meet again. The researcher may return to work and feel good about the interview. Was it an "interview," a conversation, or perhaps a dialogue? Or was it something more than that? (p. 243)

Unstructured Interviews

Corbin and Morse (2003) further explore the interactive nature of unstructured interviews as a context in which participants feel comfortable telling their stories (Ramos, 1989). When a participant feels able to express ideas that might otherwise not be forthcoming, the interviewer must struggle with a tension that is created at the boundary of conversational trust and data collection. Corbin and Morse contend that the unstructured interview provides greater control to participants because they are asked to tell their story as they see it, feel it, and experience it. They can decide how to begin the story, which topics to include or exclude, and the amount of detail to provide. While the participants may feel a sense of relief after telling their story, the purpose of the unstructured interview should not be confused with therapeutic counseling. Rather:

> The purpose of unstructured interactive interviews is . . . to gather information about topics or phenomena that happen to be of interest to researchers and at the same time are significant events or experiences in persons' lives. Although it is possible for an interviewee to feel that he or she has been coerced into being interviewed, consent forms make it clear that persons are free to choose whether to participate. Furthermore, persons may withdraw

from a study at any time without penalty. The topic of the investigation is explained clearly before persons agree to be interviewed, and once the agreement is made, researchers and participants together negotiate the time and place to meet. (Corbin & Morse, 2003, pp. 339, 341)

Focus Groups

Focus groups are popular as a means of using a group interview setting for data collection in marketing research; many textbooks are available that discuss the "how to's" of focus groups. Based on her work in the United Kingdom, where she facilitated change in health services for culturally complex communities, Chiu (2003) offers a process for the conduct of focus groups that fits within the transformative paradigm. She developed a cyclical approach integrating the steps-of-action research with focus-group methodology for the purpose of radical social transformation. The three basic stages follow:

• *Stage 1: Problem identification.* The researcher needs time to get to know the community, negotiate with stakeholders, and build relationships with participants, service providers, and funders or regulatory agencies. Focus groups are used to identify the concerns, opinions, and experiences of the participants (and other constituencies). In her study, Chiu (2003) provided opportunities for the participants to explore their perceptions and experiences with cervical and breast cancer screening. The researchers used discussion guides along with such items as a speculum and a breast model and also included video-based demonstrations of the screening procedure. This combination of stimuli enhanced the women's ability to describe their own experiences and enriched the communication between the women and the researchers. The creation of dialogue is designed to encourage critical thinking and awareness of the issues as a basis for later development of solutions.

• *Stage 2: Solution generation.* Focus groups are used to formulate solutions and identify resources needed to support the implementation of the interventions. Service consumers may be enlisted as co-researchers for the focus groups. Workshops can be offered to build the capacities of the participants and providers to implement and evaluate the proposed solutions.

• *Stage 3: Implementation and evaluation.* Staff and co-researchers implement the program, using focus groups for various purposes, such as regular problem solving during implementation and evaluation as a way to reflect on the intervention and its effectiveness. See Figure 8.1 for a depiction of Chiu's cyclical model.

Chiu (2003) developed this cyclical model of focus-group methodology on the basis of her work on the lack of participation by ethnic minority women in projects designed to promote breast and cervical cancer screening. She was concerned that previous research had been conducted from a deficit perspective, that is, by focusing on the women's deficits in communication and culture. Her intent was to uncover the barriers within the system that contributed to the low levels of participation. To this end, she found that the recommendations in focus-group books on how many participants to have in a focus group needed to be adjusted based on the size of the groups and the populations from which they came. For example, one of the breast screening projects involved bilingual women from eight language groups. Because this project was taking place in a concentrated urban setting, the focus groups had from 8 to 12 people. Another project related to cervical cancer screening involved women from isolated localities that had a low concentration of minority populations, hence the focus groups tended to number between three and four participants. She describes the factors that contributed to her access to the community members as follows:

> Working with other minority ethnic groups on the project, the importance of linguistic and cultural skills for accessing and accurately interpreting minor-

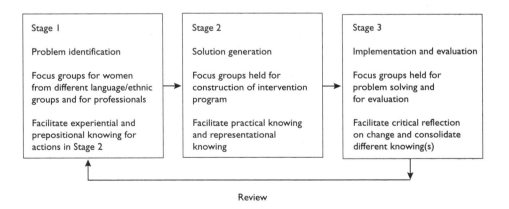

FIGURE 8.1. Cyclical model of focus groups. From Chiu (2003, p. 169). Copyright 2003 by Sage Publications, Inc. Reprinted by permission.

ity communities' experiences are paramount. By involving bilingual women from the communities as co-researchers, we had provided not only an environment where uninhibited discussion and expression of cultural nuances could take place (Egwu, 1992), but also an opportunity for community members to be actively involved in these projects. Co-researchers received intensive training to facilitate focus group discussions, in which, when possible, the use of mother tongue was actively encouraged. The co-researchers and I co-facilitated all the focus groups. Venues for these meetings varied from women's homes to health centres. (p. 172)

Mixed Methods and Focus Groups

Focus groups are effective when it is possible to get people together to discuss a topic or when individual interviews are not possible. At times, one strategy will be more feasible than another. For example, in the study of parents and their deaf children, individual interviews were used to reach parents who were deaf, had made a decision to get a cochlear implant for their child, or had a child with multiple disabilities (Meadow-Orlans et al., 2003). However, a sufficient number of parents from ethnic and racial minority groups was not represented in the individual interview data. Therefore, focus groups were held at the site of programs that served a high percentage of minority families. The participants were invited by the program director with whom they had a sustained relationship. In addition, transportation, food, and child care were provided to support the parents' participation.

Chiu (2003) found it necessary to schedule individual interviews in her study that focused on older women because the focus groups did not reflect their opinions. She also used a quasi-experimental design with pre- and postintervention interviews to determine the effectiveness of a change in the health service delivery program.

Interviews and Focus Groups with Native Americans: Using the Medicine Wheel

Cross, Earle, Echo-Hawk Solie, and Manness (2000) also combined individual interviews and focus groups in their study of mental health services for children in Native American communities. They used individual interviews with key informants such as medicine people, elders, and other important members of the community. They conducted focus groups with parents, children, service providers, community members, and staff from collaborating programs. The focus groups lasted from 2 to 3 hours and began with assurances of confidentiality and the informed consent details.

The researchers followed up with individual interviews for any tribe members who appeared to be uncomfortable in the focus-group setting. The researchers also participated in a camp-out with the staff, parents, children, and spiritual leaders. The timing of the data collection was suggested by the community members. Group interviews were either taped or recorded with handwritten notes. Individual interviews were taped, except when the participants asked that notes be taken either during or after the interview.

The specific adaptation of the focus group and individual interviews to Native American culture came in the form of the use of the four quadrants of the medicine wheel as a basis for the development of the interview questions. The four quadrants include context, body, mind, and spirit (Cross et al., 2000):

- "The *context* includes culture, community, family, peers, work, school and social history.
- The *mind* includes our cognitive processes such as thoughts, memories, knowledge, and emotional processes such as feelings, defenses and self-esteem" (p. 20).
- "The *body* includes all physical aspects, such as genetic inheritance, gender and condition, as well as sleep, nutrition and substance use.
- The *spirit* area includes both positive and negative learned teachings and practices, as well as positive and negative metaphysical or innate forces" (p. 21).

Sample questions for each quadrant include (Cross et al., 2000):

- *Context quadrant:* "How does your program draw upon extended family and kinship to help parents help their children? (for service providers)" (p. 103).
- *Body quadrant:* "Have you or your child (children) participated in any cultural activities to improve physical health? Examples include: special tribal celebrations with food served to mark the occasion, herbal or plant remedies for certain illnesses, smudging or other ways of cleansing for special occasions, or tribally-based recreational opportunities such as dancing or playing games" (p. 103).
- *Mind quadrant:* "How has the program helped you develop strategies that use Indian ways for addressing the needs of your child? (for parents)" (p. 104).
- *Spirit quadrant:* "Have you or your family participated in any rituals or ceremonies to help restore balance to your lives, either through the purging of negative forces or the development of positive forces? Do you use any Indian traditional remedies to restore balance in the spiritual area (example: sweat lodge)?" (p. 104).

The interviewers and focus-group leaders had their guiding questions; however, they encouraged community members to tell their stories in a way that was most comfortable for them. Hence, many of their comments departed from the script. The researchers believe that these departures provided invaluable data with which to measure the project's progress.

QUESTIONS FOR THOUGHT

- What approach to interviewing would you choose to employ in a research or evaluation study on a topic of interest to you?
- Using the guidance in this section of the chapter, outline your first steps in conducting an interview.
- How would you explain the importance of the study and how you plan to involve community members in the collection of data?
- What would you include in a statement of informed consent?

Gender Analysis

Gender analysis arose primarily in the world of international development with the realization that women and men experience such development efforts very differently. March et al. (1999) developed a guide to gender analysis frameworks in which they list a variety of options. However, a caveat is offered before the frameworks are examined:

> Where "gender" comes to be represented in the guise of approaches, tools, frameworks and mechanisms, these instruments become a substitute for deep changes in objectives and outcomes. The fit between the worlds they describe and any actually existing relationships between women and men is often partial. (Cornwall, Harrison, & Whitehead, 2004, p. 4)

Simply adding *gender* as a variable to the inquiry without considering the cultural and contextual factors that surround gender does not yield transformative potential. Box 8.4 lists a variety of gender analysis frameworks that are used in international development studies.

In addition to the frameworks listed in Box 8.4, two other frameworks for gender analysis merit additional mention. The women's empowerment (Longwe) framework was developed by Longwe (1991), a gender and development expert in Lusaka, Zambia. March et al. (1999) indicate that the women's empowerment framework does not consider time as a variable, addresses empowerment of women through providing them with enabling

BOX 8.4. Gender Analysis Frameworks

☐ **Harvard Proper Name Analytical Framework**[1]: designed to demonstrate that there is an economic case for allocating resources to women as well as men (Overholt, Anderson, Austin, & Cloud, 1985). March et al. (1999) describe this tool as a useful framework with which to gather and analyze information that can be used to give a clear picture of the gender division of labor. It does not consider time as a variable and focuses primarily on gender roles (i.e., who does what, who has what), treats men and women as separate groups, narrowly focuses on tangible resources (rather than including intangible resources such as friendships, credibility, status), considers the most efficient allocation of resources, and does not challenge existing gender relations.

☐ **Framework for People-Oriented Planning in Refugee Situations:** an adaptation of the Harvard analytical framework for use in refugee situations (Anderson, Howarth, & Overholt, 1992). March et al. (1999) comment that this tool is a useful framework with which to gather and analyze information that can be used to give a clear picture of the gender division of labor. It does consider time as a variable and is well suited for emergency situations in which complex assessment is not possible. It considers the most efficient allocation of resources, does not challenge existing gender relations, and shares many of the weaknesses of the Harvard analytical framework on which it is based.

☐ **Moser Framework:** a framework whose goal is to set up gender planning as an integrated planning perspective that seeks to transform all development work. Recognizing that such an analysis can lead to conflict, such conflict is reframed into a positive opportunity for debate (Moser, 1993). March et al. (1999) note that this framework considers roles in the context of relations between men and women; however, it tends to overemphasize the separation of men's and women's roles, addresses empowerment of women through providing them with enabling resources to take greater control of their lives, considers women's needs only, but could be adapted to consider men's needs, and does not consider change over time, nor does it include dimensions of diversity other than gender.[2]

☐ **Gender Analysis Matrix:** a framework that is based on participatory planning and also takes into account constraints related to time, funding, illiteracy, and lack of sufficient quantitative data on gender roles (Parker, 1993). March et al. (1999) praise this framework because it addresses empowerment of women through providing them with enabling resources to take greater control of their lives. It also includes men as one of the categories of analysis and requires trained facilitators to ensure that nonobvious categories of analysis are incorporated (e.g., resources as well as the issues of access and control) and to address dimensions of diversity other than gender.

☐ **Capacities and Vulnerabilities Analysis Framework:** based on case studies in various disaster situations around the world and focuses on providing information to facilitate response in emergency situations, as well as for long-term planning pur-

(continued)

BOX 8.4. *(continued)*

poses (Anderson & Woodrow, 1998). As the name implies, it includes both capacities (strengths in the community) and vulnerabilities (weaknesses) that could have an
impact on the occurrence of, and response to, a crisis. March et al. (1999) note that the
treatment of gender is not explicit as a differentiating factor in this framework, and thus
addressing empowerment of women through providing them with enabling resources
to take greater control of their lives requires the facilitator to consciously make a decision to implement separate analysis by gender categories.

NOTES

1. An adaptation of the Harvard and POP frameworks was developed by the Netherlands Development Assistance (NEDA), Ministry of Foreign Affairs, The Hague, Netherlands. See Lingen, Brouwers,
   Nugieren, Plantenga, and Zuidberg, (1997).
2. The Development Planning Unit at the University of London produced a methodology to analyze gender
   in all types of interventions based on the confrontation of power relations in organizations.

resources to take greater control of their lives, does not consider gender
roles and relations of both women and men, might best be looked at as a
tool rather than a full framework because it is limited in time, the concept
of equality is oversimplified (does not include the complexity of rights and
responsibilities), and there is no consideration of other dimensions of diversity. Longwe proposed the criteria noted in Box 8.5 to qualitatively assess
the level and quality of empowerment brought about by a development
project. The greater the number of levels of equality met by the project, the
more the project is judged to empower women.

The Social Relations Approach was developed by Naila Kabeer (1994)
at the Institute of Development Studies in Sussex as a collaborative effort
with stakeholders from developing countries. This approach addresses existing gender inequalities in terms of resources, responsibilities, and power to
serve as a basis for the design of policies and programs to empower women
to be agents in their own development. March et al. (1999) note that this
approach does consider time as a variable; mainly considers gender relations (i.e., "how members relate to each other: what bargains they make,
what bargaining power they have, what they get in return, when they act
with self-interest, when they act altruistically, and so on" (p. 23); explicitly considers relationships of power related to class, race, age, and gender;
addresses empowerment of women through providing them with enabling

resources to take greater control of their lives; and requires planners to critically examine their own institution and possible biases brought into the assessment process.

Key concepts from the Social Relations Approach include:

- *Development as increasing human well-being:* Concerns about survival, security, and autonomy supersede concerns about economic growth or improved productivity. Interventions must be assessed against economic and human well-being criteria.

- *Social relations:* Concerns about cross-cutting inequalities (e.g., gender, race, ethnicity, class) need to be addressed in a dynamic way with both tangible and intangible resources considered.

BOX 8.5. Longwe Criteria to Assess Empowerment

☐ **Welfare:** Does the project meet material needs or address immediate problems such as access to food, income, shelter and health-care? In other words, are these practical gender needs met in the planning, implementation and evaluation of a project?

☐ **Access:** Does the project provide better access to the means of production on an equal basis with men, such as equal access to land, labour, credit, training and all publicly available services and benefits?

☐ **Conscientisation:** Does the project enhance women's awareness of the gender roles and inequalities within communities? Are the strategic needs for creating or enhancing women's awareness and understanding considered and addressed in the planning and execution of a project?

☐ **Participation:** Are women involved in the decision-making process about the project, in policy-making in the community, in planning and administration not only of the project, but beyond its completion? A significant indication of the degree to which women's strategic needs are addressed in a project can be found in the degree to which they take part in the planning, management, implementation and assessment of a project.

☐ **Control:** Do women have control over the end product of their labour? Following on the criteria of awareness and participation, control over the end product of their labour depends on whether women's strategic needs were considered and woven into the project. The extent of women's control over the product of their input in development can also be seen as an indication of the degree to which conventional gender roles have been challenged and changed through the project.

From Longwe (1991, as cited in Sadie & Loots, 1998, pp. 2–3).

- *Institutional analysis* (four key organizations are included):
  - The state includes legal, military, and administrative organizations that pursue the national interest and welfare.
  - The market includes firms, financial corporations, farming enterprises, multinational companies, etc., that pursue profit maximization.
  - The community includes village tribunals, voluntary associations, informal networks, and nongovernment organizations (NGOs) and others involved in service provision.
  - Family/kinship includes the household, extended families, lineage groups in an altruistic, cooperative manner.

The key organizations are examined in light of:

- Rules: How do things get done? By whom will things be done? Who will benefit?
- Activities: What is done? Who does what, who gets what, and who can claim what?
- Resources: What is used and what is produced?
- People: Who is in, who is out, and who does what? Who do they allow in and whom they exclude? Who is assigned various resources, tasks, and responsibilities? Who is positioned where in the hierarchy?
- Power: Who decides and whose interests are served?
- Institutional gender policies: Are the institutional policies gender-blind ("we don't discriminate on the basis of gender"), gender-neutral ("we aim for equity for both sexes"), gender-specific (knowledge about gender is used to address needs of men and women), or gender-redistributive (existing distribution of resources will occur to establish equity based on gender)?

Effects of problems and their causes are analyzed in terms of immediate, underlying, and structural factors.

Foundations and Gender Analysis

Some foundations use standard gender-analysis approaches; others have their own specific tools. Two examples of common types are the interview protocol (ClearSighted) developed by the Chicago Women in Philanthropy and the diversity table used by the Hyams Foundation (Ryan, 2004). The ClearSighted protocol consists of a set of questions designed to facilitate discussion of gender issues with grantees. The protocol is available from the Women in Philanthropy (*www.womenphil.org*) and has been adapted for use in other organizations. The Agency Diversity table is designed to identify how inclusive an organization is in terms of both gender and race/ethnicity. This information can be used as a basis for making changes in these dimensions. The form is available as a downloadable document (*www.hyamsfoundation.org*).

QUESTIONS FOR THOUGHT

- What are your thoughts about using gender analysis in a research or evaluation study?
- Under what circumstances do you think that such a method of data collection would be advisable? What is gained if one is conducted?
- Under what circumstances do you think that use of such a method would *not* be advisable? What is lost if a gender analysis is not conducted?

Community-Based Data Collection

Hui

Maori hold day-long meetings, called *hui*, at which members of the community are invited to read papers and discuss their meaning with the authors, in this case around marginalization and research protocols (Cram et al., 2004). It is important in these gatherings not to silence voices of those who are less articulate. Some participants are very articulate and present a particular view. However, those who are living the experience, but not articulating in ways the researcher finds useful, need to be heard.

Dingaka

Another data-collection strategy from Africa is found in the *dingaka* (diviners) practices (Dube, 2001, as cited in Chilisa, 2005, p. 679). The *dingaka* use a set of up to 60 bones that symbolize divine power, evil power, foreign spirits (good or bad), elderly men and women, young and old, homesteads, family life or death, and ethnic groups (including *Makgoa*, white people) to construct a story about the consulting client's life. The client throws the bones and the resulting pattern is interpreted in reference to his or her experiences, networks, and relationships with people and the environment. The diviner proceeds to interpret the pattern of the bones, all the while asking the client to confirm or reject the story the diviner is telling. Thus, the diviner and client work together to construct knowledge that is placed within the complexity of the current context. This process yields a community-constructed story, rather than one constructed by the researcher (the diviner). Chilisa (2005) concludes: "It offers alternative ways in which researchers may work with communities to theorize and build models of research designs that are owned by the people, and restores the dignity and integrity that has [sic] been violated by First World epistemologies since colonial times" (p. 680).

Most Significant Change

The most significant change (MSC) method was developed in the mid-1990s through a collaborative partnership between the Christian Commission for Development in Bangladesh and Rick Davies to create a monitoring system that would involve the community in determining what indicators of change are important to them (Davies, 1998, as cited in Whitmore et al., 2006). The MSC method was used successfully in Bangladesh. Gujit describes the heart of this method as "the sharing of stories of lived experiences, and systematically selecting those most representative of the type of change being sought to share with others. In so doing, the method allows for an open-ended and rich discussion on a range of aspects of change, rather than snippets of reality that are defined through outsiders in the form of indicators" (Whitmore et al., 2006, p. 345). The method has two parts: First, stories of change are identified. The steps involved in the first part are displayed in Box 8.6. Second, a communication pathway is constructed to make sure that all involved parties understand the significant stories of change.
    Gujit explains:

> A key strength of the MSC method is that it allows participants to make explicit the criteria for success that they value. This occurs as a result of the built-in reflection, not just stating the most significant change but making clear why this was collectively selected as the most significant one. By allowing diverse stakeholder experiences and perspectives to meet and share, the emergent criteria for success provide important insights about what is valued about the initiative being monitored. (Whitmore et al., 2006, p. 346)

When the MSC was used with Brazilian farmers, they identified such change events as being able to prepay a loan to a micro-credit group on time and gaining title to their own land. The MSC seems to be more sus-

---

BOX 8.6. Selecting the "Most Significant Change" Story

❑ *Identify who is to be involved and how.* Who will be asked to share stories (where is the lived experience that others need to hear about)? Who will help to identify the domain(s) of change? To whom will information be communicated?

❑ *Identify the domains of change to be discussed.* These are often related to key goals of the project/organisation/initiative. (For example, in Brazil, each credit group that received money was asked to discuss three areas: changes in people's lives; changes in people's participation; and changes in the sustainability of people's institutions and their activities.) Additionally, the group can report any "other type of change" enabling field staff to report on other factors that are deemed important.

❑ *Clarify the frequency* with which stories will be shared and the most significant one selected. (For example, in Brazil, this was initially monthly but later took place less than quarterly, as this proved to be a more feasible rhythm.)

❑ *Share stories* using a simple question for each of these four types of changes: "During the last month, in your opinion, what do you think was the most significant change that took place in . . . [e.g., the lives of the people participating in the project]?"

❑ *Select the most significant one* from among the stories (per type of change).

❑ *Document the answer.* The answer has two parts: descriptive—describing what happened in sufficient detail such that an independent person could verify that the event took place—and explanatory—explaining why the group members thought the change was the most significant out of all the changes that took place over that time period.

From Davies (1998, as cited in Whitmore et al., 2006, p. 348).

---

tainable in contexts that include a stable organizational hierarchy. When changes occur in leadership, support for the method may diminish, and without support, people who are struggling to make a living may not see the benefit of expending additional time on a process that is not valued by those in power.

Visual Data

Photographs, Videos, and Web-Based Visual Presentations

Visual methods such as photographs, videos, and web-based presentations offer potentially powerful means with which to collect meaningful data, especially in visually rich cultural communities or in circumstances in which printed language is not a prevalent mode of expression (Rose, 2007; Pink, 2007; Stanczak, 2007). Extant visual materials can be analyzed or the data collection can involve the creation of visual materials by the researcher/evaluator and/or community members. If the researcher/ evaluator is taking the pictures, then he or she can plan to show changes over time, illustrate oppressive social conditions such as those experienced by immigrant farm workers, or give a human face to a global problem. A tension exists between promises of confidentiality and revelation of individual identities by showing faces and/or bodies. Rose (2007) recommends the use of a collaborative model in research that uses visual images of people because the photos are based on agreements between researchers/evaluators and community members. Permissions should be obtained both at the time of making the visual images, as well as at the point of dissemination of the images as part of the study's results in different venues. If a photo is used in a book or a video in a presentation or website, the people in the pictures should be able to grant permission for such use. The copyright for the visual materials legally rests with the person who took the pictures or video. If it is the researcher or evaluator, then a good practice is to provide copies to the people who appear in the visual materials.

Rose (2007) suggests the use of several steps in using photos that are taken by community members in research or evaluation. The researcher/ evaluator begins by interviewing community members, then gives them cameras along with guidance regarding what sort of photographs to take. Once the photos are in hand, the participants might be asked to write something about each photo. The researcher/evaluator can then interview participants again about their pictures and written remarks. Analysis and interpretation follow, based on strategies discussed for qualitative data in Chapter 9.

Visual Methods and International Development[1]

Participatory rural appraisal is associated with a number of visual data-collection strategies (Rietbergen-McCraken & Narayan-Parker, 1998). These strategies are not limited to rural areas, but they arose from a desire to engage local people in research activities in communities where written forms of literacy were not dominant. Thus, the strategies can be implemented by using paper or computer screens, but they can also be done by drawing on the ground with sticks, stones, seeds, or other local materials.

Ranking Exercises. Participants can be shown how to rank things such as problems, preferences, or solutions. The community can generate lists of problems and then rank-order them in terms of importance. If researchers develop pictures that represent the problems on cards, then community members can sort them into the categories from most to least important. In addition, the participants can generate criteria for deciding what is most and least important. A matrix can be used in which the horizontal axis plots the problems and the vertical axis plots the criteria. Participants then rank each item in a position in the matrix. Individuals can do their rankings first and then the group can compare and discuss their rankings.

Trend Analysis. Calendars or daily activity charts can be used for trend analysis. Participants can indicate their level of activity on a calendar with notations for seasonal variables such as rainfall, crop sequences, income, and food. Daily activity charts can provide a graphic way for individuals to depict how they spend their day. Such charts can provide insights into differences in time use by men and women, or those who are employed and those who are unemployed. Trend analysis is useful for identifying the busiest times of the day, month, or year as a basis for making possible changes in time use for the community members.

Mapping. The technique of mapping can be used for a number of different reasons. Historical mapping allows the participants to depict a change that has occurred in the community. Social maps can illustrate characteristics of the community such as access to resources, school attendance, or involvement in community activities. Personal maps can show different sections of the community, such as where rich and poor live or where men and women can go. Institutional maps can represent different groups and organizations in a community and their relationships. These maps can be used as a basis for facilitating participation in decision making by a wider range of constituencies.

Urban Adaptations of Visual Methods

Collins (2005) adapted the Participatory Poverty Assessment to her study of poverty among women in Niagara Falls, Ontario who participated in a food co-op. She chose her data-collection tools based on a desire to learn about the daily living experiences of those on low incomes, analyze the role of institutions in their lives, establish an agenda for action to improve their quality of life as a shared task, and give an opportunity for setting local priorities for change. Because many of the women had low literacy skills, she used visual methods such as mapping exercises, seasonality diagrams, timelines, and ranking exercises because they are nontechnical and accessible. She also used focus groups and semistructured interviews to gather data.

The visual exercises included asking the women to draw pictures of what it meant to have a good quality of life and then what it meant to have a poor quality of life. The women then used a scale to indicate the relative importance of the factors by drawing a heart around those that were most important for a good quality of life, a circle around things that were somewhat important, and a square around those that were not important. The women indicated that the most important qualities for a good life involved their relationships with family, children, and friends. The women did not indicate a need for an abundance of money, just a cushion to ensure that they would not go hungry and would have a place to live. The women used a seasonality chart to indicate that expenses and the associated stress vary throughout the month and throughout the year. As the end of the month approaches, the women expressed greater stress, wondering if they would have enough food to feed themselves and their families. Winter meant higher utility bills, siphoning off money for other needs such as food and medicine.

Children and Visual Data Collection

Barker and Weller (2003) adapted visual data-collection strategies as a means to conducting children-centered research. They used photography, diaries, drawings, in-depth interviews, and observation as multiple methods of data collection in two studies: one on children's increasing reliance on cars as a mode of transportation and the other on citizenship and social exclusion for children in rural areas in England. The researchers gave cameras to the children and asked them to photograph their experiences in the car and found that parents actually took the pictures. They discussed the importance of power relations in families and the danger in making assumptions that the intent of children-centered research will be actually operationalized. Hence, researchers should not assume that the use of a camera will result in children-centered research without monitoring by the researcher.

Community Mapping with Youths

Amsden and VanWynsberghe (2005) used a community mapping data-collection strategy with youths from two groups (a drop-in group for lesbian, gay, bisexual, transgender young people and an education and support group for youths affected by violence) to examine the quality of their health services. Their first step was to establish an atmosphere of trust by asking the youths to identify the ground rules for conduct that would be needed to garner and protect such trust. The second step was to assure the youths that their knowledge and experiences had value and that each participant would be viewed as an "expert" in his or her own experience. The researchers used two templates as visual aids to bring focus to the process. First, they showed a picture that had a baby in one corner and an adult in the other corner and used this image to generate discussion about the health challenges that youths face as they move from childhood to adulthood. Second, the youths were given a piece of paper with an empty square on it and asked to draw their ideal health service. Amsden and VanWynsberghe (2005) describe the benefits of this process as follows:

> Through this project we found that community mapping offers key strengths as a data collection technique, all of which are based on a respect and valuing of individual and collective voices. Specifically, community mapping establishes an open, unrestricted space in which youth can determine how to represent their voices; the metaphor of a map acts as a clear lens to link the research concepts to the lived, local experience of participants, and the collective nature of the mapmaking process encourages dialogue and collaboration amongst participants. Assuming, shaping, and sharing one's voice must take place within some form of community, however, and so this is the one necessary criteria of community mapping. Finding out how community is defined in each context is the challenge of research and youth facilitators. (p. 369)

Visual Data in Visitors' Studies

Visitors' studies is a field of research and evaluation that investigates the broad context of informal learning associated with zoos, museums, and historical sites. Transformative issues of salience in such contexts include the welcoming of diverse visitors; representation of relevant dimensions of diversity; addressing of critical social, historical, and environmental issues in a transformative spirit; and outreach activities that go beyond the exhibits themselves (Mertens et al., 2008). Historical analysis of the founding of many museums reveals the same hegemony of power relations as were dominant in a society at the time (Rose, 2007). Hence, museums have been criticized because they reflect the white, male, wealthy perspectives of the founders. This historical analysis is useful; however, many museums have made significant strides in addressing issues of cultural complexity and social justice (e.g., the Smithsonian displays on Japanese internment camps in the United States; the Apartheid Museum in Johannesburg, South Africa; the Holocaust Museum in Washington, DC; the National Museum of Women in the Arts in Washington, DC; the Manchester Museum in Manchester, United Kingdom). The Oregon Museum of Science and Industry has a program designed to bring youths from underrepresented racial/ ethnic groups into science fields by training them to be docents at the museum, thus increasing their knowledge and providing role models for others who visit the museum.

Concept Mapping

Concept mapping is designed to help people think more effectively as a group without losing their individuality as well as to capture the complexity of the group members' ideas (Trochim, 2006). Concept mapping is a structured process. Focusing on a topic or construct of interest, participants produce an interpretable pictorial view (concept map) of their ideas and concepts and how these are interrelated (see Box 8.7). A concept-mapping process involves six steps that can take place in a single day or can be spread out over weeks or months, depending on the situation. The process can be accomplished with everyone sitting around a table in the same room or with the participants distributed across the world using the Internet.

Social Network Analysis

Social network analysis (SNA) is the study of relationships within the context of social situations (Durland, 2005, p. 35). The collection of data for social network analysis might come from a survey or a question such as "Who are your friends?" or "Who do you work with on this project?" Data for SNA can also be collected through observations, interviews, surveys, artifacts, documents, and records. Surveys can be conducted in different formats (e.g., paper and pencil, online) and can present a list of selected options, or respondents can list names of members or categories or persons. Networks can be established in other ways, such as via snowball sampling, as discussed previously. Fredericks and Durland (2005) describe an SNA study in which the goal was to reduce gang involvement in 12-year-olds through a mentoring program. Children were asked to name their best friends and who they hung out with at the start of the program and at various intervals during the project. The SNA allowed them to use this data to determine who was cultivating friendships inside and outside of known gang members and whether leadership roles were being assumed by any of the children in the gangs. The authors used numerical data and sociograms (i.e., a social map or visual image that depicts the relationships among individuals) to explore the relationships and how they changed during the study. Analysis of data using SNA strategies is discussed in Chapter 9.

BOX 8.7. Steps in Concept Mapping

❑ **Preparation.** Step 1 accomplishes three things. The facilitator of the mapping process works with the initiator(s) (those who requested the process initially) to identify who the participants will be. A mapping process can have hundreds or even thousands of stakeholders participating, although there is usually a relatively small group of between 10 and 20 stakeholders involved. Second, the initiator works with the stakeholders to develop the focus for the project. For instance, the group might decide to focus on defining a program or treatment, or it might choose to map all of the expected outcomes. Finally, the group decides on an appropriate schedule for the mapping.

❑ **Generation.** The stakeholders develop a large set of statements that address the focus. For instance, they might generate statements describing all of the specific activities that will constitute a specific social program, or generate statements describing specific outcomes that could result from participating in a program. A variety of methods can be used to accomplish this, including traditional brainstorming, nominal group techniques, focus groups, qualitative text analysis, and so on. The group can generate between 100 to 200 statements in a concept-mapping project.

❑ **Structuring.** The participants do two things during structuring. First, each participant sorts the statements into piles of similar statements. Participants often do this by sorting a deck of index cards that has one statement on each card; but they can also do this directly on a computer by "dragging" the statements into "piles" that they create. They can have as few or as many piles as they want. Each participant names each pile with a short descriptive label. Then each participant rates each of the statements on some scale. Usually the statements are rated on a 1–5 scale for their relative importance, where *1* means the statement is relatively unimportant compared to all the rest, *3* means that it is moderately important, and *5* means that it is extremely important.

❑ **Representation.** This phase involves the analysis of the data by taking the sort, rating the input, and representing it in map form. Two major statistical analyses are used. The first— multidimensional scaling—takes the sort data across all participants and develops the basic map wherein each statement is a point on the map, and statements that were piled together by more people are closer to each other on the map. The second analysis—cluster analysis— takes the output of the multidimensional scaling (the point map) and partitions the map into groups or clusters of statements or ideas. If the statements describe program activities, the clusters show how to group them into logical units of activities. If the statements are specific outcomes, the clusters might be viewed as outcome constructs or concepts.

❑ **Interpretation.** The facilitator works with the stakeholder group to help develop its own labels and interpretations for the various maps.

❑ **Utilization.** The stakeholders use the maps to help them address the original focus. On the program side, stakeholders use the maps as a visual framework for operationalizing the program; on the outcome side, the maps can be used as the basis for developing measures and displaying results.

Surveys

Surveys can be used in many different ways, both in support of social transformation and as a tool of oppression. As we saw in Chapter 6, Irwin (2005) used surveys as transformative interventions in part of the peace process in Northern Ireland. The process of developing a survey is similar to the steps listed for generic data collection, with a few specific concerns worthy of mention. The means of delivering the survey can be phone, in person, in the mail, or electronically. The format of items on a survey can be closed-ended (e.g., multiple choice or ranking) or open-ended (short answer or essay questions). Interpretation of the meaning of items is a critical concern when the survey is conducted using a predetermined set of questions, because the researcher or evaluator may not have access to the participants to ensure that they understand the concepts being asked about in the same way that the survey designer does. The researcher/evaluator also has a choice of the design for the survey study, as was discussed in Chapter 7 (i.e., descriptive, cross-sectional, longitudinal, interventionist).

Response Rates

Survey data collection also raises issues of response rates, that is, the rate of response based on the number of surveys disseminated in relation to the number returned. Trust issues can be present in communities that have not been equal beneficiaries of prior surveys. In such cases, it may be necessary to introduce the survey through a known community member, such as a church official or a tribal leader. An advance letter explaining expected benefits to the community can be sent prior to the survey. Follow-ups with nonrespondents are often successful in raising response rates. For example, a sample of nonrespondents in a mail survey can be followed up by phone interviews in which a shorter version of the survey is presented, if logistics permit. This method allows for a comparison of respondents and nonrespondents on key questions and can give insights into any biases that might be associated with a low response rate.

Types of Questions

Dimensions of diversity, discussed in Chapter 6, have applicability in the development of demographic questions in surveys. Other types of survey questions commonly include nonthreatening behavioral questions (e.g., recent purchases, television watching habits), threatening behavioral questions (e.g., sensitive topics such as sex, alcohol, drugs, money), knowledge questions, and attitude questions.

Transformative Uses

Appreciative inquiry (AI) uses surveys during the discovery stage (Ludema et al., 2006, p. 161). Examples of survey questions in AI include:

- Think of a time in your entire experience with your organization when you have felt most excited, most engaged and most alive. What were the forces and factors that made it a great experience? What was it about you, others and your organization that made it a peak experience for you?
- What do you value most about yourself, your work and your organization?
- What are your organization's best practices (ways you manage, approaches, traditions)?
- What are the unique aspects of your culture that most positively affect the spirit, vitality and effectiveness of your organization and its work?
- What is the core factor that "gives life" to your organization?
- What are the three most important hopes you have to heighten the health and vitality of your organization for the future?

Surveys Using PAR with Youths and Health Issues

The youth researchers who participated in the Amsden and VanWynsberghe (2005) mapping exercises decided that a survey of health clinics would be a good follow-up means to gain information about the quality of available health services. The youths decided which clinics to visit and created a survey by breaking down general categories of health services into more specific questions. The youth researchers visited the doctors and asked their questions and then they completed the part of the survey form that had yes–no answers and numeric scales for attributes such as cleanliness or lighting.

Cultural Critique of Surveys

Chilisa (2005) critiques the use of surveys when they are produced from a Western perspective without acknowledgment of the potential violence embodied in such a reductive data-collection strategy. She participated in the development and implementation of a survey to ascertain Botswanans' knowledge about HIV/AIDS and its modes of transmission and prevention. The items reflected the Western scientific definition of the virus and the dominant modes of transmission, as perceived in the First World, and Botswanans' understanding of the disease was left out. "The consequences of such an instrument are that respondents play a passive role because knowledge on HIV/AIDS and its modes of transmission [are seen as] resid[ing] outside their realm" (p. 669).

The Western researchers use the term HIV/AIDS as the label for the disease (Chilisa, 2005). The Botswanans have several different ways of speaking of the disease, depending on the person's stage of life and the circumstances in which the disease was transmitted. For example:

> If it was the middle-aged and elderly who were sick, HIV/AIDS was called *Boswagadi*. In Twana culture anyone who sleeps with a widow or widower is afflicted by a disease called *Boswagadi*. For the majority of the young, HIV/ AIDS is *Molelo wa Badimo* (fire cased by the ancestral spirits), and for others it is *Boloi* (witchcraft). For Christians "AIDS is the Fire that is described in the Bible Chapter of Revelations, nobody can stop it." (Chilisa, 2005, pp. 669–670)

Western-trained researchers tend to dismiss this type of knowledge as ignorance. However, suppose researchers instead interpreted this knowledge as reflecting that the cause of HIV/AIDS is "bad social relations." Suppose this indigenous knowledge was recognized and respected and used as a basis for developing an intervention to prevent HIV/AIDS transmission. Would it consist of an intervention composed of billboards that reprimand in English: "Don't be stupid, condomise" or, "Are you careless, ignorant and stupid?"? (Chilisa, 2005, p. 673)

Computer-Based Surveying

With the emergence of more pervasive access to technology, a variety of options have been developed for conducting surveys using computer-based systems. Examples include Perseus's Survey Solutions (*www.perseusdevelopment.com*) and Survey Monkey. As this is a fast-moving area of technology, the reader is probably best advised to check updates through a search of the World Wide Web. These packages differ in terms of cost, number and type of items, number of respondents that can be handled, branching options within the survey, and analysis and reporting features. Equity issues arise because of the potential difference in access to members of populations when using computer-based technology. However, as is discussed in the section on testing in this chapter, researchers and evaluators have capitalized on the immense capacity of computers to increase the likelihood that valid data can be obtained for people whose first language is not English (in the United States) and people with disabilities.

Dillman (1999) explores the specific strategies in using web-based surveys. He makes the point that in some ways, easy access to survey software means that surveys can be conducted by a wider range of people than was possible in the past. This is good in the sense of opening up access to a method that had been available only to a privileged group; it is also cause for concern in the sense of needing to ensure that the survey results are valid. As this is a rapidly evolving area, Dillman suggests a need for a strong research agenda to explore the benefits and challenges in using web-based surveys.

QUESTIONS FOR THOUGHT

- What approach to conducting a survey would you choose to employ in a research or evaluation study on a topic of interest to you?
- Using the guidance in this section of the chapter, outline your first steps in conducting a survey.
- How would you explain the importance of the study and how you plan to involve community members in the collection of data?
- What would you include in a statement of informed consent?
- How would you incorporate the transformative paradigm's basic beliefs into your survey process?

Tests

Tests can be used for a variety of data-collection purposes to assess a wide range of knowledge, attitudes, and behaviors, including assessments of personality, cognitive skills, interests, attitudes, motivation, and neuropsychological aptitudes for various occupations. Tests can be standardized or locally constructed. They can be objective or nonobjective. Standardized tests can be used as one way to measure student learning. Also, student learning can be assessed by portfolio production, teacher-made tests, and other assessment strategies. (See *www.deafed.net* for other assessment strategies used with deaf students.) Be sure that the assessment strategy is appropriate for the study participants.

Universal Design

Universal design is a generic term describing design that is intended to "simplify life for everyone by making products, communications, and the built environment more usable by as many people as possible at little or no extra cost" (Center for Universal Design, 1997). The basic idea behind universal design is that environments and products should be created, right from the start, to meet the needs of all users rather than just an "average" user. The United Nations included commentary on the need for "universal design" in its declaration on the rights of persons with disabilities:

> "Universal design" means the design of products, environments, programmes and services to be usable by all people, to the greatest extent possible, without the need for adaptation or specialized design. "Universal design" shall not exclude assistive devices for particular groups of persons with disabilities where this is needed. (U.N. Declaration of Ad Hoc Committee on a Comprehensive and Integral International Convention on the Protection and Promotion of the Rights and Dignity of Persons with Disabilities, Eighth session, New York, 14–25 August 2006b)

Universally designed educational materials and activities have been developed for instructional purposes, and these designs have applicability in the research/evaluation process as well. In a universally designed curriculum, students are presented with a range of options for learning. When tests are used for data collection in research and evaluation studies, alternative activities allow individuals with wide differences in their abilities—to see, hear, speak, move, read, write, understand English, pay attention, organize, engage, or remember—to demonstrate their achievements. Information is presented to students through multiple means, such as audio, video, text, speech, Braille, photographs, or images. Likewise, a universal design allows students to use multiple means to express what they know through writing, speaking, drawing, or video recording.

Advances in technology have made some universal design strategies much easier to implement. Teachers have access to computers, software, assistive technology, and other tools that can be used to adapt the curriculum to suit a child's learning style. For example, textbooks and other reading materials can be made available in a digital format that includes audio, captions, and audio descriptions of visual images and charts. Box 8.8 provides a list of resources on universal design.

BOX 8.8. Resources for Universal Design Resources on UDL

☐ **Center for Applied Special Technology (CAST)** *www.cast.org.* CAST is a non-profit organization that works to expand learning opportunities for all individuals, especially those with disabilities, through the research and development of innovative, technology-based educational resources and strategies.

☐ **PACER's Simon Technology Center** (*www.pacer.org/stc*). The mission of PACER Center is to expand opportunities and enhance the quality of life of children and young adults with disabilities and their families, based on the concept of parents helping parents. The STC is dedicated to making the benefits of technology more accessible to children and adults with disabilities.

☐ **National Center on Secondary Education and Transition (NCSET)** (*www.ncset.org*) and (*www.ncset.org/topics/udl/?topic=18*). NCSET coordinates national resources, offers technical assistance, and disseminates information related to secondary education and transition for youths with disabilities in order to create opportunities to facilitate the success of their futures.

☐ **The National Center on Accessible Information Technology in Education** provides access to training for the development of fully accessible web-based materials in educational settings (*www.washington.edu/accessit/index.php*).

☐ **National Instructional Materials Accessibility Standard at CAST** contains information about a standard approach to making print resources accessible through Braille, talking books, and other strategies (*nimas.cast.org*).

Adaptive Testing

Still, other problems with computerized assessment have emerged (Trotter, 2003). One prickly issue involves the use of what is called *adaptive testing*, in which the computer adjusts the level of difficulty of questions based on how well a student is answering them. Proponents of this form of testing argue that it provides a more individualized and accurate assessment of a student's ability. Ketterlin-Geller (2005) notes that universal design for assessment is intended to increase participation by people with disabilities and students whose home language is not English (in the United States). Computer-based testing offers a mechanism for customizing the test to the student's needs. Ketterlin-Geller recommends that the degree of accommodation for each student be determined during a pretesting phase with input from teachers, parents, and student surveys, as well as student performance on basic skills tests at the start of the assessment to identify the requisite access skills needed to succeed on the test. She describes the following strategies for using universal design assessment in combination with computer-based testing:

- Write all directions and prompts in a simplified language.
- Enhance visual presentation for young learners and learners with diverse needs by placing all relevant information on the screen in an easy-to-read font.
- Use of a five-item test of mouse-maneuvering skills that mirrors those skills needed during the test itself.
- Provide additional practice using the mouse for students who need it or provide additional assistance if necessary.
- Provide additional accommodations, as needed, such as presenting math problems both visually and auditorially for students with low reading skills.
- Provide an icon on which the student can click to activate the read-aloud option.

When Ketterlin-Geller (2005) developed a computer-based test, she also sought input from the community as to the appropriateness of the computer testing process during the development period:

> Administrators, teachers, parents, child advocacy group members, and students participated in focus groups where they interacted with the test and provided direct feedback on the ease and flexibility of the computer interface. Participants responded to specific questions about the functioning of the testing system as well as the appropriateness of the test features for the diverse range of student needs. (p. 18)

She used the results to modify the test and the testing procedures. Thus, she was able to respond to the needs of the target population by developing a universally designed math test that reflected the experiences and knowledge of a variety of constituencies.

Computer-Based Testing

Much of what has been done under the auspices of universal design and accommodation for people with disabilities has relevance more generally for consideration of the feasibility and logistics of using computer-based testing. Working from a context of universal design in testing, Thompson, Thurlow, Quenemoen, and Lehr (2002) describe a five-step process for transforming a paper-and-pencil test into a computer-based test.

1. Assemble a group of experts to guide the transformation.
2. Decide how each accommodation will be incorporated into the computer-based test.
3. Consider each accommodation or assessment feature in light of the constructs being tested.
4. Consider the feasibility of incorporating the accommodation into the computer-based test.
5. Consider training implications for staff and students.

Thompson et al. raise the important issue of equity in terms of access to, and familiarity with, computer technology. The cost of the technology can be prohibitive, thus reducing opportunities for access to those with fewer resources. These individuals will then have less experience with answering questions that appear on a computer screen, using search functions, typing and composing on screen, mouse navigation, and other features unique to computer–human interaction.

The requirements of NCLB that all students receive exactly the same test item create a tension between the need to measure students against their grade levels and testing procedures that accommodate for individual differences. Because of this apparent conflict, computer adaptive testing is not integrated into the majority of large-scale testing programs by states. The U.S. Department of Education interprets the law's test-driven accountability rules as excluding so-called "out-of-level" testing. Federal officials have said the adaptive tests are not "grade-level tests," a requirement of the law. Trotter (2003) describes reaction to this stance:

> "Psychometricians regard that decision as humorous," Robert Dolan, a testing expert at the nonprofit Center for Applied Special Technology in Wakefield, Mass., says of the department's stance. Adaptive tests deliver harder or easier items, depending on how well the individual test-taker is doing. They are considered out-of-level because the difficulty range could include skills and content offered in higher and lower grades. (p. 13)

Sources of Test Information

Four ways to locate printed references for published tests are *Tests in Print* (TIP), *Mental Measurements Yearbook* (MMY), *Tests,* and *Test Critiques.*

A brief summary of these references are presented in Box 8.9. As mentioned in earlier chapters, Internet resources are also useful in searching for tests. The ERIC Clearinghouse on Assessment and Evaluation contains the "Test Locator" gateway as a source of information on tests. Simply entering the words *Test Locator* in any search engine will direct the user to the sponsoring websites: *ericae.net, www.unl.edu/buros*, or *www.ets.org/testcoll*.

The Educational Testing Service (ETS) test collection database contains records on over 10,000 tests and data-collection instruments. These records describe the instruments and provide availability information. ETS Library and Reference Services Division prepares the descriptions. The ERIC Clearinghouse on Assessment and Evaluation maintains the database and hosts the search system. The title, author, publication date, and source appear in the record. An abstract describing the instrument, intended population, and uses accompanies the record. Subject terms give

---

BOX 8.9. Resources to Search for Tests: TIP, MMY, Tests, and Test Critiques

❏ **Tests in Print (TIP;** Publisher: Buros Institute for Mental Measurements, Lincoln, NE). TIP contains information on every published (and commercially available) test in psychology and achievement. For each test, the following information is included: test title, intended population, publication date, acronym (if applicable), author, publisher, foreign adaptations, and references. Tests are listed alphabetically within subject areas and indexed in five ways: title, subject, publication date, name (of authors), and publisher.

❏ **Mental Measurements Yearbook (MMY;** Publisher: Buros Institute for Mental Measurements, Lincoln, NE). MMY contains information similar to TIP, but it also provides information about forms and prices and the extent to which reliability, validity, norming data, scoring and reporting services, and foreign language versions are available. Reviews written by qualified psychologists are generally included.

❏ **Tests** (Publisher: PRO-ED, Inc., Austin, TX). Tests contains information about tests in the fields of education, psychology, and business that are available in the English language. Similar information is included in Tests as in TIP and MMY; however, it does not include information about reliability, validity, or norms.

❏ **Test Critiques** (Publisher: PRO-ED, Inc., Austin, TX). Test Critiques provides supplemental information for the tests found in Tests, such as psychometric information and critiques.

For more information, go to *www.apa.org/science/faq-findtests.html* (American Psychological Association, 2008a).

the age and grade-level information as well as ERIC Thesaurus terms that describe the test. In addition, the ERIC Clearinghouse on Tests, Measurement, and Evaluation (ERIC/TM) processes information on approximately 2,000 documents and 2,000 journal articles per year, specifically in the area of testing and evaluation. (For more information, contact: ETS Test Collection, Educational Testing Service, Princeton, NJ 08541.)

Using the PsycINFO Database

The PsycINFO database is described in Chapter 4 as a helpful source for focusing the research or evaluation study. However, it can also be used to identify specific measurement tools because it indexes all published research in psychology since 1967. Searchers can use keywords to see if an author developed a measure in the context of the study that matches the study topic. For articles that appear relevant, use the citation to locate the study within the literature. These citations also include the university or organizational affiliation of the authors, along with an address where you can forward correspondence regarding the article. Write to the author and ask for more information on the test or measure.

Examples of How Tests Are Used

The U.S. Department of Education (2006b) secretary established the following two Government Performance and Results Act measures for evaluating the overall effectiveness of the Early Reading First program:

- The percentage of preschool-age children participating in Early Reading First programs who achieve significant gains on oral language skills as measured by the Peabody Picture Vocabulary Test–III, Receptive.
- The average number of letters that preschool-age children are able to identify as measured by the Upper Case Alphabet Knowledge subtask on the Phonological Awareness Literacy Screening (PALS) Pre-K assessment.

The secretary expects all grantees to document their success in addressing these performance measures in the required annual performance report. For example, the secretary established key performance measures for assessing the effectiveness of the Demonstration Grants for Indian Children program:

1. The percentage of preschool American Indian and Alaska Native students who possess school readiness skills gained through a scientifically based research curriculum that prepares them for kindergarten.

2. The percentage of American Indian and Alaska Native high school students successfully completing (as defined by receiving a passing grade) challenging core subjects (including English, mathematics, science and social studies).

3. The percentage of American Indian and Alaska Native high school students attaining at least the district average score in national college entrance examinations (the ACT and the SAT) and preliminary college entrance examinations (the PSAT). (U.S. Department of Education, Office of Elementary and Secondary Education, 2006b)

However, not all scholars agree that standardized tests are the best way to assess traits in ethnic and racial minority groups. Duran and Duran (2000) wrote about the Native American experience with testing in this critique:

> A good example of how some of the ideology of biological determinism affects people is seen in the field of psychometric assessment. The relevant literature is filled with studies showing cultural bias and outright racist practices, yet researchers continue to use the same racist tools to evaluate the psyche of Native American people. The very essence of Western science as applied to psychology is permeated with biological determinism[2] that has as its sole purpose the demonstration of white superiority. Many examples can be cited of Native American people losing their freedom, being sterilized, or losing their children simply because they were not able to pass the white standards of a psychometric test. (p. 93)

QUESTIONS FOR THOUGHT

- What kind of testing might you consider in a research or evaluation study on a topic of interest to you?

- Using the guidance in this section of the chapter, outline your first steps in choosing an appropriate test.

- How would you address concerns about using standardized testing in culturally diverse communities?

- How would you incorporate the basic beliefs of the transformative paradigm into your testing process?

Summary

✓ Data-collection strategies in the transformative paradigm have familiar labels, such as observations, interviews, document and artifact review, surveys, and tests. Specific adaptations of familiar strategies are necessary, however, to reflect the transformative spirit.

✓ In addition, data-collection strategies recognized as compatible with culturally diverse groups in ways that explicitly allow for addressing social justices issues are discussed. These strategies include gender analysis, community-based strategies, visual data collection, and universal design strategies.

✓ Data-collection decisions are made in conjunction with community members and are consciously selected to be culturally appropriate.

✓ Interviews are conducted with a sense of building trust with community members and awareness of differential cultural contexts, such as the need to have family members participate in the interview process.

✓ Gender analysis is used to examine discrimination on the basis of gender in communities.

✓ Visual data-collection strategies that emerged from international development projects are based on participatory rural appraisal strategies and are applied in a wide variety of settings in which human rights are a concern.

✓ Visual methods such as photographs, videos, and web-based presentations offer potentially powerful means to collect meaningful data, especially in visually rich cultural communities or in circumstances in which printed language is not a prevalent mode of expression.

✓ Surveys have great potential for use in transformative research and evaluation; however, they need to be considered with a critical eye and applied in a culturally competent manner.

✓ The same can be said for the use of tests as data-collection instruments; they are powerful if they are used in culturally appropriate manners. Universal design principles have potential to make testing accessible to many populations.

✓ Technology offers a double-edged sword in terms of advances in data collection. If used to include, rather than exclude, technology has the potential to contribute to data collection in transformative work.

MOVING ON TO CHAPTER 9 . . .

Chapter 9 considers the analysis of the data collected, whether quantitative and/or qualitative in nature. Specific issues regarding community involvement are examined in this phase of the process.

> Different facets of human experience are revealed when different methods of data collection are used. Sunlight remains undifferentiated white light until it passes through a prism and a rainbow is visible.

Notes

1. Participatory methods of data collection are commonly used in international development research and evaluation (Mikkelsen, 2005). Cost–benefit and econometric analyses are also used in this context. These topics are beyond the scope of this text; the interested reader is referred to Holland and Campbell (2005).
2. Gould (1981) characterizes biological determinism as "the practice of valuing cultural experiences that are Western and white over any other cultural experience" (p. 325, as cited in Duran & Duran, 2000, p. 93).

CHAPTER 9

Data Analysis and Interpretation

Data do not speak for themselves. You have to do the work of deciding what you take your data to mean, whether they constitute "evidence," and so whether your data are just ideas, or whether you want to claim that they can suggest connections with something else (for example, power relations, gendered inequalities, the power of ideas).

—RAMAZANOGLU AND HOLLAND (2002, p. 160)

I have to tell my Board [Foundation Board of Trustees] how many families were served. However, in this context where gentrification is causing 10 or more people to live in one apartment and the political atmosphere . . . was causing fear and distrust throughout the community, the funders' priorities were difficult, if not impossible, to achieve. This example illustrates our role as mediator between the funder and the grantee stakeholders to negotiate a modified set of outcomes that would report number of families served within an understanding of the broader contextual landscape. The final agreement reached reduced the required number of families served and made provisions for the final report to describe the impact of housing as a contextual issue affecting the project's results.

—CARDOZA CLAYSON, CASTANEDA, SANCHEZ, AND BRINDIS (2002, p. 39)

IN THIS CHAPTER . . .

▼ Theoretical frameworks are used to illustrate various approaches of using a transformative lens to analyze and interpret data.

▼ Data-analysis techniques are described for both quantitative and qualitative data and from a perspective of valuing the involvement of participants in decisions about analysis and interpretation of findings. Strategies to enhance this process are also explained.

A simplified version of advice for data analysis might read as follows:

"Gather all the data and review it. If you have quantitative data, consider putting it into a table or graph or using descriptive statistics such as frequencies or means. Then, use more complex statistical procedures as warranted by the type of data and the questions of interest. With qualitative data, read it as it is collected. When you finish data collection, read through all of it thoroughly. Develop codes (i.e., recurring concepts that arise in the data). Coding the data is somewhat of an iterative process as researchers and evaluators seek to develop codes and code data in a way that allows new codes to emerge and also allows for consistency and stability in the use of the codes. Either manually or using the computer, organize the data according to codes; analyze these to pull out themes that emerge from the data."

Transformative Theories as Guides to Data Analysis and Interpretation

When a transformative lens is applied to data analysis and interpretation, different facets of the data and their meaning emerge. Theoretical frameworks can be used to filter data in a way that brings to the fore issues of discrimination, oppression, and social justice.

Student Perspective: Filters for Interpreting Data

The paradigm filters the world for us into understandable components. Therefore it is everything when considering that a researcher filters the data and transforms it into information. The idea of subjectivity now concerns me as I wonder who can be absolutely objective when interpreting data. Are we not a product of our upbringing, culture, experiences and education?— Risa Briggs (September 2004)

Postcolonialism as an Analytic Framework

When postcolonial theory is used to frame the analysis, researchers and evaluators might focus on language as an important indicator, especially when an imperial language displaced the people's native language and thereby affected, in some way, their cultural practices. This framework might lead to questions about the use of the local language as an act of resistance or as an affirmation of identity, or the presence of cultural symbols, practices, and values from a mixture of traditions, reflecting both the colonial past and multiple ethnic groups (Madison, 2005). A second postcolonial analysis theme might relate to place and displacement, as oppressed people were often forced to migrate from one site to another or from their homeland to another place. This theme would raise issues concerning the relationship to region, land, and ethnicity among those migrating to and from other areas in the country and the cultural, social, and economic differences between, for example, rural and city life. Other themes related to postcolonialism include denigration of the indigenous cultural ways and corruption in the government and private sectors and their influence on social action.

Smith (1999) provides a detailed analysis of the theorized approach to research that was developed within the Maori community in New Zealand. The Kaupapa Maori Research approach, as mentioned in previous chapters, is based on the principles of Maori culture and self-determination. This principle also underlies the analysis and interpretation of data when working from a stance of decolonization. The process involves consultation, collective meetings, open debate, and shared decision making. Research claims need to be representative of the collective knowledge, effort, and commitment of people with diverse interests within the tribe. Given the Maori's history of betrayal by the government, avoidance of any perception that decisions were made behind closed doors is critical in order to be true to traditional Maori practices.

Marxism as an Analytic Framework

Using Marxist theory as a theoretical framework for data analysis leads researchers and evaluators to consider class issues such as the participants' articulation of class stratifications within their own country; the manner in which such stratification divisions operated in relation to degree of education, cultural capital, and moral values; and how activists focused on poverty and the political economy in their efforts to enlighten local people about class divisions (Madison, 2005, p. 53).

Feminist Theories as Analytical Frameworks

Madison (2005) suggests that feminist theories lead to questioning the data about the domains of race and gender and what effect the intersection of these variables would have on social relations, analysis of discrimination as an intermix of race and gender, and analysis of how patriarchal structures and practices position and limit women to narrow choices (p. 75). Sielbeck-Bowen et al. (2002) assert that feminist evaluators must address gender inequities that lead to social injustice at every opportunity for the possibility of reversing those inequities. They draw an interesting comparison between the Hubble Space Telescope and the feminist lens in interpretation of reality:

As the Hubble Space Telescope opened a new era in astronomy by allowing spectrographic observations of uncharted stars, planets, and galaxies, feminist approaches in evaluation can raise the evaluator's acuity and sensitivity to multiple explanations of reality where program stakeholders are the knowers and are placed at the center of evaluation activities. While the Hubble provided significant new information and discoveries about the universe, feminist inquiry has the capacity to bring into focus flaws and faults in society in order to bring about social and political change. Evaluation conducted via the lens of feminist epistemology(ies) can create equality and a more socially just society. (p. 7)

Chilisa (2005) discusses postcolonial feminisms as those that recognize as problematic Western feminism for ignoring issues of race and colonial interpretations of women and gender. In Africa, communal values are given priority. Therefore, postcolonial feminisms in Africa would seek to uncover gender inequities in a way that would not alienate men and women, but would support reasons why both men and women would benefit by addressing such inequities. In addition, the researcher needs to be aware of how language can be used to minimize the violence associated with such acts as rape by referring to them as "turning the child into a woman. . . . The language conveys messages that undermine women's right to social justice and that implicitly accept, thereby condoning, male rights to dominate women by portraying their violent acts through non-violent images" (p. 220). In African feminisms it is imperative that analysis and interpretation of data reflect a conscious awareness of the inequities in power relations between men and women and do not assume that women have the same power as men in sexual situations (as in "just say no").

Queer Theory as an Analytic Framework

According to Plummer (2005), one of the major sites of application for queer theory in the analysis of text rests in the critical analysis of how mainstream language shapes sexuality. This analysis can take the form of uncovering homosexuality and homophobia in films, videos, novels, poetry, and popular media. Ethnographic studies can focus on the world of gay men, lesbian women, and bisexual, gender queer, and transgender people, with specific focus on telling the stories of the once-silenced people in the text. Plummer (2005) writes:

What seems to be at stake, then, in any queering of qualitative research is not so much a methodological style as a political and substantive concern with gender, heteronormativity, and sexualities. Its challenge is to bring stabilized gender and sexuality to the forefront of analyses in ways they are not usually advanced and that put under threat any ordered world of gender and sexuality. (p. 369)

Critical Race Theory as an Analytic Framework

The CRT framework leads to questions such as How does race function as a barrier between the powerful and the marginalized? What is the role of racial prejudice as an explanatory lens for the research findings? How does racism operate through unconscious habit, naturalized practices, and beliefs of white supremacy? How are people in the setting constructed as racial beings and what assumptions are associated with their race and that of others (Madison 2005)? How is white privilege influencing behaviors, attitudes, and social relations in the setting? Two examples of CRT are provided here—one related to African Americans and the other to Latinos/Chicanos.

Endarkened Analysis: African American

Tillman (2006) describes culturally sensitive approaches that position experiential knowledge of African Americans as legitimate, appropriate, and necessary for analyzing, understanding, and reporting data. She proposes that the analysis and presentation of data proceed as a co-constructive process with the individuals or groups under study rooted in the cultural standpoints of African Americans to provide an "endarkened"[1] analysis of their experiences: "An endarkened analysis emanates from an identity that is centered in African American racial and cultural identity" (p. 270). She cites two examples that incorporate endarkened analysis strategies: Siddle Walker's (2003) study of African American principals in the South, and Bloom and Erlandson's (2003) study of perspectives of African American female principals in urban schools. The researchers used culturally sensitive data interpretations to present the data from the self-defined perspective of African American principals. Using theories such as feminist theory that emphasizes interpersonal caring to guide their inquiry, the researchers placed the knowledge of the participants at the center of the inquiry, rather than at the margins.

Latino CRT

Latino CRT (LatCrit) is defined as "the emerging field of legal scholarship that examines critically the social and legal positioning of Latinas/Latinos, especially Latinas/Latinos within the United States, to help rectify the shortcomings of existing social and legal conditions" (Valdes, 1998, as cited in Fernandez, 2002, p. 47). LatCrit has not been applied as widely as CRT, however, it also directs the researcher/evaluator to collect and make visible the stories, counter-stories, and narratives of marginalized people. Solórzano and Yosso (2001) extend our understanding of LatCrit through citation of the LatCrit Primer (2000), which describes a LatCrit theory in education as

> a framework that can be used to theorize and examine the ways in which race and racism explicitly and implicitly impact on the educational structures, processes, and discourses that affect people of color generally and Latinas/os specifically. Important to this critical framework is a challenge to the dominant ideology, which supports deficit notions about students of color while assuming "neutrality" and "objectivity." Utilizing the experiences of Latinas/os, a LatCrit theory in education also theorizes and examines that place where racism intersects with other forms of subordination such as sexism, classism, nativism, monolingualism, and heterosexism. (p. 38)

LatCrit is seen as a theoretical framework that extends the black–white binary perspective and emphasizes the intersection of discrimination and resistance as a means of addressing racism and its accompanying oppressions.

Application of CRT with Chicanos and Chicanas

Solórzano and Yosso (2001) use the concept of CRT as a basis for a critical race methodology that they define as a theoretically grounded approach to inquiry that (1) places race and racism in all aspects of the research process in the foregrounds; (2) challenges the traditional research paradigms by showing how race, gender, and class intersect to affect experiences of students of color; (3) makes a commitment to social justice through a transformative solution to racial, gender, and class subordination; (4) focuses on the racialized, gendered, and classed experiences of students of color; and (5) uses the interdisciplinary perspective across ethnic studies, women's studies, sociology, history, humanities, and the law to better understand the experiences of students of color.

Solórzano and Yosso (2001) recommend the use of counter-stories as a method of telling stories of people whose experiences are not often told as a means of shattering complacency, challenging the dominant discourse on race, and furthering the struggle for reform. Based on the rich storytelling traditions in African American and Native American communities, they identify three ways that counter-stories can be told to this end:

1. Personal stories or narratives: Personal stories (e.g., autobiographies) that highlight forms of racism or sexism can be juxtaposed with critical analysis of legal cases and presented in the context of a larger sociopolitical critique.

2. Third-person stories: The narrator voice can be used to highlight racism and sexism experiences in a biographical commentary of persons of color, set in the legal, historical, and political context of the United States.

3. Composite stories: Data can be combined in a composite narrative to illustrate the "racialized, sexualized, and classed experiences of people of color in social, historical, and political situations to discuss racism, sexism, classism, and other forms of subordination" (p. 32).

Solórzano and Yosso (2001) describe a process of data analysis using the concept of cultural intuition, which includes the use of personal experience and community memory (Delgado Bernal, 1998), and Strauss and Corbin's concept of theoretical sensitivity, which describes a personal quality of the researcher that permits an awareness of subtleties in the data based on readings and experience with the topic (see Box 9.1). They chose this method of analysis and interpretation because it can serve at least four functions:

(a) [Researchers] can build community among those at the margins of society by putting a human and familiar face to educational theory and practice,

(b) they can challenge the perceived wisdom of those at society's center by providing a context to understand and transform established belief systems,

(c) they can open new windows into the reality of those at the margins of society by showing possibilities beyond the ones they live and demonstrating that they are not alone in their position, and

(d) they can teach others that by combining elements from both the story and the current reality, one can construct another world that is richer than either the story or the reality alone. (p. 36)

Fernandez's (2002) extension of the notions of counter-stories and narratives takes the form of *testimonio* (first-hand testimony) as a means to transformation and empowerment. She studied the experiences of a student, Pablo, who went through the Chicago public school system, analyzing his narrative as a counter-story and supplementing her analysis with

---

BOX 9.1. Composite Counter-Stories

The researchers created counter-stories from primary data collected through focus groups and individual interviews with Chicana and Chicano undergraduate and graduate students, postdoctoral fellows, and faculty.[*] Using critical lenses of race, gender, and class, they examined concepts of self-doubt, survivor guilt, impostor syndrome, and invisibility. The next step in the analysis and construction of the counter-stories was to consider secondary sources of data, including articles in the social sciences, humanities, and legal literature. Then they decided to focus on a set of primary data on the theme of women of color and resistance in the academy. They describe the subsequent process as follows:

> Just as in the interview analysis, we listened to the voices of these women as we read and discussed the articles. We often heard varying emotions, even in traditional academic style texts. For us, literary analysis from poetry and short story segments helped tap into these emotions and challenged us to look more deeply into the humanities and social sciences to find these pained yet triumphant voices of experience. Finally, we added our own professional and personal experiences related to the concepts and ideas. Here, we not only shared our own stories and reflections but also drew on the multiple voices of family, friends, colleagues, and acquaintances.
>
> Once these various sources of data were compiled, examined, and analyzed, we created composite characters who helped us tell a story. We attempted to get the characters to engage in a real and critical dialogue about our findings from the interviews, literature, and experiences. This dialogue emerged between the characters much like our own discussions emerged—through sharing, listening, challenging, and reflecting. As the dialogue began to emerge between the characters, we started to insert the various forms of related data from fields such as literature, art, music, theatre, film, social sciences and the law. (pp. 33–34)

The researchers presented their results through a composite story of an untenured professor and a third-year graduate student at a western university, and their dialogue was used to demonstrate the critical concepts and ideas that emerged from this analysis based on CRT.

---

[*]For the original text of this study, see Solórzano and Yosso (2001).

---

quantitative data on the school. She was able to illustrate how Pablo's narrative highlighted the degradation of racist school practices toward Latina/Latino students, as well as ways in which these students resisted those practices. By using CRT as an interpretive tool, Fernandez was able to identify these themes: "race, students, and teacher expectations; vocational training; resisting and/or rejecting school; failing students; and students' lack of awareness about how the educational system operates against them" (p. 50).

Disability Theory as an Analytic Framework

Sullivan (2009) describes the power of using the perspective of people with disabilities as a socio-cultural group as an analytic lens for research with people who have disabilities. At times, the process of data analysis and interpretation can become a transformative experience for the researchers, as illustrated in Freebody and Power's (2001) description of their transformative insights that occurred in their study in which they interviewed deaf adults. When they started the study, they realized that they were portraying the deaf adults as exotic curiosities. As the study progressed, the researchers came to realize that the interviews represented a hearing community's interests, posing questions that turned the interviewee's everyday life into a series of curious, problematic speculations, making the everyday exotic as a way of consolidating the disability interpretation of deafness. Their focus was on deficiency, and its essential feature was the assumption that the salient characteristic of deafness is its restriction on people, rather than potential cultural opportunities, through association with the deaf community and culture. The researchers discovered a rich diversity within the deaf community—and ended up reporting on the many ways in which deafness is meaningful in the lives of deaf or hard-of-hearing people.

QUESTIONS FOR THOUGHT

- Identify research or evaluation studies that use a theoretical framework that is commensurate with the transformative paradigm. How does the use of this theoretical framework influence data analysis and interpretation?

- What tensions are created when a transformative theoretical framework is used at this juncture of the study?

Involving the Community in Analysis and Interpretation

Partnership and Collaboration

As described throughout this text, community involvement is a critical aspect of transformative work. This philosophy is exemplified in the work of the Middle Start Program for children in schools in high poverty areas, funded by the W. K. Kellogg Foundation (WKKF) (Rose, 2006). A holistic approach toward school improvement built a partnership among the children, teachers, school staff, and community to create a safe environment for learning. Collaborative teams reviewed data and derived goals and strategies as next steps. The impact of community participation in the data analysis and derivation of ideas for interventions is illustrated by this quotation from the WKKF website:

> Transforming a school to be more responsive to students' needs requires a culture change in which both teachers and students believe they are valued. In the midst of significant change toward school improvement, the rate of accepting change will vary from teacher to teacher, and differences in approaches and teaching philosophies will come to light. When teachers are involved in decision-making, they develop greater ownership and the partnership necessary to sustain the effort begins to unfold. (March 2, 2006)

Data Analysis and the Medicine Wheel

Cross et al.'s (2000) work in Native American communities using the medicine wheel as a mechanism to enhance cultural appropriateness in data collection was described in Chapter 8. The researchers extended the use of the medicine wheel to the analysis and interpretation of the data as a means to involve community members in that process. They took the notes from their interviews and observations and reformatted them into the four quadrants of the medicine wheel (context, body, mind, and spirit). They then sent their written materials back to the community representatives to review for accuracy and appropriateness. The comments from community members were used to illustrate the findings in each of the four quadrants of the medicine wheel.

Nichols and Keltner's (2005) study of Native American Indian families and their adjustments to their children's disabilities was also discussed in Chapter 8. Their work provides another detailed example of the use of the medicine wheel in the analysis of the data (see Box 9.2).

Analyzing Community Mapping Data

Amsden and VanWynsberghe's (2005) work with youths was also presented in the previous chapter as an example of using community mapping as a data-collection strategy in a study of health services for young people. They discussed the process of analyzing and interpreting the data as a partnership between the youths and members of the advisory committee. Their goal was to provide guidance and support to the youths and encouragement for them to take ownership of the research results. They brought together five members of the advisory committee and five youth volunteers representing the different groups who had created maps. They decided on a process

---

BOX 9.2. Nichols and Keltner's (2005) Medicine Wheel Data Analysis

The 143 interviews were transcribed and entered into the computer for analysis. The interview data were content-analyzed using ethnographic methodology. Ethnographic computer software, The Ethnograph (version 5.0; Seidel, 1998), was used in the analysis to cross-reference and categorize the data. Each piece of interview data was analyzed for the linguistic expression of cultural meaning and then compared to other pieces of interview data. Data were coded to reflect common themes and divided into domains of cultural meaning or taxonomies. The ones with common themes were merged into a central theme (cultural theme), for example, "getting services needed for the child." Cultural themes (taxonomies) about AI family adjustment were identified. Taxonomies such as: getting Social Security Income for the child with disabilities, getting counseling, learning sign language, taking long trips to medical specialists, and transporting the child with disabilities, were merged into a central theme or taxonomy of "getting services needed for the child." The taxonomies were then compared to the conceptual framework for fit. For example, the spirituality of family adjustment was "being aware of the balances in the family." The pattern of passive forbearance was the "indirect responses of accepting the child with disabilities," and some behaviors of promoting harmonious living included "getting services needed" and "altering the home environment." The researchers formulated a definition based on the properties inherent in the taxonomies using the conceptual model. Then, two patterns were formulated to describe how AI families adjust to having a child with a disability. (p. 32)

---

that involved each of the representatives coding the map from their group, a process that began by each person transferring his or her graphics and texts from the maps onto sticky notes. The group representative then sorted the stack of sticky notes into categories. In a second session, four youths and two members of the advisory committee reviewed the categories and found that many consistencies in themes emerged from the independent sorting activity. Examples of the types of categories include (Amsden & VanWynsberghe, 2005, p. 364):

- Accessibility (ease of access), e.g., wheelchair accessible buildings
- Medical practitioners (interactions with doctors), e.g., respect for privacy, nonjudgmental
- Reception (attitudes of reception staff), e.g., don't treat me like a criminal
- General (cultural diversity), e.g., acceptance of all sexualities

The researchers see value in involving the youths in the analysis and interpretation despite certain challenges that arose in the process. The coding process took a longer time and was "messier" with the involvement of the youths because time was used to discuss the meaning of the categories and to fit the images and words into the categories. Although the researchers were puzzled by some of the images and words that the youths put on their maps, the youths were able to provide meaningful interpretations of their concepts. The researchers were pleased with the open coding process and appreciated the inclusiveness that yielded rich results.

QUESTIONS FOR THOUGHT

- Locate research or evaluation studies that involve the community in the data analysis and interpretation. What strategies were used?
- What were the implications of community involvement in terms of logistics and findings?

Qualitative Data

Qualitative data takes the form of words, pictures, videos, documents, and other artifacts. Interviews typically yield transcripts (or some equivalent), observations yield field notes, and the researcher/evaluator might keep a journal. Analysis of these text-based data sources is typically done using either word-based or thematic coding analysis strategies (Jackson & Trochim, 2002).[2] Word-based analysis frequently involves computer programs to count words and co-occurrences of words to establish relationships between them. Thematic-based coding tracks codes or themes that emerge from the data and can also be done using computer program support. In discussing qualitative data analysis, the ugly head of linearity rises once again to present problems. Data analysis in qualitative studies is an ongoing process; it does not start once all the data have been collected. Hesse-Biber and Leavy (2006) provide these general steps in qualitative data analysis:

- Step 1: *Data preparation.* This step includes transcription of data and involves a number of decision points, such as: Will you transcribe all taped interviews or only portions of them? How will you do the transcription—word for word, inclusive of pauses, "you know's," laughter, hand gestures, emotions? Will you do the transcription yourself or hire someone to do it?

• Steps 2 and 3: *Data exploration and data reduction.* As mentioned previously, the qualitative researcher/evaluator begins to read through and analyze data as soon as it is collected, trying to tease out meaning, hypotheses, and personal reactions to the information that is shared. Hence, the researcher/evaluator begins to explore the data and look for codes, which will serve to reduce the data from an overwhelming pile of transcripts and notes into a meaningful depiction of the phenomenon under study.

• Step 4: *Interpretation.* Again, there is overlap in the steps here. Researchers and evaluators begin the interpretation of the data even as they are assigning codes. Often the interpretation phase takes the form of memo writing, as researchers and evaluators compose their thoughts and hypotheses during the earlier phases. Memos can be used to summarize main ideas, highlight particular quotes, formulate possible interpretations, and test out codes and themes. This is where the theoretical framework also explicitly guides the data analysis process in terms of issues to consider.

Limited generalizability is an issue that is often raised with regard to qualitative studies (as in, how can you generalize from two students or eight women or whatever?). This issue was discussed at length in Chapter 6 in relation to case studies and so will not be elaborated upon here. Erikson and Gutierrez (2002) argue that the impact of an experimental treatment cannot be determined by randomized control designs alone. Before investigators can answer the question, "Did it work?", they have to be able to document what "it" is. What treatment was actually delivered? Erickson and Gutierrez suggest that a substantial portion of the budget should be devoted to answering the question "What was the treatment as it was actually delivered?" (p. 21). Qualitative methods are suited to providing details as to the integrity of the treatment, as well as the contextual factors that might influence implementation and outcomes. Erikson and Gutierrez also suggest that qualitative methods are better suited to making causal inferences because they do not reduce complex social phenomenon to one or more numbers that can be statistically analyzed. Rather, a thorough understanding of the implementation of the treatment, contextual variables, and characteristics of the participants can be very powerful in ascertaining causal relationships between interventions and outcomes.

There is also no one right way to conduct qualitative data analysis. However, there are some useful guidelines and theoretical frameworks that are compatible with the transformative paradigm. Several strategies for qualitative data analysis are included in this section.

Grounded Theory

Charmaz (2006) provides a guide to grounded theory (a method of analysis created by Glaser and Strauss in 1967) in a social justice context. Grounded theory can be considered the method of analysis as well as the results of the analysis. As a method, it consists of a set of flexible guidelines for researchers and evaluators to focus their data collection and inductively build theories as they progress through stages of the data analysis and conceptual development. Researchers and evaluators who use grounded theory as an analytic strategy, as with most qualitative analysis strategies, begin data analysis as soon as data are collected and continue throughout the life of the study. Charmaz sees considerable compatibility between the grounded theory strategies and social justice because of the need for a close relationship with the data, to be critically self-reflective, and to provide for reciprocal benefits by increasing understanding as to conditions that support or impede the achievement of social justice.

The following description of a conceptual frame brings social justice together with grounded theory (Charmaz, 2006):

> An interest in social justice means attentiveness to ideas and actions concerning fairness, equity, equality, democratic process, status, hierarchy, and individual and collective rights and obligations. It signifies thinking about being human and about certain good societies and a better world. It prompts reassessment of our roles as national and world citizens. It means exploring tensions between complicity and consciousness, choice and constraint, indifference and compassion, inclusion and exclusion, poverty and privilege, and barriers and opportunities. It also means taking a critical stance toward actions, organizations, and social institutions. Social justice studies require looking at both realities and ideals. (p. 510)

Charmaz (2006) suggests a variety of themes and associated questions to guide data collection and analysis in grounded theory approaches. Resources such as information, control over meanings, and access to networks bring up questions about information and power, such as:

> What are the resources in the empirical world we study?
>
> Who controls the resources? Who needs them? Who determines who needs them and with what criteria is that determination made?
>
> To what extent do varied capabilities enter the discussion? (p. 513)

A second theme focuses on the nature and evolution of hierarchies that are present in social entities, raising such questions as:

Which purported and actual purposes do these hierarchies serve? Who benefits from them? Under what conditions?

How are the hierarchies related to power and oppression? How, if at all, do definitions of race, class, gender, and age cluster in specific hierarchies and/or at particular hierarchical levels? (pp. 513–514)

A third theme is associated with the social policies and practices that are part of the individual and community life under study. Charmaz (2005) proposes the following questions:

What are the rules—both tacit and explicit? Who writes or enforces them? How? Whose interests do the rules reflect? From whose standpoint?

Do the rules and routine practices negatively affect certain groups or categories of individuals? If so, are they aware of them? What are the implications of their relative awareness or lack of it?

To what extent and when do various participants support the rules and policies and practices that flow from them? When are they contested? When do they meet resistance? Who resists, and which risks might resistance pose? (p. 514)

Charmaz (2005) suggests that researchers begin by studying their data and asking:

- "What is happening? What are people doing?" (p. 514).

- "Look at each person's story and ask: What do these stories indicate? What might they suggest about social justice?" (p. 517).

- "How do grounded theory methods facilitate making sense of them?" (p. 517).

As in other qualitative analysis strategies, the grounded theorist starts with coding the data: "Grounded theory is a comparative method in which the researcher compares data with data, data with categories, and category with category" (Charmaz, 2005, p. 517). Such a constant comparison of different levels of data and emerging themes leads to an identification of similarities and differences among participants and the structures and processes that either support or impede their access to services or programs. Inductions from the data can lead to the development of theoretical structures that permit insights into the complexity of experiences. Charmaz (2006) elaborates on the uses of grounded theory as an analytic technique and a method of building theory that addresses issues of social justice in her book *Constructing Grounded Theory: A Practical Guide through Qualitative Analysis.*

Discourse Analysis

Huygens (2002) describes the process of discourse analysis as reading with an open mind and asking such questions as: "What are [participants] actually saying?", "Why did they choose to say it this way?", and "Has someone else said this?" Thus, the data analyst tries to read between the lines, taking into account images, colloquialisms, and uses of words and phrases, while looking for regularity and variation in the themes that emerge.

Christians (2005) proposes that interpretive discourse is authentically sufficient when the description is thick enough to allow the cultural complexity to be grasped by the reader and for the reader to form a critical consciousness. Using the feminist communitarian theoretical framework, he derived three conditions that would demonstrate the attainment of sufficient interpretive discourse: "[Interpretive discourse] represents multiple voices, enhances moral discernment, and promotes social transformation" (p. 152). This interpretive sufficiency forms the basis for ethics, whereby researchers and evaluators act from an authentic resonance with the context and the community members realize that they are moral agents. The outcomes of this approach to data analysis would be manifest in social criticism, political resistance, and social action on the part of those who are experiencing discrimination. In keeping with Habermas (1981, as cited in Christians, 2005, p. 155) and Freire (1970a, 1970b, 1973), transformation is possible when the oppressed become active participants rather than remaining a leader's objects of action. Through the development of critical consciousness, the oppressed gain their own voices and collaborate in transforming their culture.

Transformative Research and Evaluation as a Catalyst for Critical Consciousness

Clarke and McCreanor (2006) share their process of discourse analysis from a study of Maori responses to the grieving process when the medical examiner determines that their children died from sudden infant death syndrome (SIDS). They reiterate the need to do multiple and detailed readings of the data to develop a systematic and comprehensive description of the patterns and variations in the talk on a topic, focusing on the use of language. They note challenges associated with "objectivity" in that selection and interpretation of the data are made by the researcher and depend on his or her sensitivity and experience. They suggest that readers can make judgments for themselves on the rigor of the analysis based on the appropriateness of the results that emerge. Here is an example of their discourse analysis conducted with each of their informant groups after the researchers coded the transcripts using the emerging themes:

> The dataset under each theme were then subjected to multiple readings as a basis for developing descriptions of the general features of each. While the study identified a number of themes within the talk of participants, for the purposes of this paper, we have selected three of these themes in order to illustrate the impacts and implications of processes and practices upon grieving. These themes—police actions, post-mortem, and coroner's findings— are chosen for their likely impact on the grief processes discussed above and because each in its own way represents a modifiable influence on grieving. (pp. 31–32)

Clarke and McCreanor's goal was to provide recommendations to the professional careworkers of the national Maori SIDS prevention team.

Focus Groups and PAR

Chiu's (2003) use of focus groups as a means of data collection on the experiences of minority women and their participation in health services was described in Chapter 8. She also adds to the discussion of group involvement based on the PAR approach to the analysis and interpretation of the data. She notes that "PAR participants are often involved in data analysis to generate solutions for change actions. This involves, as good practice, the process of returning the focus group transcripts for rectification. Aided by the researcher's theoretical understanding (propositional knowing), participants are then involved in collective reflection on issues identified" (p. 179). In this instance, the researcher provided theoretical grounding in gender, sexuality, and culture. The health professionals were then able to critically reflect on their own narratives and begin to recognize their attitudes and prejudices, which serve to perpetuate problems of access to cervical screening for the women who participate in the program. As part of this analytic process, the professionals were able to suggest changes in their practice and commit themselves to critical learning. Chui attributes the success of this approach to allowing participants an opportunity to hear their own voices in a nonthreatening way by returning to the transcripts rather than challenging them in a confrontational way about their prejudice. The professionals were able to view the transcript as a collective product owned by the group and not the property of the researcher. They used the content of the focus group analysis as a basis for the development of workshops to raise critical awareness. She concludes: "It is doubtful that focus groups can become a transformational tool in the context of the more prescribed object-and-subject research relationships commonly found in conventional settings" (p. 180).

Whose Voice Is Included?

The inclusion of diverse voices, particularly the voices of people who have been pushed to the margins, is a core issue for transformative research and evaluation. In many ways, this is the topic that has dominated the discourse throughout this book. It is important to remember that not all voices are yet represented accurately—or at all—in scholarly literature. Jimerson and Oware (2006) raise questions about the dynamics of having people in the community speak for others who do not speak for themselves. Are deviants included in those who are quoted in books about deviance? Are black men included in books about whites who fear black men? Many "mainstream works on black masculinity exclude black male voices, especially those of working-class or lower-class black men. . . . A dominant theme in research about black masculinity has been to vilify, demonize, and characterize black males as dysfunctional and pathological" (Ross, 1998, as cited in Jimerson & Oware, 2006, p. 30). They conclude that the missing voice of the African American male leads us to be skeptical about who talks and what words are said by them and less skeptical about those who are talked about.

Madison (2005) suggests the following questions as a guide to analysis in a critical ethnography:

- How do we reflect upon and evaluate our own purpose, intentions, and frames of analysis as researchers and evaluators?

- How do we predict consequences or evaluate our own potential to do harm?

- How do we create and maintain a dialogue of collaboration in our projects between ourselves and others?

- How is the specificity of the local story relevant to the broader meanings and operations of the human condition?

- How—in what location or through what intervention—will our work make the greatest contribution to equity, freedom, and justice? (p. 4)

Picking up the theme of self-reflection that was addressed in Chapter 3, reflexive ethnographers ask themselves these questions:

- What are we going to do with the findings and who ultimately will benefit?
- Who gives us the authority to make claims about where we have been?
- How will our work make a difference in people's lives? What difference does it make when the ethnographer himself comes from a history of colonization and disenfranchisement? (Madison, 2005, p. 7)

QUESTIONS FOR THOUGHT

- Locate a study that includes qualitative data analysis and interpretation.
- How do the authors explain their method of data analysis?
- How do they substantiate the interpretations of the data?
- What evidence of a transformative lens is present in this section of the study report?

Quantitative Analysis

Statistical analyses are procedures that reduce many single pieces of numerical data into a form that permits a different picture to emerge— either a summary of the numbers in terms of central tendency or variation, a relationship between two or more sets of numbers, or a comparison of number sets to determine the significance of differences between or among the number sets. Definitions of common statistical terms can be found in many research and evaluation methods books, statistics textbooks, and on a variety of websites. In the transformative paradigm and more generally in the research world, it is insufficient to know how to calculate statistics with quantitative data. Transformative researchers and evaluators who use statistics raise issues related to the potential harm that can be associated with uncritically accepting results that statistical analysis show to be "statistically significant" or that rely on average scores without serious consideration of subgroup performance based on relevant dimensions of diversity.

The *Publication Manual of the American Psychological Association* serves as a guide for thousands of journals (American Psychological Association, 2001). The fifth edition echoed concerns about the way in which statistics have been calculated and reported. To address concerns about the misuse of null hypothesis testing, American Psychological Association recommended the following statistical procedures (American Psychological Association, 2001; Fidler, 2002):

1. Graphical displays of data
2. Use of descriptive statistics
3. Use of power analysis prior to data collection
4. Reporting of effect sizes
5. Reporting of confidence intervals

In keeping with the transformative spirit, the following sections describe the meaning of statistical significance, concerns about null hypothesis testing, the meaning and strategies for calculating power analysis, confidence intervals, and effect sizes—with the intent to challenge uncritical acceptance of quantitative data-analysis results. This discussion is followed by a consideration of choices of statistical techniques such as social network analysis and multilevel structural equation modeling.

Statistical Significance

In research and evaluation reports, it is very common to see results presented as being statistically significant or not statistically significant. This indication of significance or its absence is usually presented in the form of either a table, with asterisks indicating which results were significant and at what probability level (p-level); or as a parenthetical comment in the text of the report, with the name of the statistical test, the degrees of freedom, and the p-level. For example, parents who were hearing and deaf and had a child who was deaf were asked to rate their satisfaction with the early childhood services they had received (Meadow-Orlans et al., 2003). The program evaluation scores by mothers' hearing status indicated that hearing mothers' level of satisfaction was more positive than that of deaf mothers ($t(402)$, -2.73, $p = .01$). The interpretation of this is that a t-test for independent means (because the two groups of mothers did not overlap in membership) was conducted with 404 pieces of information (survey responses from the parents). Using two groups in the analysis reduces the number of independent pieces of information by 2, hence the degrees of freedom is presented as 402. The *t*-value is the statistical calculation that allows the data analyst (or the computer, as it may be) to determine if the difference between two means exceeds that expected by chance. The *p*-value of .01 associated with the *t*-test of the mothers' means indicates the probability that the difference between the hearing and deaf mothers would occur by chance with only .01 probability (or to put it another way, if the study were conducted 100 times, we would expect to see statistically significant results of this nature 99 times out of 100).

Because statistical significance is so pervasive an indicator and also controversial, I present this definition of the concept from an online statistics textbook:

> The statistical significance of a result is an estimated measure of the degree to which it is "true" (in the sense of "representative of the population"). More technically, the value of the *p-level* represents a decreasing index of the reliability of a result. The higher the *p-level*, the less we can believe that the observed relation between variables in the sample is a reliable indicator of the relation between the respective variables in the population. Specifically, the *p*-level represents the probability of error that is involved in accepting our observed result as valid, that is, as "representative of the population." For example, the *p-level* of .05 (i.e., 1/20) indicates that there is a 5% probability that the relation between the variables found in our sample is a "fluke." In other words, assuming that in the population there was no relation between those variables whatsoever, and we were repeating experiments like ours one after another, we could expect that approximately in every 20 replications of the experiment there would be one in which the relation between the variables in question would be equal or stronger than in ours. In many areas of research, the *p-level* of .05 is customarily treated as a "border-line acceptable" error level. (Retrieved September 11, 2006, from *www.statsoft.com/textbook/stathome*)

Problems with Null Hypothesis Statistical Tests

Why, then, are null hypothesis statistical tests (NHSTs) and statistical significance so controversial? Null hypothesis testing relies on particular assumptions about the size of the sample, the underlying characteristics of the population, and the accuracy with which the sample represents the population (Henson, 2006). Despite the robust nature (meaning, some of the assumptions can be violated and still yield valid results), the results of NHST can be misleading for a variety of reasons. An example of how a NHST can lead to false conclusions is presented in Box 9.3.

BOX 9.3. False Conclusions, p, and Sample Size

Henson (2006) provides a hypothetical example of a psychologist who is studying the effects of a certain cognitive treatment of depression. The psychologist randomly assigns clients with the same diagnosis to a treatment group ($n = 8$) or a wait-list control group ($n = 8$). The results on a depression measure, where a high score indicates more depression, were an average of 62 for the treatment group and 64 for the wait-list group. The researcher had hypothesized that the treatment group would show a reduction in symptoms, and so a one-way independent t-test was used. It revealed $t(14) = -1.752$, $p = .051$.

The rigid researcher would conclude that the treatment was not effective because it did not exceed the .05 alpha level set for statistical significance. The less rigid researcher might say that the results approached significance. Thompson (1992) has reminded researchers for many years that data cannot *approach* or *avoid* significance. If the study was conducted again, the p-value might be smaller or larger.

If the psychologist had added just one more client to each group and the means and standard deviations stayed the same, the results would have been statistically significant at the $p = .049$ level. Would the researcher then be justified in claiming that there was a statistically significant difference between the two groups, and then recommending this treatment as an effective way to reduce depression?

As Henson (2006) notes, the p-value from a NHST does not provide information about the practical significance of the group differences. Very small group differences can be statistically significant with a big enough sample size. Researchers and evaluators need to ask additional questions concerning the practical significance of the differences. One avenue for doing this is to look at effect sizes (discussed after the following section).

Statistical Power

Researchers and evaluators want to know how big of a sample is needed in order to make a correct decision (i.e., reject a null hypothesis when it is indeed false, or accept a null hypothesis when it is indeed true). As mentioned in Chapter 6, limiting the number of individuals in a study to the number needed to obtain an accurate estimate of effect also limits the number of people placed at potential risk. Statistical power analysis provides a way for the researcher or evaluator to calculate the sample size needed to make a correct decision. A statistical hypothesis test measures the test's ability (power) to reject the null hypothesis when it is actually false—that is, to make a correct decision more precisely:

Performing power analysis and sample size estimation is an important aspect of experimental design, because without these calculations, sample size may be too high or too low. If sample size is too low, the experiment will lack the precision to provide reliable answers to the questions it is investigating. If sample size is too large, time and resources will be wasted, often for minimal gain. (*Electronic Statistics Textbook*, 2006)

Effect Sizes

The calculation of effect size is seen as one potentially useful strategy for addressing questions about the practical importance of group differences. The general strategy for calculation is fairly straightforward: "The effect size is the experimental mean minus the control mean divided by the control group's standard deviation" (Slavin & Cheung, 2003, pp. 8–9). The fifth edition of the American Psychological Association's (2001) *Publication Manual* recommends reporting effect sizes:

> For the reader to fully understand the importance of your findings, it is almost always necessary to include some index of effect size or strength of relationship in your Results section. . . . The general principle to be followed . . . is to provide the reader not only with information about statistical significance but also with enough information to assess the magnitude of the observed effect or relationship. (pp. 25–26).

As Henson (2006) notes, there are always caveats that need mentioning when effect sizes are calculated and reported. First, the statistical strategy used to determine the effect size index needs to be made clear (e.g., standardized mean differences such as Cohen's *d* or Glass's delta, or measures of association [variance-accounted-for measures] such as R^2 for nongrouped data). Henson recommends Kline's (2004) book *Beyond Significance Testing* as a resource for such approaches to data analysis. The data analyst should also be clear about the data features that affect the statistic. Kline provides the following example:

> Reporting a mean difference effect of .30 simply does not give the reader enough information. The researcher must define this effect (e.g., Cohen's *d*, Glass's delta, etc.), maybe explain it (e.g., "divides by the control group *SD*"), and definitely interpret it within the context of the study (e.g., "The .30 effect indicates almost a one-third *SD* improvement for the treatment group, which is consistent with the average effect observed in prior related literature"). (p. 610)

Confidence Intervals

In statistical language, a confidence interval gives an estimated range of values that is likely to include an unknown population parameter, the estimated range being calculated from a given set of sample data (Easton & McColl, 2006).

In practical terms, the confidence interval is often reported in political polling as the percentage of people who favor one candidate over another, with a confidence interval around that percentage. For example: 80% of the American people are opposed to the incumbent candidate in the upcoming election, at a 90% confidence level, means that the real percentage of people who are opposed to the incumbent is thought to be between 75% and 85%. If the percentage of people who favor or oppose candidates is very close and the confidence intervals are overlapping for the two percentages, then it is usually a race that is termed "too close to call."

The width of the confidence interval gives an idea of how confident we are about the data. A very wide interval may mean that we should collect more data in order to be more precise about our conclusions. Confidence intervals can be calculated for different levels (e.g., 95%, 99%), just as p-values can be calculated from hypothesis testing. However, statisticians feel that confidence intervals are more informative than NHST because they provide a range of possible values for the variables of interest.

The American Psychological Association (2001) also recommends an increased use of confidence intervals. Henson (2006) suggests that confidence intervals be used for effect sizes as well. Thompson (2002) provides guidance on the calculation of confidence intervals around effect sizes.

Statistical Concepts and How They Come Together

Statistics such as t-tests and analysis of variance (ANOVA) are used to test for group differences. Correlational statistics are used to test for strength and direction of relationships in data sets. Because variables that represent group characteristics (e.g., gender or race/ethnicity) can be entered into statistical tests by presenting them as categorical data, in essence, the calculation of statistics can be viewed as a set of Venn diagrams in which there is considerable overlap in the choices of statistics that can be used. Given the robust nature of regression analysis in its many forms, I discuss how it can be used to bring focus to results in highly complex situations.

Balfanz, Legters, and Jordan (2004) investigated the effectiveness of an instructional program designed to bring students up to grade level whose academic achievement is below grade level when they enter high school. They examined the effects of the talent development high school's (TDHS) program on the reading and mathematics performance in ninth-grade classes from several cities in high-poverty areas. The "treatment" included 90 minutes a day of mathematics and reading—courses designed to teach strategies to approach reading and transition to advanced mathematics, and all ninth graders attended classes in a separate part of the building, called the Ninth-Grade Success Academy. Balfanz et al. used regression analysis to examine the impact of the TDHS intervention three times during the study: from eighth grade to February of ninth grade, from eighth grade to May of ninth grade, and from February to May of ninth grade. Their results indicated that "students in the experimental school significantly outperformed students in the control schools, in terms of both overall level of achievement obtained in achievement gains. This remained true when a number of control variables were entered into the equation" (p. 11). The control variables included gender, student age, ninth-grade attendance, and prior achievement. The only result that was not significant was between eighth grade and February. The researchers hypothesize that this finding might indicate the need for a lengthy intervention in order to see a turnaround in achievement. They also address the practical importance of the student changes: "The achievement impacts of the TDHS ninth grade instructional program were educationally substantive. The effect size for the eighth grade to May gain was .128 for reading and .18 for math" (p. 13). This change was enough to bring the students up to grade level.

Specific Quantitative Statistical Methods

Advances in quantitative statistical methods allow for a more refined examination of the influence of multiple variables and the importance of acknowledging the complexity of social situations. Two of these strategies are discussed in this section: social network analysis and structural equation modeling.

Social Network Analysis

Fredericks and Durland (2005) characterize social network analysis (SNA) as being focused on relationships, not categories or attributes, and on the pattern of those relationships. The structure of the patterned relationships can be partitioned into subgroups, and the researcher can focus on the limits and opportunities of that structure. Computer procedures can be used such as those that incorporate algorithms or more traditional data-analysis procedures such as factor analysis and multidimensional scaling. However, in SNA, "the differences are in the purpose of the analysis, the conceptualization of the data, and the incorporation of the results of the analysis" (p. 19). They identified the following concepts to consider in the analysis of social networks when investigating the complete network (Fredericks & Durland, 2005, p. 18):

- *Dyad:* Two actors who have a connection, a relationship
- *Clique:* A subset of actors within a network who have ties with all other actors within that subset
- *Density:* The proportion of the total available ties connecting actors
- *Centralization:* The fraction of main actors within a network
- *Reachability:* The number of ties connecting actors
- *Connectedness:* The ability of actors to reach one another reciprocally, that is, the ability to choose a relationship between both parties
- *Asymmetry:* The ratio of reciprocal relationships—those relationships that are mutual—to total relationships within a network
- *Balance:* The extent to which ties in the network are direct and reciprocated.

These concepts are analyzed through the use of algorithms (an equation that yields the relationship between components or structural elements [e.g., dyads or cliques]). For individual-level analysis, these are the important concepts (Fredericks & Durand, 2005, pp. 18–19):

- *Centrality:* The degree to which an actor is in a central role in the network
- *Homophily:* The degree to which similar actors in similar roles share information
- *Isolate:* An actor with no ties to other actors
- *Gatekeeper:* An actor who connects the network to outside influences
- *Cutpoint:* An actor whose removal results in unconnected paths in the network.

Structural Equation Modeling

Wenglinsky (2002) conducted a study of variables that influence academic success, using independent variables that were identified through previous qualitative research. The researcher was concerned about the results because ordinary least-squares regression analysis of datasets in the past had not established a link between quality of schooling (measured in terms of expenditure per pupil) and achievement. He felt that prior research had relied on somewhat simplistic factors that affect school outcomes. He identified three problems with using ordinary least-squares regression analysis:

1. The level of the data available by school and student is sometimes confounded in these studies, such that student data will be aggregated to a school level, or school-level data will be disaggregated to allow analysis at the student level.
2. Regression techniques do not take measurement error in the variables into account.
3. Regression analysis is not suited to measuring interrelationships of independent variables.

Wenglinsky (2002) suggests a two-step process to address these concerns. First, make the set of variables more inclusive by examining those that have been produced in qualitative studies of academic achievement. Thus, such classroom elements as the teacher's college major, professional development in higher-order thinking skills, professional development in diversity, hands-on learning, and higher-order thinking skills required of students are recognized as potentially important predictors of achievement. Second, he recommends using multilevel structural equation modeling (Hayduk, 1987; Jöreskog & Sörbom, 1993). This, in turn, involves generating *factor models* and *path models*. Muthén (1994) notes:

> The factor models relate a series of indicators, known as manifest variables, to a construct of those indicators, known as a latent variable. The path models then relate the latent variables to one another. The estimation procedure for both the factor and path components involves three steps. A set of hypothesized relationships is specified by the researcher. Then, through an iterative process, differences in the covariance matrix those relationships imply $(\Sigma)^3$ and the covariance matrix of observed data (S) are minimized. The resulting estimates include coefficients for the hypothesized relationships, t-tests for their statistical significance, and statistics for the goodness of fit between Σ

and S. SEM can be adapted to handle multilevel data by employing the estimation procedure separately for the two levels of analysis (see also Muthén, 1994, as cited in Wenglinsky, 2002).

Wenglinsky (2002) produced three mean square error methods (MSEMs). The first MSEM relates teacher inputs to student academic performance, taking into account student SES and class size. The second MSEM relates professional development and teacher inputs to student academic performance and one another, taking into account student SES and class size. The third MSEM relates classroom practices, professional development, and teacher inputs to student academic performance and one another, taking into account SES and class size. In schools where teachers received professional development in dealing with different student populations, students are less likely to engage in routine problem solving. And in schools where teachers received professional development in higher-order thinking skills, students are more likely to engage in hands-on learning. Also, the more time teachers engage in professional development, the more their students engage in hands-on learning and authentic assessment. These practices are associated with student achievement. Schools where students engage in hands-on learning score higher on the mathematics assessment. Schools where students solve unique problems also score higher, as do those schools that do not rely primarily on authentic forms of assessment.

Thus, using these three MSEMs, the path models help to gauge the impact of teaching on student achievement as having an overall effect size of .56. The researchers were then able to conclude that the various aspects of teacher quality are related to student achievement when class size and SES are taken into account. In particular, the following five variables are positively associated with achievement:

- Teacher major
- Teacher receives professional development in higher-order thinking skills
- Professional development in diversity
- Hands-on learning
- Teacher's ability to use higher-order thinking skills

The researchers interpreted their results by looking at the effect sizes for each of the topics and reflecting on their knowledge gained from prior qualitative and quantitative studies. They concluded that their models support the hypothesis that aspects of teacher quality and classroom practices will have the greatest effect on student performance.

QUESTIONS FOR THOUGHT

- Locate a study that includes quantitative data analysis. What specific statistical tests were used?
- To what extent do the authors address the complex issues associated with using statistics in terms of such concepts as statistical significance?
- What evidence do you see that they have attended to the American Psychological Association's recommendations with regard to
  - Graphical displays of data?
  - Use of descriptive statistics?
  - Use of power analysis prior to data collection?
  - Reporting of effect sizes?
  - Reporting of confidence intervals?
- What evidence is there that the researchers or evaluators considered the implications of the transformative paradigm in their data analysis and interpretation?

Integrating Qualitative and Quantitative Results

This topic is addressed more extensively in the next chapter in terms of reporting results. However, for now let's consider Greene, Caracelli, and Graham's (1989) five justifications for combining qualitative and quantitative results that are useful in regard to data analysis and interpretation in studies that use mixed methods:

1. *Triangulation:* Seeks convergence, corroboration, or correspondence of results from different methods.
2. *Complementarity:* Seeks elaboration, enhancement, illustration, or clarification of the results from one method with the results of another method.
3. *Development:* Seeks to use the results from one method to help develop or inform the other method, where development may include sampling, implementation, and/or measurement decisions. (This concept was discussed in Chapter 4 as the sequential design for mixed methods.)

4. *Initiation:* Seeks the discovery of paradox, contradiction, new perspectives of frameworks, and the recasting of questions or results from one method with questions or results from the other method.

5. *Expansion:* Seeks to extend the breadth and range of inquiry by using different methods for different inquiry components.

Niglas (2004) conducted an empirical study of how social science researchers integrate the results of quantitative and qualitative research, based on Greene et al.'s (1989) schema. Niglas reported that almost half of the articles reviewed were reflective of the complementarity category. The second most common strategy for combining qualitative and quantitative results was expansion, suggesting that researchers are trying to understand more facets of the prism through the use of mixed methods. She reported that the level of integration of quantitative and qualitative aspects remains relatively modest in most of the studies, especially at the stage of data analysis. More integration appears at the stage of interpretation. Very few researchers provide an explicit rationale for the use of mixed methods.

QUESTIONS FOR THOUGHT

- Locate a study that includes both quantitative and qualitative data. How do the authors combine the two types of data?

- How does the use of both types of data enhance the interpretations that are possible in this study?

- What evidence is there that the study is responsive to the principles of the transformative paradigm?

Summary

✓ Theoretical frameworks that are compatible with the transformative paradigm guide data analysis and interpretation, including postcolonial theory, Marxist theory, feminist theories, queer theory, and CRT (African American and Latino).

✓ Indigenous communities provide examples of ways to involve community members in the analysis and interpretation of data (e.g., Native American communities use the medicine wheel to vet research and evaluation findings for accuracy and appropriateness).

✓ Youths were involved in coding data, along with other community members, when analyzing data from a study of health services that used community mapping as a data-collection technique.

✓ Qualitative data analysis involves decisions about data transcription, reduction, and interpretation. These decisions can be made with guidance from such strategies as grounded theory when combined with a consciousness of social justice implications. Such an analysis includes critical reflection on such topics as available resources, control of resources, and access to power.

✓ Discourse analysis offers another data-analysis and interpretation strategy that can be used for transformative purposes.

✓ Text or visual images are read and analyzed to bring to the surface themes related to social criticism, political resistance, and social action.

✓ Participatory action researchers use community involvement to derive recommendations for action based on findings reviewed by the participants.

✓ The power dynamics associated with who speaks for whom are discussed in terms of who has access to analysis and interpretation of data.

✓ Self-reflexivity continues to be a critical part of the research and evaluation process in terms of use of the data and who benefits from such use.

✓ Quantitative data analysis is critically examined in terms of use and misuse of statistics such as statistical significance and null hypothesis testing.

✓ Remediation strategies were presented, based on recommendations from the American Psychological Association (2001), including graphic displays of data, use of descriptive statistics, use of power analysis, reporting of effect sizes, and reporting of confidence intervals. In addition, more complex statistical strategies can be used to control for sources of variance when they are warranted.

✓ Mixing quantitative and qualitative data in the analysis and interpretation phase includes such strategies as seeking convergence, identifying areas of divergence, adding clarity, raising additional questions, and expanding the breadth of the inquiry.

MOVING ON TO CHAPTER 10 . . .

Reporting results of research and evaluation studies can be done in a variety of ways. Some of the choices are associated with a higher probability that the results will be used to enhance social justice.

What do you understand if I tell you that white light is refracted at an angle between 33.39 and 33.91 degrees when it moves through glass and between 39.04 and 39.50 degrees when it moves through water (Molecular Expressions, 2007)? What do you understand when I tell you that a rainbow makes me smile, or that the bright colors from the prism in my window remind me of someone who is very important to me and who is no longer with us?

Notes

1. Dillard (2000a) used the word *endarkened* in her discussion of feminist episte-mology to reflect reality as it is rooted in black feminist thought.
2. Jackson and Trochim (2002) propose the use of concept mapping as an analytic strategy for text that takes a more concise form, such as responses to open-ended questions on a survey. The concept mapping methodology involves the respondents or their proxies in the coding process and yields a data structure through the use of multidimensional scaling and cluster analysis of the aggre-gated individual coding data. The result is a visual map of thematic clusters. (See Chapter 8 on data collection for more specifics.)
3. Σ is a statistical symbol used for the covariance matrix implied by the research-er's hypothesized relationships.

CHAPTER 10

Reporting and Utilization

Pathway to the Future

> As evaluators, we must understand how this point is important to evaluation. . . . Evaluation results ought to serve to some extent social justice functions, [and] we must be clear that if our results are culturally inappropriate, we are at risk of perpetuating or creating stereotypes of under-represented or socially oppressed groups.
>
> —GUZMAN (2003, p. 179)

> The participants gave the title, "Welcome to the Real World" to the report of their work, a title they chose because it expresses what life in poverty and on social assistance is like and it expresses the view that for someone else to understand that life, they would need to live it themselves. . . . The findings were initially summarized by the researcher and then reviewed by the women in the group who made changes and additions and decided on the title for the report.
>
> —COLLINS (2005, p. 16)

IN THIS CHAPTER . . .

▼ Options for reporting are discussed and illustrated. The value of sharing information throughout the course of the research or evaluation study is emphasized to facilitate midcourse corrections if an intervention is not moving toward the desired goal.

▼ Planning for utilization is essential during the initial design of the study; the topic of the study must be presented to participants in order to ensure that the data are gathered and disseminated in a way that they can be used to achieve the goals of social change and social justice.

▼ Policy analysis and advocacy are explained as avenues to social change from the perspective of grass-roots organizations.

▼ Closing commentary focuses on the value of putting research and evaluation side by side and integrating their pathways in the pursuit of social justice.

A simplistic explanation of reporting and utilization might look like this:

> "Plan a report that provides details of all the activities undertaken as part of the study, including:
>
>   • An introduction to the issues addressed in the study and its purpose(s). Include the questions that were answered.
>   • The strategies (interventions) used to try to achieve the desired outcomes.
>   • The methods and instruments used to collect and analyze the data.
>   • A section of the results, using both quantitative and qualitative data.
>   • A discussion of the meaning of the results and thoughts about lessons learned and/or future needs for interventions and/or additional studies.
>
> "Present the report in a format that is appropriate to the topic and the community."

The actual process of reporting and utilization is much more complex than that depicted in this brief description. Transformative researchers and evaluators address general issues related to inclusion and power, decisions about reporting timing and format, and critical analysis of dissemination and utilization strategies.

Issues of Inclusion and Power

Reporting for Whom?

In a discussion of the intended consumer of research, Lincoln (2005) asks the question, knowledge for whom? She suggests that the research dictates of the current legislative climate in the United States put greater importance on writing for producers of the knowledge (i.e., academics and scientists) than for participants in the community. Yet, local-level agencies and organizations are increasingly interested in gaining access to information and interpretations regarding their own communities and possibilities for action. According to Lincoln (2005):

> As communities acquire systematic information about themselves, they are empowered to participate in designing their own futures and to take action

where it is meaningful: Locally. If the assumption, however, is that scientific (or other systematic) social knowledge belongs to the knowledge-production community alone, then social action is curtailed in favor of official action. Democratic participation in social change, especially social change on behalf of social justice, is impaired or discouraged altogether. (p. 174)

Student Perspective: Need to Balance Reports for Producers and Communities

Is research done for the academic community or for participant communities or both? Mostly qualitative research on college/university campuses is done for academic purposes. Sometimes the research is done for the participant communities when it benefits the community to change or improve the communities themselves. I believe that the research is done for the academic community as a whole—like with Gallaudet University. The research conducted here is to "see what the deaf community is all about" or "what could we do to improve" for the sake of academics. I am not sure how much is done for or with the participant communities—maybe in several research studies, participants benefit from the research. Hmmm.—Heidi Holmes (March 4, 2006)

Student Perspective: Academic Control of Knowledge

Knowledge for the producers. In schools, academic discourse is usually encouraged, cultivated, and expanded—with white (male) students from comfortable SES. Specific academic knowledge is shared and specific skills such as vocational and homemaking skills are taught to Hispanics, African Americans, and disabled people to keep the working class large enough to serve the needs of the white-collar producers. It is our job to look for best practices in all areas of schooling, the workforce, and the research industry—which means opening up access to "knowledge" to all students, regardless of ethnicity, sex, and SES, so that they may choose to do what they want to do.

At a residential school for the deaf, we had a very oppressive white hearing woman who was responsible for "career development." She couldn't sign very well, and she had this huge lab of different "skills" such as cleaning a toilet, making jewelry, computer programming, working with tools, basket making, and so on. Students would be pulled out of class to go through all the skills (they had instructions attached) and the results would be evaluated and the career would be assigned to the student: "You're good with jewelry, so you will be making jewelry." With totally no input from the student! I remember one Hispanic deaf girl came into my class crying that she couldn't be a lawyer because that lab said she should be a computer programmer. How awful is this? And this happens everywhere, everyday—with school tracking, especially. Often, students are divided up in three tracks—college, career, and community track. The college track is usually reserved for the book-smart ones who usually were white or light skinned, career track for Native Americans and Hispanics, and the community track for those with multiple disabilities. I have so many stories to tell about "tracking" and how it really discriminates—and sets up the students for failure. They won't allow access to ACADEMIC KNOWLEDGE. It all starts before kindergarten. For ethical research, we should always aim for creating spaces for counter-hegemonic discourse as well as making sure the research is accessible to people without access, for example, writing in their preferred discourse (if research is about teaching, then write in teacher discourse, if research is about HIV/AIDS, then write in community discourse, if research is about ASL, then "write" in ASL).—Raychelle Harris (February 26, 2006)

Transformative researchers and evaluators need to be aware of the audience for whom the study findings have implications. Reporting can take a variety of forms, and the choice of presentation has implications for the furtherance of social justice.

A sample of the interpretation and conclusions of a study of bilingual reading instruction is presented in Box 10.1. The data are analyzed using a meta-analytic strategy that combines results from a number of different experimental studies. The researchers (Slavin & Cheung, 2003) focused on high-quality quantitative studies to reach a conclusion that bilingual education appears to be effective when it pairs the native language with English.

BOX 10.1. Interpretation and Conclusion for Meta-Analysis of Reading Strategies

This report reviews experimental studies of reading for English language learners, focusing both on comparisons of bilingual and English-only programs and on specific, replicable models that have been evaluated with English language learners. The review method is best-evidence synthesis, which uses a systematic literature search, quantification of outcomes as effect sizes, and extensive discussion of individual studies that meet inclusion standards. The review concludes that while the number of high-quality studies is small, existing evidence favors bilingual approaches, especially paired bilingual strategies that teach reading in the native language and English at the same time. Whether taught in their native language or English, English language learners have been found to benefit from instruction in comprehensive reform programs using systematic phonics, one-to-one or small group tutoring programs, cooperative learning programs, and programs emphasizing extensive reading. Research using longitudinal, randomized designs is needed to understand how best to ensure reading success for all English language learners.

From Slavin and Cheung (2003, p. v).

They also concluded that additional research is necessary to further the goal of successful reading for all students in U.S. schools.

Inclusion of Voices with "Bad Language"

Barker and Weller (2003) note that complex issues around the dissemination of results are commonly overlooked in the research literature. Dissemination is usually the responsibility of adults, even when the research is focused on children. Hence, when children feel very strongly about a situation and express their feelings in what might be considered "bad language," the researcher is faced with a decision regarding whether or not to report the exact words that the children used. These researchers struggled with a crisis of representation in that they worried that if the children's bad language was perceived as being offensive to the people in power, then they might dismiss the findings. "Thus, accurately portraying the graphic views of some children may well place the researcher in a position of conflict of interests. There is a conflict between representing the views of some children and maintaining relationships with other significant adults such as parents or teachers" (p. 221). The researchers chose not to include the bad language during their reporting to the local authorities; however, they did include it in the article in which they discuss their dilemma.

Shared Authorship

Miskovic and Hoop (2006) worked with two participatory research action projects in Chicago that were designed to empower youths to become active researchers and to design a project that addressed social inequities in their schools and neighborhoods. At the completion of the projects, the question arose as to who was responsible for writing the research reports. In the end, the university center's staff members were named as the sole authors because:

> It seemed that this role was expected and welcomed by the community partners, because the writing phase may be seen as less "active," more analytical and, therefore, less interesting. The underlying message from the community partners was "After all, you are trained to write, and we'll gladly let you do it." The question, then is, what should be the research product and who owns it? (p. 284)

Greenwood, Brydon-Miller, and Shafer (2006) discuss the challenges in decisions about authorship of reports resulting from research. Greenwood describes a process that he used in an action research project in Mondragon (a town in the Basque area of Spain) that involved over 40 participants throughout the course of the research. The general manager wanted a report after the first month of the project in order to decide if the project should go forward or be terminated. Greenwood worked with two others to write a quick report to address the manager's information needs. The report went forward without a named author because it was viewed as an internal document. When the time came for a more extensive report in the final year of the project, a variety of reactions was expressed by the participants, from high appeal to fear. A small writing group was formed, composed mainly of the leaders of the human resource groups in the central service area. Greenwood developed outlines that were then revised by the writing group. Each person accepted responsibility for writing his or her section. The group members also agreed to publish one monograph in Spanish through a local publisher and another in English through a university press.

Greenwood et al. (2006) encountered resistance from the writers to putting their names on the final document. The community members did not want to represent themselves as "a cult of personality inimical to the concept of cooperation" (p. 84). Greenwood asked them to examine their motives: "Were they not willing to own up publicly to what they had concluded or [did they wish] to avoid being confronted by others about their interpretations?" (p. 84). The writers then decided to include their names on the document. Greenwood and his principal collaborator and initiator of the project, José Luis Gonzalez Santos, were listed as first and second author, respectively. They assisted other writers who had had less experience in this type of writing. They then came to realize that they needed to reach a general agreement concerning authorship and review process for different types of project-based writing. They identified three types of documents: (1) internal-use documents could be written by stakeholders and used as they saw fit; (2) collaborative documents needed to be reviewed and agreed upon by the group (this review process resulted in the elimination of some of the writing that Greenwood wanted to include but the group did not); and (3) Greenwood wrote for the action research community about his experiences from a methodological point of view, did not review these papers with the community, and published them under his own name.

Who Owns the Data?

As noted in an earlier chapter, Chilisa (2005) reported that the contract to conduct the HIV/AIDS research in Botswana was given to a European university, with ownership of the data and all subsequent reports from that data belonging to said university. The contract language represents hegemony in action: "Any and all intellectual property including copyright in the final and other reports arising from the work under this agreement will be the property of the University X" (p. 676). Chilisa describes this practice as exploitation of the researcher. Under the transformative paradigm, ownership should go to the community.

Student Perspective: Ownership of Data and Dissertations

This should be interesting! I have no idea, really. I hope Gallaudet will allow me to transfer the ownership of this project to the participants, but I'm sure there's some bunch of political hoopla to argue with first. I know I can dedicate my dissertation to the participants, but is that enough? That's not an official "property" ownership statement, though.—Raychelle Harris (February 23, 2006)

Issues of Power

Since the purpose of the transformative paradigm is to transform society based on research and evaluation results, we need to revisit the issues of power discussed throughout this text. Social change for the good of people without power, for oppressed people, can be liberating. However, power redistribution is not necessarily appreciated by those currently in power, and can also be confusing for people currently without power. The role of the researcher or evaluator in this paradigm is to share information in a way that empowers those who are oppressed. What if those without power do not know what to do with the new elevation in power or status and the new information? Also, what if those with power scramble to cover their bases, to prevent the power redistribution from happening? The researcher or evaluator should also include suggestions, guidance, and tools to help oppressed people use the information proactively as well as to help the people in power safely redistribute their own power without compromising themselves or their employment (Mertens, 2005). The research I did on court system accessibility provides examples of how this can be done (Mertens, 2000).

I asked my PhD students to comment explicitly on how they would deal with issues of power in their own research plans. Raychelle Harris is preparing to write her dissertation on the use of ASL in the classroom.

Student Perspective: Issues of Power in Dissertation Reports

That's a very good question—how will I deal with issues of power in my dissertation topic? I'm not sure. I don't want to get too political with my dissertation, specifically, I do not want to discuss the politics of who should teach, although I do want to open doors for people who are fluent ASL users and show how exceedingly complex it is for fluent ASL users to mediate academic ASL discourse, classroom management, and learning. Showing that much will hopefully encourage readers to give them the same respect we give other top-notch teachers. I hope this will also encourage teachers to learn from each other the techniques and skills they use while teaching. This dissertation, hopefully, will specify some techniques and skills that can be taught to teachers who are not as fluent in ASL to help them increase their skill in academic ASL discourse by making this discourse explicit.—Ray-chelle Harris (February 26, 2006)

Power and Suppression

Power can be used either to suppress research findings or to allow their dissemination. In my experience as a researcher and evaluator, I have had only one report suppressed completely. It dealt with the use of alcohol and drugs by college students. The university did not want such "bad news out," even though it is a problem recognized on many college campuses. My earlier example of the power struggles around reporting about sexual abuse in a residential school for deaf students was another example of an attempt to subvert the focus of the research away from the central topic of sexual abuse, which was seen as a public relations nightmare for the school. I chose to report to the state department of education that commissioned the study the conditions that permitted the occurrence of the sexual abuse and those that might reduce the probability of recurrence. However, in wider dissemination, I chose not to reveal the name of the particular school. In the end, I believe that this was the right decision, as I have had numerous people from different areas of the country contact me to ask if the study was conducted at their school. I assure them that I will not reveal the name of the school, but their inquiries reinforce my belief that the results from that study have a certain type of generalizability. An example of how power can be used to suppress research is presented in Box 10.2.

Reporting Schedule

The topics of dissemination and utilization are discussed further toward the end of this chapter. However, it seems important to point out in this section on general issues that reporting is not seen as something that happens only at the end of a project. "Dissemination is present at the very moment of conceptualizing research and . . . it continues in ways we have

BOX 10.2. Suppression of Data about Worker Illnesses

After a four-year ordeal, a long-suppressed report by a Boston University researcher of elevated cancer rates among semiconductor workers at IBM factories was published online in the open-access peer-reviewed journal *Environmental Health: A Global Access Science Source* (Clapp, 2006). "Mortality among U.S. Employees of a Large Computer-Manufacturing Company: 1969–2001," a paper describing the study, by Richard W. Clapp, is available on the journal's website.

Clapp (2006) analyzed data about employee deaths and work histories obtained from IBM's company files as part of a lawsuit over worker illnesses. He was a consultant for the plaintiffs in that trial. His analysis was revealed during a deposition; however, it was not allowed in the trial itself. IBM claimed that the company data were provided in confidence and could not be made public. The company also contended that the data that Mr. Clapp used were not appropriate for his analysis.

Interestingly, peer reviewers disagreed three times with IBM's assertion. Clapp submitted and then withdrew the first submission to *Medical Clinics of North America*, after receiving a stern legal warning from lawyers for IBM.

The submission to *Clinics in Occupational and Environmental Medicine* was accepted by peer reviewers, but was rejected by Elsevier, the company that publishes that journal. Elsevier representatives said the journal publishes only reviews and that Clapp's article contained original, previously unpublished results. To protest the journal's rejection of Clapp's paper, a guest editor and other authors whose work was scheduled to appear in the same issue withdrew their papers. Finally, Clapp went to court to establish his right to publish the paper. A judge issued a ruling in March 2006 that gave Clapp the legal right to publish his research.

The online journal that made Clapp's paper available is published by BioMed Central, which has more than 150 peer-reviewed open-access journals. In the article, Clapp concludes that men and women involved in manufacturing at the company died of cancer more frequently than people in the general population, although he was unable to draw any conclusions about what chemicals might be responsible.

Clapp hopes the information will help to protect future workers from harmful exposure.

Adapted from Brown (2006).

yet to explore well after the formal stages of research are complete" (Barnes, Clouder, Pritchard, Hughes, & Purkis, 2003, p. 147).

Reynolds (2006) explores the theme of transparency in ongoing reporting. He describes his work in Botswana in which he produced three interim reports for a 2-year study. He began each report by acknowledging his own role and purpose in the evaluation, explaining the limitations of the methods in terms of scientific criteria, and focusing on the main issues of the evaluation. He used language that was specifically geared to address the values and purpose of the project, including the issues of power, decision making, and moral underpinnings. Reynolds invited all stakeholders to comment on the interim reports either in written or verbal form, whether privately or publicly. One seminar was held for a government committee and one public seminar was convened in Botswana for feedback. The underlying theme in each of these reporting venues was that the data were being presented as a basis for discussion and comment.

QUESTIONS FOR THOUGHT

- Who would you include in the preparation and dissemination of findings?
- How would you include members of the community in this process?
- What challenges might you anticipate encountering at this stage of your study?
- How would you deal with power differences among those involved in these activities?
- What is your thinking about ownership of the data and how would you handle this issue?
- What aspects of the transformative paradigm are most salient at this point in the study?

Reporting Options

Written Formats

While writing might seem as natural as breathing for some in the academic community, the territory around writing as a means of communication is contested. In this section, options for reporting formats are discussed in terms of mode of transmission, including written, visual, and oral forms of communication. I begin with reflections from Charmaz (2006), who places her discourse on how writing is a process of discovery in the context of grounded theory and social justice:

Our written works derive from aesthetic principles and rhetorical devices—in addition to theoretical statements and scientific rationales. The act of writing is intuitive, inventive, and interpretive, not merely a reporting of acts and facts, or in the case of grounded theory, causes, conditions, categories, and consequences. Writing leads to further discoveries and deeper insights; it furthers inquiry. Rather than claiming silent authorship hidden behind a scientific facade, grounded theorists—as well as proponents of social justice—should claim audible voices in their writings. (Charmaz, 2006, pp. 528–529; see also Charmaz & Mitchell, 1996; Mitchell & Charmaz, 1996)

Cummins (2000) continues this notion that report writing is, in essence, a "dialogue . . . that brings together what is seen from outside and what is felt from inside as necessary to articulate understandings. These understandings are always partial, and subject to expansion and refinement through further dialogue. Theory expresses this ongoing search for understanding. As such, theory itself is always dialogical" (p. 1).

I asked my PhD students to comment on the implications of viewing writing and theory construction as a dialogue and how they would address this aspect of their work in their research proposals.

Student Perspective: Writing as Dialogue

I think power will be potentially redistributed if we all look at theory as dialogical and build a relationship from outside the researched community and inside the researched community and with knowledge that we are not all geniuses and that nothing is finalized even with a published dissertation or book, and we can always use new understandings and perspectives to increase our understandings of what is happening. This meditative perspective is more empowering for the researched because it allows for their voices/signs to be heard/seen rather than the "scientist knows all" habit of white, hearing, First World researchers.—Raychelle Harris (February 26, 2006)

In a discussion of the importance of avoiding the promotion of hegemonic discourse, Ladd (2003) notes that a discourse system:

contains its own unspoken rules as to what can or cannot be said and how, when and where. Each, therefore, constructs canons of "truth" around whatever its participants decide is "admissible evidence," a process that in the case of certain prestigious discourse, such as those found in universities, medical establishments and communication medias, can be seen as particularly dangerous when unexamined, for these then come to determine what counts as knowledge itself. (p. 76)

Chilisa (2005) also critiqued the act of privileging the written format when she wrote the following:

> First World researchers have enjoyed the privilege of the written word and have used the written text as the forum for debate and for legitimizing knowledge. Unfortunately, the majority of the researched, who constitute two-thirds of the world, are left out of the debate and do not, therefore, participate in legitimizing the very knowledge they are supposed to produce. The end result has been that ethics protocols of individual consent and notions of confidentiality have been misused to disrespect and make value judgements that are psychologically damaging to communities and nations at large. But, above all, the production of knowledge continues to work within the framework of colonizer/colonized. The colonizer still strives to provide ways of knowing and insists on others to use these paradigms. In the postcolonial era, however, it is important to move beyond knowledge construction by the Western First World as the knower. Resistance to this domination continues and it is attested, among other things, by the current African Renaissance. (p. 677)

Student Perspective: Reflection on Chilisa's Article

I also enjoyed learning about the different ways the information is disseminated—through songs, plays, poems, dance, theater, and storytelling (as opposed to Western ways—through demeaning billboards—in ENGLISH!). I wonder how the information should be disseminated to the deaf community. Like with the "ASL" journal being experimented with by the Deaf Studies Department, would it be accessible to all Deaf? Even those who aren't into academics? Would plays and presentations at NAD [National Association of the Deaf] be more far-reaching into the deaf community as opposed to the "ASL" journal? Just wondering . . . Raychelle Harris (February 8, 2006)

Researchers and evaluators need to be conscious of the fact that academic knowledge/discourse is powerful (Harris et al., 2009). Gilmore and Smith (2005) argue that academic genre/discourse is not "simply academic writing, but also knowledge of traditional rules for creating and disseminating knowledge" (p. 71). Academic discourse is not only powerful but also colonizing, as pointed out by bell hooks: "I know that it is not the English language that hurts me, but what the oppressors do with it, how they shape it to become a territory that limits and defines, how they make it a weapon that can shame, humiliate, colonize" (1990, p. 37).

The very concept of introducing alternative reporting formats, such as visual sign language to depict the deaf experience into academic research, may be inconceivable to some people. However, Lincoln and Denzin (2005) argue that journals and conferences now accept "experimental, 'messy' layered poetic and performance texts" (p. 1121). More researchers are now "increasingly preparing research papers and dissertations that are, at a minimum, bilingual—writings that address the needs of multiple rather than singular audiences. . . . It is no longer unheard of, or even strange, for students to produce doctoral dissertations that include portions that some of the members of their dissertation committees may not be able to translate" (Lincoln & Denzin, 2005, p. 1121). Bienvenu (2003) published Chapter 5 of her dissertation, on linguistics in ASL, entirely in a video format in ASL, even though some members on her dissertation committee did not know ASL.

On the other hand, Gilmore and Smith (2005) say that "research not conforming to the prevailing academic genres still risks being either patronized or denigrated as 'not real scholarship'" (p. 78). However, taking the risk of blending academic genre with conventions by the researched is an indication of community solidarity. Those who take risks in research that detract from the conforming standards imposed by those with academic power teach those in power a thing or two (Lincoln & Denzin, 2005). In fact, researchers have much to learn from the researched. Much work lies ahead for us, to *re-write and reright* existing and often damaging academic research" (Gilmore & Smith, 2005, p. 71, emphasis in original).

Writing a Case Study

The complexity of conducting case studies and making inferences toward building theoretical and practical knowledge are discussed in Chapter 6 in the context of Flyvbjerg's (2006) article about myths and misunderstandings about case studies. He expanded on the myth related to the difficulty of summarizing and developing general propositions and theories on the basis of a specific case study in the following passage:

> It is correct that summarizing case studies is often difficult, especially as concerns case process. It is less correct as regards case outcomes. The problems in summarizing case studies, however, are due more often to the properties of the reality studied than to the case study as a research method. Often it is not desirable to summarize and generalize case studies. Good studies should be read as narratives in their entirety. (p. 221)

Flyvbjerg (2006) suggests that violence is done when writers summarize factual findings or condense the findings into a high-level generalization of theory. He recommends presentation of the case study results in their full complexity. He writes:

> First, when writing up a case study, I demur from the role of omniscient narrator and summarizer. Instead, I tell the story in its diversity, allowing the story to unfold from the many-sided, complex, and sometimes conflicting stories that the actors in the case have told me. Second, I avoid linking the case with the theories of any one academic specialization. Instead, I relate the case to broader philosophical positions that cut across specializations. In this way, I try to leave the scope for readers of different backgrounds to make different interpretations and draw diverse conclusions regarding the question of what the case is a case of. The goal is not to make the case study be all things to all people. The goal is to allow the study to be different things to different people. (p. 239)

Thus, readers are left to determine the path to truth by bringing their own interpretations to answer the questions presented in the case study.

Theory and Writing

Parker and Lynn (2002) discuss the usefulness of the rich data provided by interviews and observations in case study research. They examine how CRT can be used to illuminate issues of institutional and overt racism by using interview quotations to illustrate discriminatory practices. In Villenas et al.'s (1999) research in education, CRT was used as a lens through which to report on discriminatory practices and policies such as tracking, operating dual school systems based on race, and failing to provide bilingual services. They describe the use of CRT in this context as follows:

> The use of narrative in CRT added a different dimension to the purposes of educational research by taking on a different potential dimension as an integral part of legal testimony. In this case, expert witness testimony and personal narratives of discrimination played a key role in proving the school district's intent to discriminate and neglect the legal rights of Navajo children with respect to equal educational opportunity through an inequitable distribution of education services. Deyhle (Villenas et al., 1999) connected this testimony to *social justice validity*, a term used by Deyhle and Swisher (1997) in their review of research on Native American tribal nations and education. Social justice validity posits a research validity that is seriously grounded in social justice and commitment on tribal nation terms and long-term involvement in challenging White supremacy over tribal nation affairs. (Parker & Lynn, 2002, p. 11)

Feminist Theory

Cornwall et al. (2004) talk about the way gender is reframed in the international development community by changing language, for example, the use of terms such as *poverty, empowerment, rights, exclusion*, and *citizenship*. At times, bringing *women* and *poverty* into the same conversation has had the effect of enabling some women to gain better access to resources. However, in other instances, myths and stereotypes operate to control the gendered power relations. They explain that:

> discursive position as perpetually poor, powerless and pregnant works to place African women as illiterate victims of national systems of resource distribution and disadvantage, putting them in such abject positions that only development can rescue them. It represents its objects as so lacking in the resources that underpin agency, and in such political and economic deficit, that they will never be able to get into a position on their own from which they can make claims. Powerlessness described in this way by outsiders simply serves to reinforce it. (p. 6)

Cornwall et al. (2004) continue their insights into the use of feminist theory in reporting research results by bringing the myth of empowerment under a critical lens. They see the use of the term *empowerment* as a way of making the need for radical transformation more palatable to a mainstream audience. The wrong-headed interpretation of empowerment of women by giving them a little more money leads to a deflection of their energies away from the political action needed to reach a truly transformative state. Choices made in terms of discourse can have powerful effects in the consequences of research work. They (Cornwall et al., 2004) write:

> Discourses are not just tactical, but are powerful forms of interpretation for ourselves as well as others. They enable us to act. If we discard the notion of interests in favour of a language of rights and citizenship, or displace the language of conflict with the language of trade-offs, is this only, or even primarily, an opportunistic response? Do we spot a potential discursive space that will unlock resources or get us to the table with the powerful and adopt it mainly for these reasons? We think not. We adopt different languages about how we explain the routes to gender justice and equality to ourselves because we have learnt from experience. (p. 6)

Experience with political encounters around women's rights has led to an understanding that struggle is necessary and forthrightness is a quality to be nurtured.

Self-Reflection and Writing

Transformative researchers are encouraged to keep an eye on themselves from beginning to end of an inquiry. We discussed this most explicitly in Chapter 3, on knowing ourselves as researchers and in relation to our communities. We also saw the recommendation that researchers keep a journal or diary as a way of tracking their changing perceptions, hypotheses, and understandings throughout the course of a study. Marshall (2006) addresses the use of self-reflective data in the writing of the report. She frames the use of this self-reflective data as a decision point that needs to be revisited throughout the development of the report. How much of the personal reflections should be reported? Reporting all of it might be viewed as too much self-absorption; reporting too little of it removes the richness and context that make it worthy of inclusion. She concludes: "No rules of practice can resolve these dilemmas; they must be engaged in the process of inquiring" (p. 337).

Interpretation and Supportive Data

Chiu's (2003) work with the women in the health services project provides a good example of how excerpts of dialogue can be used in a report to bring to the professionals' attention their stereotypes of minority ethnic women. During work with initial focus groups with professionals, Chiu asked them to comment on their own perceptions of reasons for the lack of participation by the minority ethnic women in the cervical screening services. She later presented these quotes from their focus group to them:

> They don't keep appointments always. And they come in the wrong date and they want one yesterday. That is how their system works and that is how their mind set is. . . .
>   Their culture is that you can't see any point in preventative medicine. They don't deal with preventative medicine or any preventative measures. That isn't how they see it. And the other thing is, that time matters very little. [All nodded.] (p. 178)

Chiu used these quotations as a way to make visible the professional's use of stereotypes, such as lack of a sense of time and fear of medical procedures, and their tendency to generalize these stereotypes to all members of the cultural groups. She explains the purpose of returning the transcripts to the professionals and using them as a basis for a second focus group:

Rather than being challenged on the spot, participants were allowed to confront their own prejudice through *hearing their own voices* in a non-threatening way. The transcript as a collective product owned by the group, rather than as "data" primarily belonging to the researcher, turned out to be a useful tool in supporting critical reflection and facilitating critical awareness. . . . This experience highlights the complexity involved in the process of facilitating critical awareness. It is doubtful that focus groups can become a transformational tool in the context of the more prescribed object-and-subject research relationships commonly found in conventional settings. (p. 178)

Group Processes as Part of Reporting

Group discussion was explored in earlier chapters in relation to focusing the research and collection of data. It is also a relevant strategy in terms of reporting results. Cram et al. (2004) reported their results of the series of *hui* related to understanding the meaning of research and relations in the Maori community by describing the progression of ideas and illustrating the points by citing quotations from the community members. A sample that illustrates the synthesis and presentation of specific quotations appears in Box 10.3.

Student Perspective: Reaction to Cram et al.'s Paper

I loved how this paper was written—I could see the voices of many Maori coming through the hui *gatherings and quoted throughout the paper. I felt this really was reflective of their thoughts and feelings. I also enjoyed how it was easily read (I hate it when people write so complicated, making everything harder to read).—Raychelle Harris (February 8, 2006)*

Chilisa and Preece (2005) recommend the use of group discussion so that researched communities can validate findings that are generalized or extrapolated to them. Such an exercise can enable the researched to participate more fully in the construction of knowledge that is produced about them. Moving away from writing as a form of reporting, the next section extends group interaction strategies and examines the use of visual presentation of data.

Visual Presentations

Visual presentation of results can be useful for all participants, but especially for those who are more comfortable with forms of communication

---

BOX 10.3. Structural Change and the Marginalization Project Report

Linda Smith suggests that we "return to some of the foundation of principles of Kaupapa Maori research, . . . which do argue that our role as Maori researchers is to deal with structural relations of power [and] to attempt to address those [tensions]. It is about trying to seek transformation and it is about being Maori as a given, and not having to apologise for that and being a Maori researcher" (Wellington Hui, May 31, 2004).

HUI TUARUA: STRUCTURAL CHANGE

Desires for social change usually have repercussions within a wider society and are often fought because they have resource implications. And so often it's around multiple levels of why we do research, being very clear about what research can achieve and being honest about why we may be committed to social change. Sometimes it's very difficult for research to achieve social change because when research challenges a power structure, it's invariably looked at really, really closely and unpicked by those who want to dispute the findings and the [resulting] request for social change. We've seen that time and time again. . . . So I think that it's a tricky thing that we do sometimes . . . (Wellington Hui, May 31, 2004.

From Cram et al. (2004, p. 162).

---

other than writing, whether this is because of low literacy levels or because the community's communication is more orally or visually based. Chiu (2003) provides an example of visual presentation of data in her work with focus groups composed of women from a variety of minority populations in England whose home language was not English. The focus groups were used not only to identify issues related to access and delivery of health services, but also as a venue for developing materials to be used in reporting to the professionals who served this community and the funding agency. The women produced photo stories in which they took part in the portrayal of the health screening services. Through this process, they not only produced materials for the purpose of enlightening the professionals, but they also gained knowledge about the medical procedures themselves. The production of the materials also made visible the cultural codes of modesty to which health professionals need to attend with these clients in order to allay their fears during the procedures. The materials from the focus group's production were later used in training materials for the professionals.

Recall the earlier description of Collins's (2005) research and how she used visual methods in her study of poor women in the food co-op study. She asked the women, as a group, to draw a picture that depicted a good quality of life. They drew a house and then surrounded it with words that reflected qualities they felt were part of that picture. The group took a vote on which of the qualities were very important, somewhat important, or not as important. They then drew a heart shape around the very important qualities, a circle around the somewhat important ones, and a square around the less important qualities. In this way a visual depiction was created in which factors deemed to be very important became very visible. (These included relationships with friends, family, and children.) While tangible assets such as a car, fresh water, and a full cupboard were mentioned as part of the good quality of life, the women emphasized more intangible qualities such as love, happiness, religion, success, freedom from stress, and a sense of community.

They drew another picture depicting sources of stress in their lives. The factors that contributed to stress were more tangible and included lack of money, food, housing, and health care services. They also drew a picture that revealed the cyclical nature of stress. In the beginning of the month when they got their social assistance, they were less stressed than at the end of the month, when bills went unpaid and the cupboard was bare. The results of this use of a visual presentation to convey information are discussed further in a later section of this chapter about working for change.

Performance: Slide Show

Cardoza Clayson et al. (2002) provide an example of how they adopted the role of storyteller and used a 20-minute bilingual, bicultural slide presentation to present results of their work to an audience of Latino community members, staff, non-Latino community-based organizations, and funders. The use of Spanish and English as two languages of equal importance guided the development of the presentation. In addition, the slide presentation included graphics such as Aztec imagery and an owl to symbolize wisdom and education. As part of the development process, a team of evaluators, one a native Spanish speaker from Mexico and the other a native English speaker from California, created a story board that depicted concepts related to how civic engagement was reflected in Mexico and the United States. The goal was to inform all the groups as to ways in which the members of the Latino U.S. community could navigate civic participation in this country. The slide show included information about how city halls and public utilities function and how parents participate in schools. The presentation addressed the feeling of distrust that often surrounds Latino communities in relation to issues of documentation. In order to make a smooth presentation, the evaluators rehearsed before their first formal appearances. Comments from that first presentation were solicited in order to make the next presentation more responsive to the stakeholders.

Additional information related to translation in research and evaluation contexts is presented in Chapter 8 on data collection and Chapter 9 on data analysis.

Ethnodrama

Mienczakowski and Morgan (2006) and Mienczakowski (2000) raise a point that many researchers are unwilling to acknowledge or do not see as problematic in terms of the number of people who actually read their research reports. Mienczakowski (2000) wrote: "As an ethnographer and teacher of social science research methodologies and the performing arts, I have been only too aware of how small the readership of most academic ethnographic reports can be and how receptive and yet *unchallenged* the audiences of most theatrical productions remain" (p. 127). Cherryholmes (1993) amplifies concerns about the use (or nonuse) of reports by commenting that it is most uncommon for research participants to have the opportunity to comment on an academic ethnographic report once it has been published.

Mienczakowski (2000) suggests a blend of ethnographic research and critical drama in creating an ethnodrama approach to sharing data with relevant constituencies. He wrote:

> The processes of critical ethno-drama attempt to offer emancipatory insights by telling informants' stories, largely narrated in their own words, to wide audiences inside and outside the confines of the academy. By combining research process with theatrical narratives constructed by informants, it is hoped that research becomes relevant to both its informants and those outside the academy. (p. 127)

Mienczakowski and Morgan (2006) used ethnodrama to translate the results of action research with a variety of audiences, including teachers, nurses, and medical students. After they completed the informant-led data-collection process and validation of that data with informants, they used the derived themes to develop a script, based on views of the stakeholders, for dissemination in the form of an ethnodrama. They shared the script with the stakeholders as a means of validation. The second phase (dissemination) is the actual performance of the script and provision of opportunities for interaction between the performers and the audience.

The script consists primarily of verbatim narrative. In order to keep the repertoire company to a reasonable size *and* reflect the wider issues of the stakeholder groups, the researchers combined the words and thoughts of more than one participant for a character. However, no fictional characters or language were added. The scripts were returned to the stakeholders on an ongoing basis in order to further validate the data presentation. To prevent misunderstandings or false expectations, the researchers provided a detailed program book that staff could use to prepare the audience, guide discussion after the performance, and serve as an educational tool for further reflection. The first performance is always made to the informant group, prior to any public performances, providing yet another opportunity to incorporate the voices of the relevant stakeholders. Revisions are made as necessary based on this "piloting" of the performance piece. Box 10.4 provides excerpts from scripts that were part of an ethnodrama based

---

BOX 10.4. Excepts from Scripts from a Study of Recovery from Sexual Assault

From a scene in which the police explain their attitudes toward victims:

COL: The [forensic] evidence can be got in a couple of hours. . . . We need to get this done quickly in order to get the baddy before he gets a story lined up or gets away.

ROB: So we have a female cop for this interview then?

COL: No. Not one available today. Look, I might as well put you straight on this. I reckon that this woman—woman stuff is all bullshit. I am a professional person and so are you, the lawyer, the doctor even. . . .

From a scene in which a woman tells her story:

When I went to the police . . . it wasn't offered to me to see a woman, and retelling the whole saga took eight hours. . . . He . . . didn't record or anything. . . . I had to come back the next day and make my statement in a public office and you could have heard a pin drop—so it was quite intimidating really. . . . I would have much preferred to talk to someone . . . a woman in an office in a sexual assault clinic.

From Mienczakowski and Morgan (2006, p. 180).

on Mienczakowski and Morgan's (2006) study of recovery from sexual assault.

The opportunity for the cast and audience members to discuss the implications of the performance is a crucial part of ethnodrama. Audience members are encouraged to draw implications from the performance for their professional practice. In some cases, a follow-up survey is used to gather data about the audience members' reflections after the performance. Mienczakowski and Morgan (2006) report that medical personnel have declared that they modify their professional behaviors, and other audiences have been stimulated to modify the way health education takes place.

Ethnodrama provides one strategy for increasing the dissemination to targeted audiences. Mienczakowski and Morgan (2006) write: "When a theatre auditorium is nightly crowded with people who are about to hear a research report, we think back to our first ethnographies (no less weighty in construction or so we then thought) that were probably read by no more than a handful of people" (p. 181). However, ethnodrama also introduces new ethical complexities.

Ethical concerns arise because of the potentially psychologically harmful thoughts, feelings, or behaviors that can emerge in the discussion. Relevant counselors are available in private meeting rooms, if needed. Concerns emerge related to the impact of witnessing emotionally painful scenes on both the performers and the audience members. Mienczakowski and Morgan (2006) provide an example of a stakeholder who committed suicide soon following a performance that depicted a schizophrenic person who had also committed suicide. They cannot establish a causal path from the performance to the subsequent suicide, but they raise it as an ethical concern of which researchers should be aware.

Mienczakowski and Morgan (2006) raise other ethical issues based on the potential of performances to impact audiences.

> Research ethics are a well-trammeled tenet of most research activity. However, the ethical dilemmas of performed research are less well recognized or understood. Performance, ethnodrama and health theatre are important facets of health education and health promotion and to embrace their worth fully researchers need to embrace and develop a fuller understanding of the ethical ramifications and potentials of this emerging mode of research performance. Beyond the containment of action research this mode of performance of research represents a challenge to audiences' emotions. Consequently we are in new territory and this is the ethical dilemma. (p. 183)

Zines and Web-Based Dissemination

Derived from the word *magazines*, zines are noncommercial booklets that can be published in paper or electronic form. In a study of youths and health services, Amsden and VanWynsberghe (2005) report that the youths lost interest when the researchers indicated a need to write a report to share their experiences. The youths met and decided that a zine would provide a better format than a traditional report to express their feelings and experiences. The zine used a photo essay that depicted their experiences when they visited the health clinics, as well as a clinic rating system (much like a movie rating system) on specific criteria such as hours of operation. These youths also participated in presentations at a child and youth health conference.

Additional web-based dissemination outlets are emerging as technology rapidly expands such options. Blogs, a form of web-based chat rooms, are used to disseminate information quickly and provide an opportunity to obtain feedback from a large audience almost immediately. As technology continues to develop, ethical issues around the use of these modes for disseminating research and evaluation findings surface (see Burbules, 2009).

QUESTIONS FOR THOUGHT

- What modes of reporting would you use in your study?
- If you are considering using a written mode of reporting, what steps would you take to be responsive to the transformative paradigm?
- What is the potential for ethnodrama, visual methods, or electronic means as reporting modes in your field of interest?

Utilization

Patton (2002) set "utilization" at the top of the pinnacle as a goal to achieve in his book *Utilization Focused Evaluation*. He presents an approach to evaluation that infuses concerns about utilization throughout the process of inquiry. The beginning of utilization is the identification of the intended users. This topic was covered in previous chapters and brings to light, once again, the nonlinear nature of transformative research and evaluation. As was noted in Collins's (2005) study, discussed earlier in this chapter, the principle of participation needs to underlie the research rather than a mere technique applied at the end of a study. Participation needs to occur at every stage of a study: focusing the research or evaluation, making decisions about designs and methods, engaging in dialogues, gathering data and analyzing it, as well as at the reporting and utilization stages.

Amsden and VanWynsberghe (2005) recognized that they had separated the two concepts of action and participation, with the consequence that they did not maximize either one in their study. In retrospect, they realized that action and participation need to come together in a continual reflection, or praxis, within the research process. They also realized that their study could have benefited by including health professionals as participants as a means of creating service changes that the youths had identified.

Collins (2005) discussed this idea further in reflecting on her study of the poor women who were part of the food co-op. She had an initial goal of social change, and as she progressed through the inquiry process, she came to realize that social change must be a shared, communal goal. Researchers with a goal of social change need to ask themselves: What kind of power does participation in my study give and to whom? While the women in her study gained in their insights as to what was wrong with the system, and they gained in their ability to work for change in the food co-op, they did not necessarily gain in power to make changes to the national welfare system. Just as Amsden and VanWynsberghe (2005) also found—that the youths did not have the power to change the health clinic services—Collins realized that participation in such a study did not necessarily imbue poor women with political power.

Researchers need to be honest about their expectations for social change and realize the unfairness of shifting responsibility for such change onto the backs of those who have little political power. It is important for academic researchers to share their power by sharing their links to networks of agencies or policymakers and to share the experiences of those who are traditionally not heard in those corridors and offices.

The food co-op members used their understandings of poverty and the effects of cutbacks in social assistance to transform the co-op into a place of social support (Collins, 2005). Two of the women ran for the executive position in the co-op and won. They implemented such changes as soliciting and reviewing member suggestions and holding parties for the children. They also produced a report that was shared with a local committee that works for improvements to the social assistance system and to the advisory committee that administers social assistance in the region.

Policy and Advocacy

Two important uses of research and evaluation studies are to develop, critique, and refine policy and to advocate actions that support changes in policy. Cornwall et al. (2004) recognize that many feminists work to change policies that were not of their own making. Such work demands cognizance of complex processes of policymaking and being able to provide the appropriate types of information to be seen as a credible player at the policy table. Yet, feminists realize that radical social change requires engagement with those who hold power in the national and international arenas.

Policy analysis is a discipline unto itself, and thus it is not possible to give a full rendition of the topic in this book. Instead, I offer some resources related to the use of research to influence policy and strategies for advocacy that were developed by the California Endowment, a foundation that supports equity in access to health services, and a grass-roots organization, the Work Group on Health Promotion and Community Development at the University of Kansas in Lawrence.

Guthrie, Louie, David, and Foster (2005) authored a report for the California Endowment and other foundations to guide their work in assessing projects that addressed policy change and advocacy. I adapted their principles to focus more on the community members' role in policy and advocacy projects:

• Step 1: Adopt a conceptual model for understanding the process of policy change. Involvement of key stakeholders is critical to ensure that contextual factors are understood and strategies for making change are articulated through a communal effort.

• Step 2: Develop a theory about how and why planned activities lead to desired outcomes (often called a "theory of change"). Continued stakeholder involvement is needed to clarify how the group's activities are expected to lead to the desired change, to build a common language, and to reach consensus on the desired outcomes.

• Step 3: Select benchmarks to monitor progress (benchmarks are outcomes that indicate change or progress). Because policy change is a complicated process, benchmarks need to be developed that address such issues as constituency and coalition building, conduct of necessary research, education of policymakers, and media and public information campaigns. In addition, outcomes need to be included that indicate the capacity building of the community members themselves in their role in policy and advocacy projects.

- Step 4: Prepare a policy change proposal and bring it to the attention of the policymakers. Recognize the complexity of the policy environment and the many factors that influence policy decisions. Because timing is of the essence in the policy world, policy initiatives need to be introduced at the right time of the policy-making cycle.

- Step 5: Collect data and measure progress toward benchmarks. Additional capacity building and resources may be needed to (a) support the collection of data that documents changes in policy or (b) create advocacy activities to that end.

The following links provide additional information on the California Endowment's resources on policy and advocacy:

www.calendow.org/reference/publications/Policy.stm (California Endowment publications)

www.calendow.org/policy/advocacy_info.stm (California Endowment and advocacy)

The Work Group on Health Promotion and Community Development at the University of Kansas developed a toolbox for community development in collaboration with AHEC/Community Partners in Amherst, Massachusetts. Their information is available at a website that contains a list of core competencies and toolboxes (*ctb.ku.edu/tools/tk/en/corecompetencies.jsp*). These toolboxes are organized to help communities gain access to frameworks with which to organize their work. They can also provide examples of how the work could be accomplished and links to specific tools in the Community Tool Box and to the CTB Learning Community, which includes forums and chat rooms for individual support. Their toolbox begins with a framework for community development and includes many steps that are useful in terms of agenda setting, promotion of ideas through the media, development of a strategic plan, and leadership skill building. A list of their core competencies appears in Box 10.5.

Their web links include:

A list of core competencies for community development and change and links to resources to that end (*ctb.ku.edu/tools/tk/en/corecompetencies.jsp*).

A link to a full table of contents for the core competencies and the resources associated with those (*ctb.ku.edu/tools/en/tools_toc.htm*).

BOX 10.5. Community Tool Box Core Competencies

1. Creating and maintaining coalitions and partnerships

2. Assessing community needs and resources

3. Analyzing problems and goals

4. Developing a framework or model of change

5. Developing strategic and action plans

6. Building leadership

7. Developing an intervention

8. Increasing participation and membership

9. Enhancing cultural competence

10. Advocating for change

11. Influencing policy development

12. Evaluating the initiative

13. Implementing a social marketing effort

14. Writing a grant application for funding

15. Improving organizational management and development

16. Sustaining the work or initiative

Retrieved February 11, 2008, from *ctb.ku.edu/tools/tk/en/corecompetencies.jsp.*

The next section focuses on resources for advocacy and policy change.

Advocating for Change

Advocacy starts with a goal and mission for the intended social action. These include identification of the community or system changes that the advocacy group hopes to accomplish, such as initiate new programs or modify existing policies or practices. Action steps need to be developed that specify who will do what when to bring about what specific change. The advocacy group needs to include those who can contribute to making the change and how the group can support them in that effort. Specific strategies for carrying out the advocacy work need to be developed, such as writing letters to the newspaper or public officials, arranging for media exposure, offering proposals for new laws or policies, conducting a letter-writing campaign, organizing public demonstrations, or initiating legal action. Strategies should be chosen to match the goal and to fit the group's style and available resources.

Advocacy groups need to identify the resources and assets that they possess in terms of people, finances, and communication technologies and facilities. Allies and potential opponents need to be identified in the broader community. Opponents are known to use a variety of strategies to resist or oppose advocates' efforts, such as delaying by calling for additional review, denying that there is a real problem, dividing by trying to get group members to oppose each other, or discrediting by labeling advocates as agitators or socialists. These tactics can be turned around to serve positive purposes for advocates if they can turn the discrediting into an issue or publicize the opponent's strategy (e.g., denial).

Influencing Policy Development

The Community Tool Box provides additional insights into ways to influence public policy. For example, it begins with the identification of reasons why the policy needs to be developed or changed, based on basic needs not being met or inequities in terms of access, distribution, or implementation of current policies. Transformative research and evaluation can be conducted that provides data to support the type and extent of the problem and who is affected by it. Potential solutions can be framed in terms of changes to public laws or business policies and organizational rules.

Community group members need to delineate the steps they will take to accomplish their goals. These might include bringing the issue to the attention of the public and decision makers in a way that frames it in terms of policy options. Lobbyists can be used to bring the message to decision makers. The community group should also have plans to monitor the implementation of changes to verify that the group is having the desired effect.

Just as with advocacy work, communities trying to influence policy need to know who their people are and what financial, communication, and facility resources they have available. Identification of allies and opponents is also necessary in this process. The specific targets of attention are the people who have the power to change the policy, as well as those who implement policies and those who would be affected by this specific policy. To influence policy, the community needs to know the chain of command, who answers to whom, and who supports whom. What would another group gain by choosing to work alongside your group? How would their members benefit? How would your issue affect them? Answering such questions provides insights into which strategies will work and who will support you in your efforts.

The following advice is adapted from the Community Tool Box:

- Review whether the planned policy goals, strategies, and actions fit the situation. Consider whether they:
  - Are timed well (i.e., Is this a good time to raise the issue?)
  - Use available resources and allies (i.e., Do they take advantage of the group's strengths? Engage its allies? Deter opponents?)
    - Fit the group's style (i.e., Are group members comfortable with the approach?)
    - Are flexible (i.e., Do they permit adjustments with changing situations?)
    - Are likely to work (i.e., Do they correct the original problem or inequalities?)
- Create an action plan to carry out your policy efforts (who is going to do what, by when), describing:
  - What specific action will occur (e.g., conduct a letter-writing campaign)
  - Who will carry it out
  - When the plan will be completed or for how long it will be maintained
  - Resources (money and staff) needed
  - Who should know what about this (e.g., local media will be informed of your efforts in order to increase your visibility)

Dissemination and Sustainability

Smith (2000) expresses concerns about the silencing of voices because of the lengthy process that is often associated with conducting and reporting on a research study. She notes that researchers in the Maori community are called upon to make a commitment to report back to the people concerned:

> It is partly a commitment of reciprocity and partly a process of accountability. Students who have written theses, for example, have taken a copy back to the families whom they interviewed; other researchers have invited people into their centre for a presentation; still others have made use of an occasion to publicly thank the participants concerned. The significance of these acts is

that sometimes a written piece of work is passed around the *whanau*, other people phone and ask for their own copies, and others put it alongside the photos of family members that fill their sitting rooms. This final reporting closes off one part of an activity; it does not close off the relationships established. (pp. 243–244)

Gaventa and Cornwall (2006) identify several factors that need attention in order to increase the probability that a societal change will be made and sustained:

1. The importance of organizational and institutional change: Organizational culture and structure need to change; often these changes come in the form of strengthening the capacity of local organizations to develop a culture of learning through institutionalizing participatory research approaches.

2. The importance of personal attitudes and behavior change: Organizations tend to drift toward rote practice of participatory inquiry if their people have not changed their personal attitudes and behaviors. Training and dissemination that focus on changing personal values, ethics, and commitments can be implemented.

3. Taking time to go slow: Going too fast in making changes can be a shock to the system. Gaventa and Cornwall (2006) suggest starting with smaller-scale demonstration projects and allowing them to grow, giving sufficient time to learning and revisions, as necessary.

4. Links to social movements and local capacity: Organizations that support the movement of different voices into the openings created by the increased consciousness of a need for social change are more likely to be successful at making substantive changes. Without this commitment, openings tend to be filled with voices that reflect the status quo, thus negating the opportunity for real and sustained change.

5. Creating vertical alliances and networks: Organizations need to create mechanisms for processes and networks that cut vertically across the hierarchies. Thus, creating processes that facilitate meaningful representation across levels is critical.

6. The importance of monitoring for quality and accountability: Organizations need to evolve ways to measure the validity of research processes and the knowledge produced by the research.

Gujit's reflections on the use of the most significant change method (MSC; described in Chapter 8) provide insights into issues involved in the sustainability of change (Whitmore et al., 2006). She used MSC in two different settings with farmer trade unions. Participants initially reported a very positive response to the MSC process because it helped them track their progress and highlight problems they needed to address to make a significant local impact. However, neither group continued to use the process because:

> In Paraíba, after the change of presidency following trade union elections in one of the unions, there was little interest in using this method that was associated with their ousted opponents. The sharing between the two unions and the NGO quickly fell by the wayside. Furthermore, the participants were extremely busy with their everyday farming tasks, besides their union- and NGO-related volunteer activities. Any extra task was viewed with skepticism. As union members said during our evaluation of the Minas Gerais process: "Monitoring, even with this relatively simple method without indicators, is still perceived as one more task." (p. 348)

The Community Tool Box (2006) offers guidance on sustaining initiatives. First, discuss the worthiness of sustaining the effort:

- How long does the initiative need to be in place to accomplish your goals?
- Is there a reasonable time frame in which to expect closure without adverse effect on the community?
- Is there sufficient support in the community to sustain the project?

If the community and conditions are supportive of sustaining the effort, then it is important to take some time to examine the current status and determine if this status is the course for continuation or if modifications are needed. Answers to these questions will vary depending on the structure of the community. For example:

- Is this a stand-alone initiative, or is it the product of a collaborative?
- How does the current leadership and membership view the prospect of continuation?
- What resources are available to continue support over a period of time?
- How long will funding from the current sources be available and what alternative sources exist?
- Who will contact other funding sources?

If the community decides to continue the project, then its members need to develop a business plan that lays out the needed resources, services and/or products, competition, and potential audience. A budget needs to be developed that includes personnel, salaries, expenses, and projected income. The Community Tool Box suggests the following strategies for generating financial resources and sustaining programs:

- Share positions and resources. Collaborate with other organizations with similar philosophical and practical foundations.

- Become a line item in an existing budget of another organization. Convince another organization to pick up part of the expenses of running the initiative (e.g., have a local church provide rent by allowing the initiative to work out of its physical facility or provide basic office and mailing expenses).

- Incorporate the initiative's activities or services into another organization with a similar mission, either by planning for incorporation within a few years of being established (e.g., plan an after-school program and have the local YMCA start sponsoring it after several years) or by initially including representatives from a community group that will eventually become responsible for the program (e.g., start a food pantry with several representatives from an interfaith council that has committed to supporting and continuing it).

- Apply for grants at either the local or federal level—Consider the length of time and depth of resources that will be necessary for success and the need for reapplication.

- Tap into personnel resources that are shared or in training—Recruit people or positions in other organizations that can be shared at low or no cost (e.g., clerical staff). Take advantage of volunteers, internships, college work–study programs.

- Solicit in-kind support—Utilize resources other than direct financial contributions that provide goods and services the organization would otherwise have to purchase (e.g., donations of paint or office supplies from a local business, requesting plumbing or roof repair as a form of support).

- Develop and implement a fundraiser. Identify products, services, or events that will inspire others to contribute money to the organization and determine the scope of the fundraiser (e.g., Does the organization plan to conduct such a fundraiser on a regular basis or should it plan to raise funds for multiple years?).

- Pursue third-party funding. Solicit third parties not actually involved with the initiative and not directly benefiting from it to provide resources for two other parties to interact. Choose organizations or businesses that have an interest in the outcome of the interaction (e.g., providing job training for adolescents to create a better prepared workforce in the community).

- Develop a fee-for-service structure. Require clients who access services to pay for them. Sliding-fee scales can be used to help those with little money who need the services and to support the organization's philosophy, which is opposed to refusing those in need.

- Acquire public funding from state legislature or city council. Successful relationship building with legislators could result in regular or annual financial support if the organization's goals are perceived to align with local interests.

- Secure endowments or planned giving arrangements. Use interest from funds as annual income.

- Establish membership fees and dues. Making dues a condition of membership will probably yield less financial resources than outside sources, but doing so may allow the organization to initially forecast expected income.

QUESTIONS FOR THOUGHT

- What methods make sense to you for the utilization of study findings?
- How would you approach linking your findings with social action?
- What further involvement would you foresee with the community in furthering their concerns for social justice?

Future Directions

Most studies end with the identification of future directions for researchers and evaluators. The following list is suggestive of possible future directions for studies conducted in the transformative paradigm:

- Identify specific research topics that relate to human rights and social justice.
- Further explore the development of a transformative approach to research and evaluation.

- Encourage multilateral explorations of the meaning of the concept of cultural competence in research and evaluation contexts.
- Provide a forum for the expression of ideas concerning the meaning of cultural competence in specific national/regional organizations of research and evaluation.
- Advocate for a broader base of those who understand the meaning of cultural competence within organizations.
- Explore the link between social justice issues and cultural competence in multinational contexts (e.g., Rights Based Approach/UNI-CEF/ UNDP).
- Examine ways that client-based perspectives can be accessed to provide greater insights into how researchers and evaluators can become more culturally competent.
- Explore implications for training programs to further this end.
- Use web-based resources and pathways to support these activities.
- Develop training on how to increase the cultural competence of communities to deal with outside professional researchers and evaluators to ensure that they are doing something useful for the community.

Student Perspective: Training Researchers and Evaluators

Why not add a course or training for researchers (and evaluators)—especially for graduate and doctoral students? The ethics, the methods, the procedures for building partnerships with indigenous communities while doing research.—Heidi Holmes (February 8, 2006)

Bringing It Together to Take It Apart to Shake Things Up

Social science research and evaluation have a complicated relationship. Social science research has a much longer history involving formal disciplines such as psychology, sociology, and anthropology. Program evaluation emerged in the 1960s and was seen at first as a "child" of applied social science (Mark, Greene, & Shaw, 2006). However, early experiences with program evaluation suggested a need to separate it from social science in order for its unique character and identity to develop. I have been witness to that evolutionary process since the 1960s, having participated in program evaluation since the time that it was defined in education as measuring the attainment of established behavioral objectives through the awareness of the broader political context in which evaluation lives and breaths. As a professor of research and evaluation, I fully recognize those features that are uniquely associated with these two disciplines. However, I have also grown increasingly aware that it is time for these two (whether we see them as estranged parent and child or younger and older siblings) to fully embrace and converse respectfully about their journeys. There is much to be learned by putting their stories side by side and integrating them at certain points. Evaluation took many pathways as it struggled to address political contexts and multiple stakeholders. Yet, applied social science researchers also struggle with these concepts, often in the absence of the insights evaluators have to offer. This book offers pathways that intersect in the interest of expanding our understanding of the role of research and evaluation in social transformation and the furtherance of social justice.

Summary

✓ Complexities associated with the reporting and utilization of research and evaluation in transformative studies are addressed by considering several critical issues, such as who the intended audience is for the reports and the tensions that arise in preparing reports for communities and academic audiences.

✓ Power is a concern when the more powerful dictate that reports be written in academic parlance that, in essence, excludes community members who do not work in such settings.

✓ The crisis of representation of voice is also illustrated in decisions that need to be made regarding how to present "bad language."

✓ Coauthorship, with researchers/evaluators sharing responsibility with community members, is one avenue for collaboration at this stage of the process.

✓ Data ownership is another critical issue that merits discussion in the transformative spirit. If community members provide the data, then how can they be included in the ownership of that data?

✓ Power also needs to be examined when results are suppressed that might not reflect positively on any segment of the population of interest.

✓ Continuous and transparent reporting is commensurate with transformative research and evaluation.

✓ The use of theoretical frameworks that are commensurate with transformative research and evaluation are explored in terms of their potential contribution to the analysis and interpretation of data.

✓ Case study reports are singled out for attention because of their central importance as an approach in transformative work.

✓ A multitude of options for reporting can be used, including different formats for written reports; visual modalities such as videos, photographs, web-based media, or graphics; group discussions; and performance media such as slide shows and ethnodramas.

✓ Utilization of the findings to further social justice is the most critical factor in transformative work. Possible strategies include the use of collaborative planning to establish the next steps and the use of the findings to work toward policy change and advocacy.

✓ The Community Tool Box provides a number of strategies and actions for working toward policy change.

✓ The sustainability of change needs to be addressed by building alliances and networks from the perspective of institutions, organizations, and local capacity. Seeking additional funding to continue efforts is also a key consideration.

 Reporting and dissemination activities may reflect different facets of the findings for different people. It is all good if each facet serves to further social justice.

How Prisms Work

How do prisms work? When light goes into a piece of glass it bends, unless it goes straight into the surface. (You've seen something just like this when you look at things under water from above the water.) Now the interesting thing is that different colors of light bend different amounts. . . . You don't notice that because in a window the light bends back on the way out, so the different colors are just barely shifted from another. Because the prism faces aren't parallel, the bending on the way out doesn't just reverse the bending on the way in. So different colors of light come out at different angles, and gradually spread apart. Since a beam of white light is actually made up of all the colors, you can see the different colors because they all come out moving in different directions.

Why do different colors bend different amounts? The amount the light bends depends on how much it slows down in the glass. How much it slows down depends on how much its electromagnetic field shakes the electrons in the glass. The electrons respond a little differently to different frequencies of shaking, and different frequencies of light means the same thing as different colors.

Prisms normally have a triangular cross-section and extend in the direction perpendicular to the plane of the triangle. But prisms can bend around in a curve, they can have four or more sides, and just about any shape will work.

Refraction—The word comes from the fact that light can change direction, or *refract,* when it passes from one medium to another. Why does light do this? . . . Fundamentally it has to do with the fact that the light, an electromagnetic wave, is

From Physics Van, University of Illinois, Department of Physics (*van.physics.uiuc.edu*) and Queen's University Astronomy Research Group (*www.astro.queens.ca*).

moving from a medium of one kind, which consists of atoms arranged in some way, into a new medium in which the atoms are disposed differently. Since all atoms contain charged particles (their electrons and protons), the way in which electro-magnetic radiation passes through the new material—and in particular the *speed* at which it does so—may be different because of the way in which the wave inter-acts with and influences those particles. . . . The focus is on the essential fact that refraction is caused because of the change in speed of the wave as it enters the new medium. In a beam of sunlight, the red and the blue (and the yellow and the green . . .) waves travel together through space, all at exactly the same speed. But when they pass into some new medium, like glass, they slow down to various extents, in a way which depends on the wavelength—or equivalently the color—of the light. What this means, of course, is that the light gets *dispersed*: red light is slowed somewhat and (unless it lands perpendicularly) changes direction a little; blue light is slowed quite a bit more, and changes direction more appreciably; and so on. That is why a prism forms a spectrum, with the light spread out from blue to red.

Physicists usually pass light through a narrow slit before it hits the prism. Why do we do this? Why not just allow a broad beam of light from a lamp to fall onto the prism? The main reason is that it allows us to examine one particular wave-length in detail, without light of other wavelengths mixed in with it. We talk about the *spectral purity* of the spectrum we produce in this way. . . . [The slit] defines a narrow location from which light can enter the prism, and then the red light and the blue light are dispersed by the action of the prism to different spots. There will be no blue light mixed in with the red light, and vice versa, and we can study one particular wavelength in detail if we like.

By the way, Isaac Newton used a fairly wide hole to admit sunlight into his prism, so he had rather poor spectral purity. To his eye, then, the spectrum was completely continuous: he failed to detect the "missing" bits of light which define the *absorption lines*. . . . It is a real pity that a scientist of his powers missed out on this fundamental discovery—what might he have made of it?

In the Spirit of Self-Disclosure

My family was poor when I was very young. My parents, Theodore James and Mona Ann Mertens, had 12 children. My father worked as a traveling salesman to make enough money to support our basic needs, traveling extensively throughout the United States. My mother, I now realize, worked long days and nights taking care of us, raising a garden, putting food by, and making our clothes. Despite those early hardships, I have, in many respects, lived a life of privilege. My family valued hard work, education, and each other. We were taught to love one another and to reach out to those in need. We were also taught to live our values, even when it was difficult to do so. Through the end of sixth grade, I lived in Spokane Washington, and I do not have a recollection of seeing any people in my immediate environment who looked much different than I. In seventh grade I moved to Lexington, Kentucky (1963). Although the adjustment to a new place was challenging, I credit that move into an overtly different cultural milieu as the starting point of my consciousness of racial inequality. All of a sudden, I saw a world with many black people who were clearly living in less fortunate economic circumstances than I was. However, I did not see any black people at the schools that I attended or at the swimming pool where my family went for recreation. When I asked the teacher why there were no black people at my school, she patted my head and said, "They just prefer to be with their own kind."

I share this with you because it is my earliest recollection of becoming aware of social injustice. It gnawed at me such that I used my assignments at school to investigate such topics as the economic effects of the civil rights movement for African Americans. As I matured, I gradually became aware that race was not the only basis for discrimination in the United States. I became a lifelong feminist and found in that literature much to inspire me with regard to strategies of resistance. I also became aware that the feminist movement had not been inclusive of the concerns of women of color and that it was perceived by some women as reflective of white privilege, a haven for lesbians, and by others as women who hate men.

My professional career started in the University of Kentucky's College of Medicine as an educational researcher and program evaluator. I moved on from there to evaluate a professional development program using one of NASA's first satellites for social purposes, to deliver continuing education for people who lived in isolated rural areas along the Appalachian Mountain chain. As the funding for that endeavor wound down, I found employment at Ohio State University's National Center for Research in Vocational Education in the evaluation and policy analysis division. Based primarily on extant data (read: large data tapes gathered by someone else), I investigated the effects of vocational education for women in the workforce, people with disabilities, high school dropouts, and those in isolated rural areas, to name a few populations.

I felt discomfort based on my distance from, and lack of involvement with, the people in the programs described in the reports that I was sending to the U.S. Congress for policy hearings. Consequently, I looked around for a place where I could be *in* the community *with the people*. I was reading the *Washington Post* and saw a classified ad for an assistant professor at Gallaudet University, the world's only university specifically for deaf people. The fact that I had never met a deaf person did not dissuade me from applying. Nearly 30 years ago, they hired me and there I remain to this day. I studied deaf culture and sign language intensely. I passed the faculty sign competency test at an advanced level, although I am still learning more about sign language and deaf culture almost everyday. I realized that deaf people are a heterogeneous group with many dimensions of diversity and that to live and research/evaluate with this community meant that I needed to revise my understanding of methodology as I had learned it. Working in the deaf community provided me with the challenge of looking at intersections of inequity on the basis of not just hearing status, but also race/ethnicity, gender, socioeconomic status, and other characteristics that are relevant, depending on the specific context of the research or evaluation.

My work of integrating dimensions of diversity has not always followed a smooth path. Walking into unfamiliar territory is associated with risks, and I have at times stumbled inadvertently by breaking cultural mores. These experiences sometimes take a heavy toll, but I have a vision of the world as a better place, and that vision helps me get up and learn from my experiences.

One of the great rewards that I associate with my struggles to integrate diversity in my personal and scholarly work is the development of the transformative paradigm. My work around the transformative paradigm led to opportunities outside the world of deafness and into worlds where other dimensions of diversity were more salient. When I found myself invited to participate in a training session with the UNIFEM (United Nations Development Fund for Women) initiative in South Africa (November 2004), at first I suggested that they might better invite someone from Africa. After some back and forth, my hosts became a bit angry with me and suggested that I was insulting them by questioning their judgment as to whom they needed at this moment in their process. After I arrived, I felt that it was best to get the issue of my origins and their implications for my credibility in Africa out on the table directly. I explained that I was a hearing, able-bodied woman from the United States, with a PhD in educational psychology, professor at Gallaudet University with over 30 years of experience in research and evaluation, and a mother of two sons. Based on those characteristics, it was not immediately apparent why I should address them. I then shared with them a picture of myself with a statue of my mentor-in-spirit, Eleanor Roosevelt, along with these words that are inscribed in stone:

> The structure of world peace cannot be the work of one man, or one party, or one nation ... It must be a peace which rests on the cooperative effort of the whole world.
> —FRANKLIN DELANO ROOSEVELT

I did not go to Africa as a Western imperialist expert, but as a willing partner, if they would have me, to share our experiences and expertise as we worked together toward the goal of a better world.

References

Abbott, G., Bievenue, L., Damarin, S., & Kramarae, C. (2007). Gender equity in the use of educational technology. In S. Klein (Ed.), *Handbook for achieving gender equity through education* (2nd ed., pp. 191–214). Mahwah, NJ: Erlbaum.

Altschuld, J. (1999). *From needs assessment to action.* Thousand Oaks, CA: Sage.

American Anthropological Association. (2004). *Statement on ethnography and institutional review boards.* Retrieved December 14, 2006, from *www.aaa-net.org/stmts/irb.htm*.

American Educational Research Association, American Psychological Association, & National Council on Measurement in Education. (1999). *Standards for educational and psychological testing.* Washington, DC: American Educational Research Association.

American Evaluation Association. (2003). American Evaluation Association Response to U.S. Department of Education, notice of proposed priority, Federal Register RIN 1890-ZA00, November 4, 2003, "Scientifically Based Evaluation Methods." Retrieved October 25, 2004, from *www.eval.org/doestatement.htm*.

American Evaluation Association. (2004). *American Evaluation Association's guiding principles.* Retrieved August 26, 2006, from *www.eval.org/Publications/GuidingPrinciples.asp*.

American Psychological Association. (1991a). Avoiding heterosexual bias in language. *American Psychologist, 46*(9), 973–974.

American Psychological Association. (1991b). Avoiding heterosexual bias in psychological research. *American Psychologist, 46*(9), 957–963.

American Psychological Association. (2000a). *Guidelines for psychotherapy with lesbian, gay, and bisexual clients.* Washington, DC: Author.

American Psychological Association. (2000b). *Guidelines for research in ethnic minority communities.* Council of National Psychological Associations for the Advancement of Ethnic Minority Interests, Washington, DC: Author.

American Psychological Association. (2001). *Publication manual of the American Psychological Association* (5th ed.). Washington, DC: Author.

American Psychological Association. (2002). *Guidelines on multicultural education, training, research, practice, and organizational change for psychologists.* Washington, DC: Author.

American Psychological Association. (2008a). *APA government relations: Public interest policy.* Retrieved January 16, 2008, from *www.apa.org/ppo/pi.*

American Psychological Association. (2008b). *Answers to your questions about transgender individuals and gender identity.* Retrieved January 21, 2008, from *www.apa.org/topics/transgender.html#whatis.*

Amsden, J., & VanWynsberghe, R. (2005). Community mapping as a research tool with youth. *Action Research, 3*(4), 357–381.

Anderson, E. (1999). *Code of the street: Decency, violence, and the moral life of the inner city.* New York: Norton.

Anderson, L. (2006). Analytic autoethnography. *Journal of Contemporary Ethnography, 35*(4), 373–395.

Anderson, M. B., Howarth, A. M., & Overholt, C. (1992). *A framework for people-oriented planning in refugee situations taking account of women.* Geneva: United Nations High Commission on Refugees.

Anderson, M. B., & Woodrow, P. J. (1998). *Rising from the ashes: Development strategies in times of disaster* (2nd ed.). Boulder, CO: Rienner.

Ashcroft, B., Griffiths, G., & Tiffin, H. (1998). *Post-colonial studies: The key concepts.* London: Routledge.

Association of Canadian Universities for Northern Studies. (1997). *Ethical principles for the conduct of research in the North Yukon College.* Retrieved September 16, 2002, from *www.yukoncollege.yk.ca/~agraham/82comp97.htm.*

Attenborough, K. (2007). Soft systems in a hardening world: Evaluating urban regeneration. In B. Williams & I. Iman (Eds.), *Systems concepts in evaluation* (pp. 75–88). Point Reyes, CA: Edge Press of Inverness.

Balch, G., & Mertens, D. M. (1999). Focus group design and group dynamics: Lessons from deaf and hard of hearing participants. *American Journal of Evaluation, 20*(2), 265–277.

Balfanz, R., Legters, N., & Jordan, W. (2004). *Catching up: Impact of the Talent Development ninth grade instructional interventions in reading and mathematics in high poverty high schools.* Retrieved December 14, 2006, *www.csos.jhu.edu/crespar/techReports/Report69.pdf.*

Bamberger, M., Rugh, J., & Mabry, L. (2006). *Real world evaluation.* Thousand Oaks, CA: Sage.

Barker, J., & Weller, S. (2003). "Never work with children?": The geography of methodological issues in research with children. *Qualitative Research, 3*(2), 207–227.

Barnes, V., Clouder, D. L., Pritchard, J., Hughes, C., & Purkis, J. (2003). Deconstructing dissemination: Dissemination as qualitative research. *Qualitative Research, 3*(2), 147–164.

Battiste, M. (Ed.). (2000a). *Reclaiming indigenous voice and vision.* Vancouver: University of British Columbia Press.

Battiste, M. (2000b). Maintaining aboriginal identity, language, and culture in modern society. In M. Battiste (Ed.), *Reclaiming indigenous voice and vision* (pp. 192–208). Vancouver: University of British Columbia Press.

Bawden, R. (2006). A systemic evaluation of an agricultural development: A focus on the worldview challenge. In B. Williams & I. Iman (Eds.), *Systems concepts in evaluation* (pp. 35–46). Point Reyes, CA: Edge Press of Inverness.

Beebe, J. (2001). *Rapid assessment process: An introduction.* Walnut Creek, CA: Altamira Press.

Bell, L. A. (2001, May–June). *Self-awareness and social justice pedagogy.* Paper presented at the National Conference on Race and Ethnicity in Higher Education, Seattle, WA.

Bennis, W. G., & Thomas, R. J. (2002). Crucibles of leadership. *Harvard Business Review, 80*(9), 39–45.

Bienvenu, M. (2003). *Developing a prototype for a monolingual ASL dictionary.* PhD dissertation, Union Institute and University, Cincinnati, OH. Retrieved April 29, 2007, from ProQuest Digital Dissertations database.

Bishop, R. (1996). Addressing issues in self-determination and legitimation in Kaupapa Maori research. In B. Webber (Ed.), *He paipai korero.* Wellington: New Zealand Council for Educational Research.

Bishop, R. (2005). Freeing ourselves from neocolonial domination in research: A Kaupapa Maori approach to creating knowledge. In Y. S. Lincoln & N. K. Denzin (Eds.), *The Sage handbook of qualitative research* (3rd ed., pp. 109–138). Thousand Oaks, CA: Sage.

Bledsoe, K. (2001). Why I believe theory-driven evaluation is useful in program development for underserved and diverse populations. *Mechanisms: The Newsletter of the Program Theory and Theory-Driven Evaluation Topical Interest Group, 5,* 3–6.

Bledsoe, K. (2005). Using theory-driven evaluation with underserved communities: Promoting program development and program sustainability. In S. Hood, R. Hopson, & H. Frierson (Eds.), *The role of culture and cultural context* (pp. 175–196). Greenwich, CT: Information Age.

Bledsoe, K., & Graham, J. A. (2005). Using multiple evaluation approaches in program evaluation. *American Journal of Evaluation, 26*(3), 302–319.

Bloom, C. M., & Erlandson, D. A. (2003). African-American women principals in urban schools: Realities, (re)constructions, and resolutions. *Educational Administration Quarterly, 39*(3), 339–369.

Blow, F. C., Zeber, J. E., McCarthy, J. F., Valenstein, M., Gillon, L., & Bingham, C. R. (2004). Ethnicity and diagnostic patterns in veterans with psychoses. *Social Psychiatry and Psychiatric Epidemiology, 39*(10), 841–851.

Booth, D. (1998). Coping with cost recovery in Zambia: A sectoral policy study. In J. Holland & J. Blackburn (Eds.), *Whose voice?: Participatory research and policy change* (pp. 28–30). London: Intermediate Technology.

Boyer, D. (2004). *Initiating partnerships: Gathering the players.* Retrieved May 9, 2008, from *www.uml.edu/centers/CFWC/Community_Tips/Research%20 Ethics/Research%20Ethics%20Tipsheets.pdf.*

Boykin, A. W. (2000). The Talent Development Model of Schooling: Placing students at promise for academic success. *Journal of Education for Students Placed at Risk, 5*(1/2), 3–25.

Brabeck, M. M. (Ed.). (2000). *Practicing feminist ethics in psychology.* Washington, DC: American Psychological Association.

Brainerd, J. (2003). Federal agency says oral history is not subject to rules on human research volunteers. *Chronicle of Higher Education.* Retrieved October 21, 2003, from *chronicle.com/daily/2003/10/2003102101n.htm.*

Brooks, P. (2006, July). *Racism, ethics, and research.* Paper presented at the International Sociological Association World Congress, Durban, South Africa.

Broom, M. F., & Klein, D. C. (1999). *Power: The infinite game.* Ellicott City, MD: Sea Otter Press.

Brown, S. (2006). Disputed report on IBM workers is finally published, in peer-reviewed online journal. Chronicle of Higher Education (online version). Retrieved May 9, 2008, from *chronicle.com/daily/2006/10/2006102002a. htm.*

Bryman, A. (2004). *Social research methods* (2nd ed.). Oxford: Oxford University Press.

Burbules, N. (2009). Privacy and new technologies: The limits of traditional research ethics. In D. M. Mertens & P. Ginsberg (Eds.), *Handbook of social research ethics* (pp. 537–549). Thousand Oaks, CA: Sage.

Butty, J. L. M., Reid, M. D., & LaPoint, V. (2004). A culturally responsive evaluation approach applied to the Talent Development School-to-Career Intervention Program. In V. G. Thomas & F. I. Stevens (Eds.), *Co-constructing a contextually responsive evaluation framework* (pp. 37–47). San Francisco: Wiley.

Caldwell, J. Y., Davis, J. D., Du Bois, B., Echo-Waek, H., Erickson, J. S., Goins, R. T., et al. (2005). Culturally competent research with American Indians and Alaska Natives: Findings and recommendations of the First Symposium of the Work Group on American Indian Research and Program Evaluation Methodology. *American Indian and Alaska Native Mental Health Research, 12*(1), 1–21.

Campbell, D. T., & Stanley, J. C. (1966). *Experimental and quasi-experimental designs for research.* Skokie, IL: Rand McNally.

Cardoza Clayson, Z., Castaneda, X., Sanchez, E., & Brindis, C. (2002). Unequal power—changing landscapes: Negotiations between evaluation stakeholders in Latino communities. *American Journal of Evaluation, 23*(1), 33–44.

Carvello, S., & White, H. (2004). Theory based evaluation: The case of social funds. *American Journal of Evaluation, 25*(2), 5–12, 18.

Center for Universal Design. (1997). What is universal design? Retrieved October 12, 2004, from www.*design.ncsu.edu/cud/univ_design/ud.htm.*

Centers for Disease Control. (2006). *Identifying ground-breaking behavioral interventions to prevent human immunodeficiency virus (HIV) transmission in high-risk groups center for disease control.* Retrieved February 23, 2006, from *www.grants.gov/search/search.do?mode=VIEW&oppId=8140.*

Charmaz, K. (2005). Grounded theory in the 21st century. In N. K. Denzin & Y. S. Lincoln (Eds.), *The Sage handbook of qualitative research* (3rd ed., pp. 507–535). Thousand Oaks, CA: Sage.

Charmaz, K. (2006). *Constructing grounded theory: A practical guide through qualitative analysis.* London: Sage.

Charmaz, K., & Mitchell, R. G., Jr. (1996). The myth of silent authorship: Self, substance, and style in ethnographic writing. *Symbolic Interaction, 19*(4), 285–302.

Cheek, J. (2005). The practice and politics of funded qualitative research. In N. K. Denzin & Y. S. Lincoln (Eds.), *The Sage handbook of qualitative research* (3rd ed., pp. 387–410). Thousand Oaks, CA: Sage.

Cherryholmes, C. H. (1993). Reading research. *Journal of Curriculum Studies, 25*(1), 1–32.

Chiev, S. (2004). *Everything you always wanted to know about IRBs.* Retrieved May 9, 2008, from *www.uml.edu/centers/CFWC/Community_Tips/Research%20Ethics/Research%20Ethics%20Tipsheets.pdf.*

Chilisa, B. (2005). Educational research within postcolonial Africa: A critique of HIV/AIDS research in Botswana. *International Journal of Qualitative Studies in Education, 18,* 659–684.

Chilisa, B., Bennell, P. S., & Hyde, K. (2001). *The impact of HIV/AIDS on the University of Botswana: Developing a strategic response.* London: Department for International Development (Serial Number 44).

Chilisa, B., & Preece, J. (2005). *Research methods for adult educators in Africa.* Cape Town, South Africa: Pearson.

Chiu, L. F. (2003). Transformational potential of focus group practice in participatory action research. *Action Research, 1*(2), 165–183.

Christians, C. (2005). Ethics and politics in qualitative research. In N. K. Denzin & Y. S. Lincoln (Eds.), *The Sage handbook of qualitative research* (3rd ed., pp. 139–164). Thousand Oaks, CA: Sage.

Clapp, R. W. (2006). Mortality among U.S. employees of a large computer-manufacturing company: 1969–2001. *Environmental Health: A Global Access Science Source, 5*(30).

Clarke, E., & McCreanor, T. (2006). *He wahine tangi tikapa . . . :* Statutory investigative processes and the grieving of Maori families who have lost a baby to SIDS. *Kotuitui: New Zealand Journal of Social Sciences Online, 1,* 25–43.

Cleaver, F. (2000). Institutions, agency and the limitations of participatory approaches to development. In B. Cooke & U. Kothari (Eds.), *Participation: The new tyranny?* (pp. 36–55). London: Zed Books.

Clewell, B. C., & Campbell, P. B. (2002). Taking stock: Where we've been, where we are, where we're going. *Journal of Women and Minorities in Science and Engineering, 8,* 255–284.

Cohn, D. (2005, June 9). Hispanic growth surge fueled by births in U.S. *The Washington Post,* A1–A7.

Collins, S. B. (2005). An understanding of poverty from those who are poor. *Action Research, 3*(1), 9–31.

Community Tool Box. (2006). Community Tool Box. Retrieved December 14, 2006, from *ctb.ku.edu/tools/tk/en/corecompetencies.jsp.*

Cook, T. D. (1985). Postpositivist critical multiplism. In R. L. Shotland & M. M. Mark (Eds.), *Social science and social policy* (pp. 21–62). Thousand Oaks, CA: Sage.

Cooper, H. M. (1998). *Synthesizing research* (3rd ed.). Thousand Oaks, CA: Sage.

Cooper, H. M., & Hedges, L. V. (Eds.). (1994). *The handbook of research synthesis.* New York: Sage.

Corbin, J., & Morse, J. M. (2003). The unstructured interactive interview: Issues of reciprocity and risks when dealing with sensitive topics. *Qualitative Inquiry, 9*(3), 335–354.

Corn, A. L., & Spungin, S. J. (2003). *Free and appropriate public education and the personnel crisis for students with visual impairments and blindness.* Gainesville, FL: Center on Personnel studies in Special Education. Retrieved September 21, 2004, from *www.copsse.org.*

Cornwall, A., Harrison, E., & Whitehead, A. (2004). *Repositioning feminisms in gender and development.* Brighton, Sussex, UK: University of Sussex Press.

Costello, M. (2004). *Ethical considerations in participatory research: The researcher's point of view.* Retrieved May 9, 2008, from *www.uml.edu/centers/CFWC/Community_Tips/Research%20Ethics/Research%20Ethics%20Tipsheets.pdf.*

Cram, F., Ormond, A., & Carter, L. (2004). *Researching our relations: Reflections on ethics and marginalization.* Paper presented at the Kamehauneha Schools 2004 Research Conference on Hawaiian Well-being, Kea'au, HI. Retrieved September 15, 2006, from *www.ksbe.edu/pase/pdf/KSResearchConference/2004presentations.*

Creswell, J. W., & Plano Clark, V. L. (2007). *Designing and conducting mixed methods research.* Thousand Oaks, CA: Sage.

Cross, T., Earle, K., Echo-Hawk Solie, H., & Manness, K. (2000). *Cultural strengths and challenges in implementing a system of care model in American Indian communities. Systems of Care: Promising Practices in Children's Mental Health, Vol. I.* Washington, DC: Center for Effective Collaboration and Practice, American Institutes Research.

Cummins, J. (2000). *Language, power and pedagogy: Bilingual children in the crossfire.* Buffalo, NY: Multilingual Matters.

Davies, R. (1998). An evolutionary approach to organizational learning: An experiment by an NGO in Bangladesh. *Impact Assessment and Project Appraisal, 16*(3), 243–250.

Davis, F., Greeno, J. G., & West, M. M. (2000). *Improvement of mathematics literacy in African-American students: Preparation for algebra and higher mathematics.* Technical report for the National Science Foundation.

De Jesus, M., &. Lykes, M. B. (2004). Racism and "whiteness" in transitions to peace: Indigenous peoples, human rights, and the struggle for justice. In L. Weis & M. Fine (Eds.), *Working method: Research and social justice* (pp. 331–344). New York: Routledge.

Delgado Bernal, D. (1998). Using a Chicana feminist epistemology in educational research. *Harvard Educational Review, 68,* 555–582.

Denzin, N. K., & Lincoln, Y. S. (Eds.). (2005). *The Sage handbook of qualitative research* (3rd ed.). Thousand Oaks, CA: Sage.

Development Planning Unit, University of London. (1997). *DPU gender policy and planning programme training materials.* London: Author.

Devereux, S. (Ed.). (2006). *The new famines.* New York: Routledge.

Deyhle, D., & Swisher, K. (1997). Research in American Indian, Alaskan, and Native American education: From assimilation to self-determination. In M. Apple (Ed.), *Review of research in education* (pp. 113–147). Washington, DC: American Educational Research Association.

Diamond, M. (2000). Sex and gender: Same or different? *Feminism and Psychology, 10*(1), 46–54.

Dillard, C. (2000a). The substance of things hoped for, the evidence of things not seen: Examining an endarkened feminist epistemology in educational research and leadership. *Qualitative Studies in Education, 13*(6), 661–681.

Dillard, C. (2000b, March). *Cultural considerations in paradigm proliferation.* Paper presented at the annual meeting of the American Educational Research Association, New Orleans.

Dillman, D. (1999). *Mail and Internet surveys: The tailored designed method* (2nd ed.). New York: Wiley.

Dodd, S. J. (2009). LGBTQ: Protecting vulnerable subjects in *all* studies. In D. M. Mertens & P. Ginsberg (Eds.), *Handbook of social research ethics* (pp. 474–488). Thousand Oaks, CA: Sage.

Donaldson, S. (2001). Mediator and moderator analysis in program development. In S. Sussman (Ed.), *Handbook of program development for health behavior research* (pp. 470–496). Thousand Oaks, CA: Sage.

Dube, M. W. (2001). Divining Ruth for international relations. In M. W. Dube (Ed.), *Other ways of reading the Bible* (pp. 67–79). Geneva: WCC Publications.

DuBois, W. E. B. (1920). The souls of white folk (from Darkwater.) In N. Huggins (Ed.), *W. E. B. DuBois: Writings* (pp. 357–547). New York: Library of America.

Duran, B., & Duran, E. (2000). Applied postcolonial clinical and research strategies. In M. Battiste (Ed.), *Reclaiming indigenous voice and vision* (pp. 86–100). Vancouver, BC: University of British Columbia Press.

Duran, E. (1990). *Transforming the soul wound.* Berkeley: Folklore Press.

Durland, M. M. (2005). Exploring and understanding relationship. In M. M. Durland & K. A. Fredericks (Eds.), Social network analysis in program evaluation: New directions for evaluation (pp. 25–40). San Francisco: Wiley.

Easton, V. J., & McColl, J. H. (2006). *Statistics glossary.* Retrieved September 11, 2006, from *www.cas.lancs.ac.uk/glossary_v1.1/confint.html#confinterval.*

Eichler, M. (1991). *Nonsexist research methods.* New York: Routledge.

Electronic Statistics Textbook. (2006). Tulsa, OK: StatSoft. Retrieved May 9, 2008, from *www.statsoft.com/textbook/stathome.html.*

Elze, D. (2003a). Gay, lesbian, and bisexual youths' perceptions of their high school environments and comfort in school. *Children and Schools, 25, 4,* 225–239.

Elze, D. (2003b). 8,000 miles and still counting. . . . researching gay, lesbian, and bisexual adolescents for research. *Journal of Gay and Lesbian Social Services, 15*(1/2), 127–145.

Elze, D. (2005). Research with sexual minority youths: Where do we go from here? *Journal of Gay and Lesbian Social Services: Issues in Practice, Policy and Research, 18*(2), 73–99.

Endo, T., Joh, T., & Yu, H. C. (2003). *Voices from the field: Health and evaluation leaders on multicultural evaluation.* Oakland, CA: Social Policy Research Associates.

Erickson, F., & Gutierrez, K. (2002). Culture, rigor, and science in educational research. *Educational Researcher, 31*(8), 21–24.

Fals Borda, O. (2006). Participatory (action) research in social theory. In P. Reason & H. Bradbury (Eds.), *Handbook of action research* (pp. 27–37). London: Sage. (Original work published 2001)

Feller, B. (2006, September 23). Audit finds ethical lapses in U.S. reading program. *Washington Post*, p. A02. Retrieved September 10, 2008, from *http://www.washingtonpost.com/wp-dyn/content/article/2006/09/22/AR2006092201356.html*

Fernandez, L. (2002). Telling stories about school: Using critical race and Latino critical theories to document Latina/Latino education and resistance. *Qualitative Inquiry, 8*(1), 45–65.

Ferrell, K. A., Luckner, J. L., Jackson, L., Correa, S. M., Muir, S. G., Howell, J. J., et al. (2004). *All learners, all the time: Including students with low-incidence disabilities.* Paper presented at the Council for Exceptional Children annual convention, New Orleans. Retrieved September 21, 2004, from *www.nclid.unco.edu/Presentations/CEC/index.html.*

Fidler, F. (2002). The fifth edition of the APA publication manual: Why its statistics recommendations are so controversial. *Educational and Psychological Measurement, 62*(5), 749–770.

Fine, M., Weis, L., Pruitt, L. P., & Burns, A. (Eds.). (2004). *Off white* (2nd ed.). New York: Routledge.

Firme, T. (2006, November). *Improved community conditions in a Brazilian slum: A significant consequence of its evaluation.* Paper presented at the annual meeting of the American Evaluation Association, Portland, OR.

Fisher, C. B. (2003). *Decoding the ethics code: A practical guide for psychologists.* Thousand Oaks, CA: Sage.

Flyvbjerg, B. (2006). Five misunderstandings about case study research. *Qualitative Inquiry, 12*(2), 219–245.

Foa, U., & Foa, E. (1974). *Societal structures of the mind.* Springfield, IL: Charles C Thomas.

Foucault, M. (1979). *The history of sexuality: Part 1.* London: Lane.

Foucault, M. (1980). Power/knowledge: Selected interviews and other writings (1972–1977) (C. Gordon, Ed.). New York: Pantheon Books.

Frable, D. E. S. (1997). Gender, racial, ethnic, sexual, and class identities. *Annual Review of Psychology, 48*, 139–162.

Fredericks, K. A., & Durland, M. M. (2005). The historical evolution and basic concepts of social network analysis. In M. M. Durland & K. A. Fredericks

(Eds.), *Social network analysis in program evaluation: New directions for evaluation* (pp. 15–24). San Francisco: Wiley.

Freebody, P. & Power, D. (2001). Interviewing deaf adults in postsecondary settings: Stories, cultures and life histories. *Journal of Deaf Studies and Deaf Education, 6*(2), 131–142.

Freire, P. (1970a). *Education as the practice of freedom: Cultural action for freedom.* Cambridge, MA: Harvard Educational Review/Center for the Study of Development.

Freire, P. (1970b). *Pedagogy of the oppressed.* New York: Seabury.

Freire, P. (1973). *Education for critical consciousness.* New York: Seabury.

Frierson, H. T., Hood, S., & Hughes, G. B. (2002). Strategies that address culturally responsive evaluation. In J. Frechtling (Ed.), *The 2002 user friendly handbook for project evaluation* (pp. 63–73). Arlington, VA: National Science Foundation.

Garbani, P. (2004). Knowledge creation in research partnerships. Retrieved May 9, 2008, from *www.uml.edu/centers/CFWC/Community_Tips/Research%20 Ethics/Research%20Ethics%20Tipsheets.pdf.*

Gaventa, J., & Cornwall, A. (2006). Power and knowledge. In P. Reason & H. Bradbury (Eds.), *Handbook of action research* (pp. 71–82). London: Sage. (Original work published 2001)

Geertz, C. (1973). Thick description: Toward an interpretive theory of culture. In C. Geertz (Ed.), *The interpretation of cultures* (pp. 3–30). New York: Basic Books.

Gerner de Garcia, B. (2004). Literacy for Latino deaf students: A socio-cultural approach. *Gallaudet Newsletter*, Washington, DC, Gallaudet University.

Gill, C. (1999). Invisibility ubiquity: The surprising relevance of disability issues in evaluation. *American Journal of Evaluation, 29*(2), 279–287.

Gilmore, P., & Smith, D. (2005). Seizing academic power: Indigenous subaltern voices, metaliteracy, and counternarratives in higher education. In T. McCarty (Ed.), *Language, literacy, and power in schooling* (pp. 67–88). Mahwah, NJ: Erlbaum.

Glaser, B. G., & Strauss, A. L. (1967). *The discovery of grounded theory.* Chicago: Aldine.

Glod, M. (2008, May 2). Study questions "No Child" Act's reading plan: Lauded program fails to improve test scores. *Washington Post*, p. A01. Retrieved May 9, 2008, from *http://www.washingtonpost.com/wp-dyn/content/article/2008/05/01/AR2008050101399_pf.html.*

Gordon, B. (1990). The necessity of African-American epistemology for educational theory and practice. *Journal of Education, 172*(3), 88–106.

Graveline, F. J. (2000). Circle as methodology: Enacting an aboriginal paradigm. *Qualitative Studies in Education, 13*(4), 361–370.

Greene, J. C. (2008). *Mixed methods in social inquiry.* San Francisco: Jossey-Bass.

Greene, J. C., Caracelli, V. J., & Graham, W. F. (1989). Toward a conceptual framework for mixed-methods evaluation designs. *Educational Evaluation and Policy Analysis, 11*(3), 255–274.

Greene, J. C., & Pranis, K. (2007). *Gang wars: The failure of enforcement tactics and the need for effective public safety strategies.* Washington, DC: Justice Policy Institute.

Greenwood, D. J., Brydon-Miller, M., & Shafer, C. (2006). Intellectual property and action research. *Action Research, 4*(1), 81–95.

Greenwood, D. J., & Levine, M. (2007). *Introduction to action research.* Thousand Oaks, CA: Sage.

Grove, J. T., Kibel, B. M., & Haas, T. (2005). *EVALULEAD guide.* Oakland, CA: Public Health Institute.

Guba, E. G., & Lincoln, Y. S. (1989). *Fourth generation evaluation.* Newbury Park, CA: Sage.

Guba, E. G., & Lincoln, Y. S. (1994). Competing paradigms in qualitative research. In N. K. Denzin & Y. S. Lincoln (Eds.), *Handbook of qualitative research* (pp. 105–117). Thousand Oaks, CA: Sage.

Guba, E. G., & Lincoln, Y. S. (2005). Paradigmatic controversies, contradictions, and emerging confluence. In N. K. Denzin & Y. S. Lincoln (Eds.), *The Sage handbook of qualitative research* (3rd ed., pp. 191–215). Thousand Oaks, CA: Sage.

Gubrium, J., & Holstein, J. (Eds.). (2002). *Handbook of interview research: Context and method.* Thousand Oaks, CA: Sage.

Gustavsen, B. (2006). Theory and practice: The mediating discourse. In P. Reason & H. Bradbury (Eds.), *Handbook of action research* (pp. 17–26). London: Sage. (Original work published 2001)

Guthrie, K., Louie, J., David, T., & Foster, C. C. (2005). *The challenge of assessing policy and advocacy activities: Strategies for a prospective evaluation approach.* Los Angeles: The California Endowment. Retrieved December 14, 2006, from *www.calendow.org/reference/publications/pdf/npolicy/51565_CEAdvocacyBook8FINAL.pdf.*

Guzman, B. L. (2003). Examining the role of cultural competency in program evaluation: Visions for new millennium evaluators. In S. I. Donaldson & M. Scriven (Eds.), *Evaluating social programs and problems: Visions for the new millennium* (pp. 167–182). Mahwah, NJ: Erlbaum.

Habermas, J. (1981). *The theory of communicative action* (T. McCarthy, Trans., 2 vols.). Cambridge, MA: Polity.

Habermas, J. (1996). *Postmetaphysical thinking: Philosophical essays* (W. M. Hohengarten, Trans.). Cambridge, MA: MIT Press.

Hall, M., & Hood, D. W. (2005). Persuasive language, responsive design: A framework for interculturally responsive evaluation. In S. Hood, R. Hopsonh, & H. Frierson (Eds.), *The role of culture and cultural context* (pp. 39–58). Greenwich, CT: Information Age.

Harris, R., Holmes, H., & Mertens, D. M. (2009). Research ethics in sign language communities. *Sign Language Studies, 9*(2).

Hartsock, N. (1974). Political change: Two perspectives on power. *Quest: A Feminist Quarterly, 1*(1). (Reprinted in *Building Feminist Theory: Essays from Quest.* [1981]. New York: Longman, pp. 3–19.)

Hayduk, L. A. (1987). *Structural equation modeling with LISREL: Essentials and advances.* Baltimore: Johns Hopkins University Press.

Henderson, J. Y. (2000). Postcolonial ledger drawing: Legal reform. In M. Battiste

(Ed.), *Reclaiming indigenous voice and vision* (pp. 161–171). Vancouver: University of British Columbia Press.

Henson, R. (2006). Effect-size measures and meta-analytic thinking in counseling psychology research. *Counseling Psychologist, 34*(5), 601–629.

Heron, J., & Reason, P. (2006). The practice of co-operative inquiry: Research "with" rather than "on" people. In P. Reason & H. Bradbury (Eds.), *Handbook of action research* (pp. 144–154). London: Sage. (Original work published 2001)

Hesse-Biber, S., & Leavy, P. (2006). *The practice of qualitative research.* Thousand Oaks, CA: Sage.

Hill, N. S., Jr. (Ed). (1994). *Words of power: Voices from Indian America.* Golden, CO: Fulcrum.

Holland, J., & Campbell, J. (Eds.). (2005). *Methods in development research.* Warwickshire, UK: ITDG.

Hood, S., Hopson, R., & Frierson, H. (Eds.). (2005). *The role of culture and cultural context.* Greenwich, CT: Information Age.

hooks, b. (1990). *Yearning: Race, gender, and cultural politics.* Boston: South End.

Husserl, E. (1970). *Logical investigation.* New York: Humanities Press.

Huygens, I. (2002, June). *Journeys away from dominance: Dissonance, struggle, and right relationships—the journey to accepting indigenous authority.* Paper presented at the 8th biennial conference of the Society for Community Research and Action, Atlanta, GA.

Irwin, C. (2005, September). *Public opinion and the politics of peace research: Northern Ireland, Balkans, Israel, Palestine, Cyprus, Muslim world and the "war on terror."* Paper presented at the WAPOR 58th annual conference, Cannes, France.

Jackson, K., & Trochim, W. (2002). Concept mapping as an alternative approach for the analysis of open-ended survey responses. *Organizational Research Methods, 5*(4), 307–336.

Jimerson, J. B., & Oware, M. K. (2006). Telling the code of the street: An ethnomethodological ethnography. *Journal of Contemporary Ethnography, 35*(1), 24–50.

Johnson, H. A. (2003). *U.S. deaf education teacher preparation programs: A look at the present and a vision for the future.* Gainesville, FL: Center on Personnel Studies in Special Education. Retrieved September 21, 2004, from *www. copsse.org.*

Johnson, H., & Mertens, D. M. (2006). New strategies to address old problems: Web based technologies, resources, and applications to enhance K–20 deaf education. In D. Martin & D. Moores (Eds.), *Deaf learners: Developments in curriculum and instruction.* Washington, DC: Gallaudet Press.

Jones, S. H. (2005). Autoethnography: Making the personal political. In N. K. Denzin & Y. S. Lincoln (Eds.), *The Sage handbook of qualitative research* (3rd. ed., pp. 763–792). Thousand Oaks, CA: Sage.

Jöreskog, K. G., & Sörbom, D. (1993). *Structural equation modeling and the SIM-PLIS command language.* Chicago: Scientific Software International.

Kabeer, N. (1994). *Reversed realities: Gender hierarchies in development thought.* London: Verso.

Kahn, M. J. (1991). Factors affecting the coming out process for lesbians. *Journal of Homosexuality, 21*(3), 47–70.

Kawakami, A. J., Aton, K., Cram, F., Lai, M., & Porima, L. (2008). Improving the practice of evaluation through indigenous values and methods. In N. L. Smith & P. R. Brandon (Eds.), *Fundamental issues in evaluation* (pp. 219–242). New York: Guilford Press.

Kellogg Foundation, W. K. (2006). *Competence: Confidence in the middle years.* Retrieved March 2, 2006, from *www.wkkf.org/default.aspx?tabid=55&CID=3&ProjCID=40&ProjID=63&NID=28&LanguageID=0.*

Kemmis, S. (2006). Exploring the relevance of critical theory for action research: Emancipatory action research in the footsteps of Jurgen Habermas. In P. Reason & H. Bradbury (Eds.), *Handbook of action research* (pp. 94–105). London: Sage. (Original work published 2001)

Kendall, F. E. (2006). *Understanding white privilege.* New York: Routledge.

Kershaw, T. (1992). Afrocentrism and the Afrocentric method. *Western Journal of Black Studies, 16*(3), 160–168.

Ketterlin-Geller, L. R. (2005). Knowing what all students know: Procedures for developing universal design for assessment. *Journal of Technology, Learning, and Assessment, 4*(2). Available at *www/jtla.org.*

King, J. A., Nielsen, J. E., & Colby, J. (2004). Lessons for culturally competent evaluation from the study of a multicultural initiative. In M. Thompson-Robinson, R. Hopson, & S. SenGupta (Eds.), *In search of cultural competence in evaluation* (pp. 67–80). San Francisco: Wiley.

King, J. E. (Ed.). (2005). *Black education: A transformative research and action agenda for the new century.* Washington, DC: American Educational Research Association Commission on Research in Black Education.

Kirkhart, K. (1995). Seeking multicultural validity: A postcard from the road. *Evaluation Practice, 16*(1), 1–12.

Kirkhart, K. (2005). Through a cultural lens: Reflections on validity and theory in evaluation. In S. Hood, R. Hopson, & H. Frierson (Eds.), *The role of culture and cultural context* (pp. 21–38). Greenwich, CT: Information Age.

Kline, R. B. (2004). *Beyond significance testing: Reforming data analysis methods in behavioral research.* Washington, DC: American Psychological Association.

Kosciw, J., Byard, E., Fischer, S. N., & Joslin, C. (2007). Gender equity and lesbian, gay, bisexual, and transgender issues in education. In S. Klein (Ed.), *Handbook for achieving gender equity through education* (2nd ed., pp. 553–572). Mahwah, NJ: Erlbaum.

Kozol, J. (2005). Still separate, still unequal: America's educational apartheid. *Harper's Magazine, 311*(1864). Retrieved December 13, 2005, from *www.mindfully.org/Reform/2005/American-Apartheid-Education1sep05.htm.*

Kret, N. (2004). *Questions to ask about community based research partnerships.* Retrieved May 9, 2008, from *www.uml.edu/centers/CFWC/Community_Tips/Research%20Ethics/Research%20Ethics%20Tipsheets.pdf.*

Kuhn, T. (1962). *Structure of scientific revolutions.* Chicago: University of Chicago Press.

Kumar, R., & Saidah, C. (2005). *Disability and early tsunami relief efforts in India, Indonesia, and Thailand.* International Disability Rights Monitor.

Washington, DC: Center for International Rehabilitation. Available at *www. disability.ws/idrm*.

Ladd, P. (2003). *Understanding deaf culture: In search of deafhood*. Tonawanda, NY: Multilingual Matters.

Ladson-Billings, G. (2000). Racialized discourses and ethnic epistemologies. In N. K. Denzin & Y. S. Lincoln (Eds.), *Handbook of qualitative research* (2nd ed.). Thousand Oaks, CA: Sage.

Ladson-Billings, G. (2006). From the achievement gap to the education debt: Understanding achievement in U.S. schools. *Educational Researcher, 35*(7), 3–12.

LaFrance, J. (2004). Culturally competent evaluation in Indian Country. In S. SenGupta, R. Hopson, & M. Thompson-Robinson (Eds.), *In search of cultural competence in evaluation toward principles and practices: New directions for evaluation* (pp. 39–50). San Francisco: Jossey-Bass.

LaPoint, V., & Jackson, H. J. (2004). Evaluation of the co-construction of the Family, School, and Community Partnership Program in a low-income urban high school. In V. G. Thomas & F. I. Stevens (Eds.), *Co-constructing a contextually responsive evaluation framework: New directions for evaluation* (pp. 25–36). San Francisco: Wiley.

LatCrit Primer. (2000, May 4–7). *Fact sheet: LatCrit*. Paper presented at the 5th annual LatCrit conference, Breckenridge, CO.

Lather, P. (1992). Critical frames in educational research: Feminist and post-structural perspectives. *Theory and Practice, 31*(2), 1–13.

Lee, K. (2004). *The meaning and practice of civic participation among four immigrant communities*. Unpublished doctoral dissertation, Graduate College of the Union Institute and University, Cincinnati, OH.

Lincoln, Y. S. (1995, April). *Standards for qualitative research*. Paper presented at the annual meeting of the American Educational Research Association, San Francisco.

Lincoln, Y. S., & Denzin, N. K. (2005). The eighth and ninth moments: Qualitative research in/and the fractured future. In Y. S. Lincoln & N. K. Denzin (Eds.), *The Sage handbook of qualitative research* (3rd ed., pp. 1115–1126). Thousand Oaks, CA: Sage.

Lincoln, Y. S., & Guba, E. G. (1985). *Naturalistic inquiry*. Beverly Hills, CA: Sage.

Lincoln, Y. S., & Guba, E. G. (2000). Paradigmatic controversies, contradictions, and emerging confluences. In N. K. Denzin & Y. S. Lincoln (Eds.), *Handbook of qualitative research* (2nd ed., pp. 163–188). Thousand Oaks, CA: Sage.

Lingen, A., Brouwers, R., Nugieren, M., Plantenga, D., & Zuidberg, L. (1997). *Gender assessment studies: A manual for gender consultants*. The Hague: Netherlands Development Assistance, Ministry of Foreign Affairs.

Little Bear, L. (2000). Jagged worldviews colliding. In M. Battiste (Ed.), *Reclaiming indigenous voice and vision* (pp. 77–85). Vancouver: University of British Columbia Press.

Longwe, S. H. (1991). Gender awareness: The missing element in the Third World development project. In T. Wallace & C. March (Eds.), *Changing perceptions: Writings on gender and development* (pp. 151–153). Oxford, UK: Oxfam.

Losen, D. J., & Orfield, G. (Eds.). (2002). *Racial inequity in special education*. Boston: Harvard Education Press.

Ludema, J. D., Cooperrider, D. L., & Barrett, F. J. (2006). Appreciative inquiry: The power of the unconditional positive question. In P. Reason & H. Bradbury (Eds.), *Handbook of action research* (pp. 155–165). London: Sage. (Original work published 2001)

Lyotard, J.-F. (1984). *The postmodern condition: A report on knowledge* (G. Bennington & B. Massumi, Trans.). Manchester, UK: Manchester University Press.

Madison, A. M. (Ed.). (1992). *Minority issues in program evaluation*. San Francisco: Jossey-Bass.

Madison, D. S. (2005). *Critical ethnography*. Thousand Oaks, CA: Sage.

Maguire, P. (2006). Uneven ground: Feminisms and action research. In P. Reason & H. Bradbury (Eds.), *Handbook of action research* (pp. 60–70). London: Sage. (Original work published 2001)

March, C., Smyth, I., & Mukhopadhyay, M. (1999). *A guide to gender-analysis frameworks*. Oxford, UK: Oxfam.

Mark, M. M., & Gamble, C. (2009). Experiments, quasi-experiments and ethics. In D. M. Mertens & P. Ginsberg (Eds.), *Handbook of social research ethics* (pp. 198–213). Thousand Oaks, CA: Sage.

Mark, M. M., Greene, J. C., & Shaw, I. F. (2006). The evaluation of policies, programs, and practices. In I. F. Shaw, J. C. Greene, & M. M. Mark (Eds.), *The Sage handbook of evaluation* (pp. 1–30). Thousand Oaks, CA: Sage.

Marshall, J. (2006). Self-reflective inquiry practices. In P. Reason & H. Bradbury (Eds.), *Handbook of action research* (pp. 335–342). London: Sage. (Original work published 2001)

Martinelli, M. (2004). *Overcoming the roadblocks to partnership*. Retrieved May 9, 2008, from *www.uml.edu/centers/CFWC/Community_Tips/Research%20 Ethics/Research%20Ethics%20Tipsheets.pdf*.

Mathison, S. (2008). What is the difference between evaluation and research—and why do we care? In N. L. Smith & P. R. Brandon (Eds.), *Fundamental issues in evaluation* (pp. 183–196). New York: Guilford Press.

McCaskill, C. (2005). *Critical race theory and black deaf Americans at the time of school desegregation*. Doctoral dissertation, Gallaudet University, Washington, DC.

McCreanor, T., & Nairn, R. (2002). Tauiwi general practitioners' explanations of Maori health: Colonial relations in primary healthcare in Aotearoa/New Zealand. *Journal of Health Psychology, 7*(5), 509–518.

McCreanor, T., Tipene-Leach, D., & Abel, S. (2004). The SIDS careworkers study: Perceptions of Maori SIDS families. *New Zealand Journal of Social Policy, 23*, 154–166.

McCreanor, T., Watson, P., & Denny, S. (2006). "Just accept us how we are more": Experiences of young Pakeha with their families in Aotearoa New Zealand. *Social Policy Journal of New Zealand, 27*, 156–170.

McIntosh, T. (2004). *Theorising marginality and the processes of marginalization*. Unpublished manuscript.

McKenzie, J. (2001, June). Maori children with special abilities: Taking a broader perspective. *New Zealand Principals' Federation Magazine*, p. 1. Retrieved February 11, 2008, from *www.nzpf.ac.nz/resources/papers.htm*.

Meadow-Orlans, K., Mertens, D. M., & Sass-Lehrer, M. (2003). *Parents and their deaf children: The early years*. Washington, DC: Gallaudet University.

Mertens, D. M. (1994). Training evaluators: Unique skills and knowledge. In J. Altschuld & M. Engle (Eds.), *The preparation of professional evaluators: Issues, perspectives, and current status* (pp. 17–28). San Francisco: Jossey-Bass.

Mertens, D. M. (1996). Breaking the silence about sexual abuse of deaf youth. *American Annals of the Deaf, 141*(5), 352–358.

Mertens, D. M. (1998). *Research and evaluation in education and psychology: Integrating diversity with quantitative and qualitative approaches.* Thousand Oaks, CA: Sage.

Mertens, D. M. (2000). Deaf and hard of hearing people in court: Using an emancipatory perspective to determine their needs. In C. Truman, D. M. Mertens, & B. Humphries (Eds.), *Research and inequality* (pp. 111–125). London: Taylor & Francis.

Mertens, D. M. (2003). Mixed methods and the politics of human research: The transformative-emancipatory perspective. In A. Tashakkori & C. Teddlie (Eds.), *Handbook of mixed methods in social and behavioral research* (pp. 135–164). Thousand Oaks, CA: Sage.

Mertens, D. M. (2005). *Research and evaluation in education and psychology: Integrating diversity with quantitative, qualitative and mixed methods* (2nd ed.). Thousand Oaks, CA: Sage.

Mertens, D. M. (2007). Transformative paradigm: Mixed methods and social justice. *Journal of Mixed Methods Research, 1*(3), 212–225.

Mertens, D. M. (2008). Representation of stakeholders in culturally complex communities. In N. Smith & P. Brandon (Eds.), *Fundamental issues in evaluation* (pp. 41–60). New York: Guilford Press.

Mertens, D. M., Fraser, J., & Heimlich, J. E. (2008). M or F?: Gender, identity and the transformative research paradigm. *Museums and Social Issues, 3*(1), 81–92.

Mertens, D. M., & Ginsberg, P. (Eds.). (2009). *Handbook of social research ethics* (pp. 580–613). Thousand Oaks, CA: Sage.

Mertens, D. M., Holmes, H., & Harris, R. (2009). Transformative research and ethics. In D. M. Mertens & P. Ginsberg (Eds.), *Handbook of social research ethics* (pp. 85–102). Thousand Oaks, CA: Sage.

Mertens, D. M., & Hopson, R. (2006). Advancing evaluation of science, technology, engineering, and mathematics efforts through attention to diversity and culture. In D. Huffman & F. Lawrenz (Eds.), *New directions in evaluation* (pp. 35–52). San Francisco: Jossey-Bass.

Mertens, D. M., & McLaughlin, J. (2004). *Research and evaluation methods in special education.* Thousand Oaks, CA: Corwin Press.

Mertens, D. M., Wilson, A., & Mounty, J. (2007). Gender equity for people with disabilities. In S. Klein et al. (Eds.), *Handbook for achieving gender equity through education* (pp. 583–604). Mahwah, NJ: Erlbaum.

Messick, S. (1995). Validity of psychological assessment. *American Psychologist, 50,* 741–749.

Mienczakowski, J. (2000). People like us: Ethnography in the form of theatre with emancipatory intentions. In C. Truman, D. M. Mertens, & B. Humphries (Eds.), *Research and inequality* (pp. 126–142). London: Taylor & Francis.

Mienczakowski, J., & Morgan, S. (2006). Ethnodrama: Constructing participatory, experiential and compelling action research through performance. In P.

Reason & H. Bradbury (Eds.), *Handbook of action research* (pp. 176–184). London: Sage. (Original work published 2001)

Mikkelsen, B. (2005). *Methods for development work and research* (2nd ed.). Thousand Oaks, CA: Sage.

Miskovic, M., & Hoop, K. (2006). Action research meets critical pedagogy. *Qualitative Inquiry, 12*(2), 269–291.

Mitchell, R. G., Jr., & Charmaz, K. (1996). Telling tales, writing stories. *Journal of Contemporary Ethnography, 25*, 144–166.

Molecular Expressions. (2007). *Science optics and you.* Retrieved August 23, 2007, from *micro.magnet.fsu.edu/primer/java/scienceopticsu/refraction/index.html.*

Moran, D. (2000). *Introduction to phenomenology.* London: Routledge.

Morse, J. (2006). The politics of evidence. *Qualitative Health Research, 16*(3), 415–422.

Morsillo, J., & Fisher, A. (2007). Appreciative inquiry with youth to create meaningful community projects. *Australian Community Psychologist, 19*(1), 47–61.

Moser, C. (1993). *Gender planning and development: Theory, practice and training.* Routledge: London.

Moses, R. P., & Cobb, C. E. (2001). *Radical equations: Math literacy and civil rights.* Boston: Beacon Press.

Moses, R. P., Kamii, M., Swap, S. M., & Howard, J. (1989). The algebra project: Organizing in the spirit of Ella. *Harvard Educational Review, 59*(4), 423–443.

Mukhopadhyay, M. (2004). Mainstreaming gender or "streaming away": Feminists marooned in the development business. In A. Cornwall, E. Harrison, & A. Whitehead (Eds.), *Repositioning feminisms in gender and development* (pp. 4–8). Brighton, Sussex, UK: University of Sussex Press.

Muthén, B. O. (1991). Multilevel factor analysis of class and student achievement components. *Journal of Educational Measurement, 28*, 338–354.

Muthén, B. O. (1994). Multilevel covariance structure analysis. *Sociological Methods and Research, 22*(3), 399–420.

Myers, C. (2004). Differences from somewhere: The normativity of whiteness in bioethics in the United States. *The American Journal of Bioethics, 3*, 1–11.

Myers v. the Board of Education of San Juan County. (1995). 905 F.Supp. 154 (D. Utah 1995).

Nairn, R., & McCreanor, T. (1991). Race talk and common sense: Patterns in Pakeha discourse on Maori/Pakeha relations in New Zealand. *Journal of Language and Social Psychology, 10*(4), 245–262.

National Commission for the Protection of Human Subjects of Biomedical and Behavioral Research. (1979). *The Belmont Report: Ethical principles and guidelines for the protection of human subjects of research* (DHEW Publication No. OS 78-0012). Washington, DC: Government Printing Office.

National Education Association. (2003). *Letter to Rod Paige, U.S. Department of Education, Secretary.* Available at *www.eval.org/doe.nearesponse.pdf.*

National Institutes of Health. *Certificates of confidentiality kiosk.* Retrieved January 21, 2008, from *www.grants.nih.gov/grants/policy/coc.*

National Institutes of Health, Office of Behavioral and Social Science Research. (1999). *Qualitative methods in health research.* Washington, DC: Author. Retrieved January 17, 2008, from *obssr.od.nih.gov/.*

Newman, C. (2001). *Gender, time use, and change: Impacts of agricultural export employment in Ecuador.* Policy research report on gender and development, Working Paper Series No. 18. Poverty Reduction and Economic Management Network/Development Research Group, The World Bank. Available at *www. worldbank.org/gender/prr.*

Nichols, L. A., & Keltner, B. (2005). Indian family adjustment to children with disabilities. *Journal of the National Center: American Indian and Alaska Native Mental Health Research, 12*(1), 22–38.

Niglas, K. (2004). *The combined use of qualitative and quantitative methods in educational research.* Doctoral dissertation, Educational Sciences of the Tallinn Pedagogical University, Tallin, Estonia.

O'Connor, C., & Fernandez, S. D. (2006). Race, class, and disproportionality: Reevaluating the relationship between poverty and special education placement. *Educational Researcher, 35*(6), 6–11.

Okie, S. (2000, November 24). Health officials debate ethics of placebo use. *The Washington Post,* p. A3.

Open University. (2007). *Systems thinking and practice: Diagramming.* Retrieved June 30, 2007, from *systems.open.ac.uk/materials/t552/index.htm.*

Opfer, V. D. (2006). Evaluating equity: A framework for understanding action and inaction on social justice issues. *Educational Policy, 20*(1), 271–290.

Ormond, A., Cram, F., & Carter, L. (2004). *Researching our relations: Reflections on ethics and marginalization—protocols for research with vulnerable and marginalised Mäori'.* Unpublished manuscript, University of Auckland, New Zealand.

Overholt, C. A., Anderson, M. B., Austin, K., & Cloud, J. E. (1985). *Gender roles in development projects* (2nd ed.). West Hartford, CT: Reinner.

Painter, N. I. (2003, November). *Why are white people called Caucasian?* Paper presented at the fifth annual Gilder Lehrman Center International Conference, Yale University, New Haven, CT.

Parker, A. R. (1993). *Another point of view: A manual on gender analysis training for grassroots workers.* New York: UNIFEM. Available at *www.womenink. org.*

Parker, L., & Lynn, M. (2002). What's race got to do with it?: Critical race theory's conflicts with and connections to qualitative research methodology and epistemology. *Qualitative Inquiry, 8*(1), 7–22.

Parsons, B. A., Hammond-Hanson, Z., & Bosserman, C. (1998). *Partnerships: A powerful tool for improving the well-being of families and neighborhoods.* Battle Creek, MI: W. K. K. Kellogg Foundation.

Patton, M. Q. (2002). *Utilization focused evaluation.* Thousand Oaks, CA: Sage.

Pharmer, K. (2004). "Science shops" in Lowell? Retrieved May 9, 2008, from *www.uml.edu/centers/CFWC/Community_Tips/Research%20Ethics/ Research%20Ethics%20Tipsheets.pdf.*

Pink, S. (2007). *Doing visual ethnography* (2nd ed.). Thousand Oaks, CA: Sage.

372 References

Plummer, K. (2005). Critical humanism and queer theory. In N. K. Denzin & Y. S. Lincoln (Eds.), *The Sage handbook of qualitative research* (3rd ed., pp. 357–373). Thousand Oaks, CA: Sage.

Pomare, E., Keefe-Ormsby, C., Pearce, H., Reid, P., Robson, B., & Watene-Hayden, N. (1995). *Hauora: Maori standards of health* (3rd ed.). Wellington, New Zealand: Te Ropu Rangahau Hauora a Eru Pomare.

Raghavan, S., & Paley, A. R. (2005, August 8). Montgomery long ignored gang, some say stabbings called result of lax prevention effort. *Washington Post*, p. A01.

Ramazanoglu, C., & Holland, J. (2002). *Feminist methodology*. Thousand Oaks, CA: Sage.

Ramos, M. C. (1989). Some ethical implications of qualitative research. *Research in Nursing and Health, 12,* 57–63.

Reason, P., & Bradbury, H. (Eds.). (2006a). *Handbook of action research*. London: Sage.

Reason, P., & Bradbury, H. (2006b). Introduction: Inquiry and participation in search of a world worthy of human aspiration. In P. Reason & H. Bradbury (Eds.), *Handbook of action research* (pp. 1–14). London: Sage.

Reddy, S. (2005, August 13). State is given some control of city schools. *Baltimore Sun*. Available at *www.baltimoresun.com/news/education/bal-te.md.special13aug13,1,7596697.story?coll=bal-education-k12.*

Reina, D., & Reina, M. (2006). *Trust and betrayal in the workplace* (2nd ed.). San Francisco: Berrett-Koehler.

Reynolds, M. (2006). Evaluation based on critical systems heuristics. In B. Williams & I. Imam (Eds.), *Using systems concepts in evaluation: An expert anthology* (pp. 101–122). Point Reyes, CA: EdgePress.

Richardson, L., & St. Pierre, E. A. (2005). Writing: A method of inquiry. In N. K. Denzin & Y. S. Lincoln (Eds.), *The Sage handbook of qualitative research* (3rd ed., pp. 959–978). Thousand Oaks, CA: Sage.

Rietbergen-McCraken, J., & Narayan-Parker, D. (1998). *Participation and social assessment: Tools and techniques*. Washington, DC: World Bank.

Ros, D., & Craig, Y. (1997). Participation begins at home. *Gender and Development, 5*(3), 35–44.

Rose, G. (2007). *Visual methodologies* (2nd ed.). Thousand Oaks, CA: Sage.

Rose, L. W. (2006). *Middle Start schools striving for excellence*. New York: Academy for Educational Development. Retrieved August 14, 2007, from *www.middlestart.org/resources/Striving_for_Excellence.pdf.*

Roulston, K., deMarrais, K., & Lewis, J. B. (2003). Learning to interview in the social sciences. *Qualitative Inquiry, 9*(4), 643–668.

Rousso, H., & Wehmeyer, M. L. (2001). *Double jeopardy*. Albany: State University of New York.

Ruddin, L. P. (2006). You can generalize stupid!: Social scientists, Bent Fylvbjerg, and case study metholodogy. *Qualitative Inquiry, 12*(4), 797–812.

Ryan, W. (2004). *Grant making with a gender lens*. New York: GrantCraft, Ford Foundation. Retrieved February 11, 2008, from *www.grantcraft.org.*

Sadie, Y., & Loots, E. (1998). RDP projects in South Africa: A gender perspective analysis. *Security, Development and Gender in Africa*, Monograph No.

27. Retrieved September 15, 2006, from *www.iss.org.za/pubs/Monographs/No27/rdp.html.*

Savedoff, W. D., Levine, R., & Birdsall, N. (2006). *When will we ever learn?* Washington, DC: Center for Global Development.

Saylor, B., Apaza, J., & Austin, M. (2005, September). *Using data to "make a case" for mathematics reform within a K–12 district.* Paper presented at the National Science Foundation Evaluation Summit, Minneapolis.

Schalet, A., Hunt, G., & Joe-Laidler, K. (2003). Respectability and automony. *Journal of Contemporary Ethnography, 32*(1), 108–143.

Scheurich, J., & Young, M. (1997). Coloring epistemologies: Are our research epistemologies racially biased? *Educational researcher, 26*(4), 4–16.

Scheurich, J., & Young, M. (1998). Rejoinder: In the United States of America, in both our souls and our sciences, we are avoiding white racism. *Educational Researcher, 27*(9), 27–32.

Schutz, A. (1970). *On phenomenology and social relations.* Chicago: University of Chicago Press.

Scriven, M. (1967). The methodology of evaluation. In M. E. Gredler (Ed.), *Program evaluation* (p. 16). Englewood Cliffs, NJ: Prentice-Hall.

Seelman, K. D. (1999). *Testimony to the Commission on Advancement of Women and Minorities in Science, Engineering, and Technology.* Washington, DC: National Institute on Disability and Rehabilitation Research.

Seelman, K. D. (2000). *The new paradigm on disability: Research issues and approaches.* Washington, DC: National Institute for Disability and Rehabilitative Research.

Segone, M. (Ed.). (2006). *New trends in development evaluation.* Geneva: UNICEF Regional Office for CEE/CIS and IPEN, Issue #5. Available at *www.unicef.org/ceecis/resources_1220.html.*

Seidel, J. (1998). *The ethnographic interview.* New York: Holt, Rinehart & Winston.

Selener, D. (1997). *Participatory action research and social change.* Ithaca, NY: Cornell University Press.

Seligman, M. E., Steen, T. A., Park, N., & Peterson, C. (2005). Positive psychology progress. *American Psychologist, 60*(5), 410–421.

Seligman, M. E. P. (2006). Breaking the 65 percent barrier. In M. Csikszentmihalyi & I. S. Csikszentmihalyi (Eds.), *A life worth living: Contributions to positive psychology* (pp. 230–236). New York: Oxford University Press.

Sen, A. (1999). *Development as freedom.* New York: Anchor Books.

SenGupta, S., Hopson, R., & Thompson-Robinson, M. (Eds.). (2004). *In search of cultural competence in evaluation: Toward principles and practices.* San Francisco: Jossey-Bass.

Serait, G. M. (2004). *Partnership-based research: How the community balances power within a research partnership.* Retrieved May 9, 2008, from *www.uml.edu/centers/CFWC/Community_Tips/Research%20Ethics/Research%20Ethics%20Tipsheets.pdf.*

Sherman, C. (2004).Yahoo!: Birth of a new machine. *SearchEngineWatch,* February 18. Retrieved December 13, 2006, from *searchenginewatch.com/showPage.html?page=3314171.*

Siddle Walker, V. (2003). The architects of black schooling in the segregated South: The case of one principal leader. *Journal of Curriculum and Supervision, 19*(1), 54–72.

Sieber, J. (1992). *Planning ethically responsible research.* Newbury Park, CA: Sage.

Sielbeck-Bowen, K. A., Brisolara, S., Seigart, D., Tischler, C., & Whitmore, E. (2002). Exploring feminist evaluation: The ground from which we rise. In D. Seigart & S. Brisolara (Eds.), *Feminist evaluation: Explorations and experiences* (pp. 3–8). San Francisco: Jossey-Bass.

Silka, L. (2002). Immigrants, sustainability and emerging roles for universities. *Development, 45*(3), 119–123.

Silka, L. (2005, August). *Building culturally competent research partnerships.* Paper presented at the annual meeting of the American Psychological Association, Washington, DC.

Simons, H. (2006). Ethics in evaluation. In I. Shaw, J. Greene, & M. Mark (Eds.), *The Sage handbook of evaluation* (pp. 243–265). Thousand Oaks, CA: Sage.

Slavin, R. E. (1986). Best-evidence synthesis: An alternative to meta-analytic and traditional reviews. *Educational Researcher, 15*(9), 5–11.

Slavin, R. E., & Cheung, A. (2003). *Effective reading programs for English language learners: A best-evidence synthesis.* Baltimore, MD: Center for Research on the Education of Students Placed at Risk (CRESPAR), Johns Hopkins University. Available at *www.csos.jhu.edu.*

Smith, G. H. (1995). Whakaoho whānau. *He Pukenga Korero, 1*, 18–36.

Smith, L. T. (1999). *Decolonizing methodologies: Research and indigenous peoples.* London: Zed Books.

Smith, L. T. (2000). Kaupapa Maori research. In M. Battiste (Ed.), *Reclaiming indigenous voice and vision* (pp. 225–247). Vancouver: University of British Columbia.

Smith, L. T. (2004). *Researching in the margins: Issues for Maori researchers.* Unpublished manuscript.

Smith, L. T. (2005). On tricky ground: Researching the native in the age of uncertainty. In N. K. Denzin & Y. S. Lincoln (Eds.), *The Sage handbook of qualitative research* (3rd ed., pp. 85–108). Thousand Oaks, CA: Sage.

Smith-Maddox, R., & Solórzano, D. G. (2002). Using critical race theory, Paulo Freire's problem-posing method, and case study research to confront race and racism in education. *Qualitative Inquiry, 8*(1), 66–84.

Solórzano, D. G., & Yosso, T. J. (2001). Critical race and LatCrit theory and method: Counterstorytelling Chicana and Chicano graduate school experiences. *International Journal of Qualitative Studies in Education, 14*, 471–495.

Spivak, G. C. (1988). Can the subaltern speak? In C. Grossberg & N. L. Grossberg (Eds.), *Marxism and the interpretation of culture* (pp. 271–313). Urbana: University of Illinois Press.

Spry, T. (2007, July). *Performing autoethnography.* Paper presented at the Mixed Methods Conference, Homerton School of Health Sciences, Cambridge, United Kingdom.

Stake, R. E. (2005). Qualitative case studies. In Y. S. Lincoln & N. K. Denzin (Eds.), *The Sage handbook of qualitative research* (3rd ed., pp. 443–466). Thousand Oaks, CA: Sage.

Stanczak, G. C. (Ed.). (2007). *Visual research methods.* Thousand Oaks, CA: Sage.

Stein, G. (1922). Sacred Emily. In *Geography and plays* (pp. 178–188). Boston: Four Seas. (Original work published 1913)

Stufflebeam, D. L. (2001). Evaluation models. In G. Henry (Ed.), *New Directions for Evaluation, 89,* 7–105. San Francisco: Jossey-Bass.

Sue, D. W., & Sue, D. (2003). *Counseling the culturally diverse: Theory and practice* (4th ed.). New York: Wiley.

Sullivan, M. (2009). Philosophy, ethics and the disability community. In D. M. Mertens & P. G. Ginsberg (Eds.), *Handbook of social research ethics* (pp. 69–84). Thousand Oaks, CA: Sage.

Symonette, H. (2004). Walking pathways toward becoming a culturally competent evaluator: Boundaries, borderlands, and border crossings. In M. Thompson-Robinson, R. Hopson, & S. SenGupta (Eds.), *In search of cultural competence in evaluation* (pp. 95–110). San Francisco: Wiley.

Szarkowski, A. (2002). *Positive aspects of parenting a deaf child.* Doctoral dissertation, Gallaudet University, Washington, DC.

Tashakkori, A., & Teddlie, C. (Eds.). (2003). *Handbook of mixed methods in social and behavioral research.* Thousand Oaks, CA: Sage.

Thomas, V. G. (2004). Building a contextually responsive evaluation framework: Lessons from working with urban school interventions. In V. G. Thomas & F. I. Stevens (Eds.), *Co-constructing a contextually responsive evaluation framework* (pp. 3–24). San Francisco: Wiley.

Thompson, B. (1992, April). *The use of statistical tests in research: Some criticisms and alternatives.* Paper presented at the annual meeting of the American Educational Research Association, San Francisco.

Thompson, B. (2002). What future quantitative social science research could look like: Confidence intervals for effect size. *Educational Researcher, 31*(3), 25–32.

Thompson, S. J., Thurlow, M. L. L., Quenemoen, R. F., & Lehr, C. A. (2002). *Access to computer-based testing for students with disabilities.* Minneapolis: University of Minnesota, National Center on Educational Outcomes.

Tillman, L. C. (2006). Researching and writing from an African-American perspective: Reflective notes on three research studies. *International Journal of Qualitative Studies in Education, 19*(3), 265–287.

Tippens, D. J., Veal, W. R., & Wieseman, K. C. (1995). *An exploratory study of the role of proverbs in the construction of knowledge teaching and learning about science.* Paper presented at the annual meeting of the National Association for Research in Science Teaching, San Francisco.

Todorov, T. (1995). *The morals of history.* Minneapolis: University of Minnesota Press.

Towns, D. P., & Serpell, Z. (2004). Successes and challenges in triangulating methodologies in evaluations of exemplary urban schools. In V. G. Thomas & F. I. Stevens (Eds.), *Co-constructing a contextually responsive evaluation framework* (pp. 49–62). San Francisco: Wiley.

Trochim, W. M. (2006). *The research methods knowledge base* (2nd ed.). Ithaca, NY: Author. Retrieved February 11, 2008, from *www.socialresearchmethods. net/kb/index.php*.

Trochim, W. M., Milstein, B., Wood, B., Jackson, S., & Pressler, V. (2004). Setting objectives for community and systems change: An application of concept mapping for planning a statewide health improvement initiative. *Health Promotion Practice, 5*(1), 8–19.

Trotter, A. (2003). A question of direction. *Editorial Projects in Education, 22*(35), 17–18, 20–21. Retrieved February 11, 2008, from *counts.edweek.org/sreports/tc03/article.cfm?slug=35adaptive.h22*.

TwoTrees, K. (1993). Mixed blood, new voices. In J. James & R. Farmer (Eds.), *Spirit, space, and survival: African American women in (white) academe* (pp. 13–22). New York: Routledge.

Ulrich, W. (2000). Reflective practice in the civil society: The contribution of critically systemic thinking. *Reflective Practice, 1*(2), 247–268.

United Nations. (1948). *Universal declaration of human rights.* Retrieved February 11, 2008, from *www.un.org/Overview/rights.html*.

United Nations. (1969). *The international convention on the elimination of all forms of racial discrimination.* New York: Author. Retrieved February 11, 2008, from *www.ohchr.org/english/law/pdf/cerd.pdf*.

United Nations. (1975). *The declaration on the rights of disabled persons.* Retrieved February 11, 2008, from *www.ohchr.org/english/law/res3447.htm*.

United Nations. (1979). *The convention on the elimination of all forms of discrimination against women (CEDAW).* Retrieved February 11, 2008, from *www.un.org/womenwatch/daw/cedaw/text/econvention.htm*.

United Nations. (1990a). *Convention on the rights of the child.* Retrieved February 11, 2008, from *www.ohchr.org/english/law/pdf/crc.pdf*.

United Nations. (1990b). *International convention on the protection of the rights of all migrant workers and members of their families.* Retrieved February 11, 2008, from *www.un.org/millennium/law/iv-13.htm*.

United Nations. (2003–2004). *The United Nations and disabled persons: The first fifty years.* Retrieved June 19, 2007, from *www.un.org/esa/socdev/enable/dis50y00.htm*.

United Nations. (2006a). *Report to the General Assembly on the first session of the Human Rights Council.* Retrieved February 11, 2008, from *daccessdds.un.org/doc/UNDOC/LTD/G06/128/65/PDF/G0612865.pdf?OpenElement*.

United Nations. (2006b). *Declaration of ad hoc committee on a comprehensive and integral international convention on the protection and promotion of the rights and dignity of persons with disabilities.* Retrieved May 10, 2008, from *www.un.org/disabilities*.

United Nations. (2006c). *Declaration of rights of indigenous peoples.* Retrieved March 21, 2007 from *http://www.un.org/esa/socdev/unpfii/en/declaration. html*

U.S. Census Bureau. (2001). *Census 2000 shows America's diversity*. Washington, DC: Author.

U.S. Department of Education. (2002). *Twenty-fourth annual report to Congress on the implementation of the Individuals with Disabilities Education Act*. Retrieved June 17, 2005, from *www.ed.gov/about/reports/annual/osep/2002/index.html*.

U.S. Department of Education. (2004). *The facts about . . . investing in what works*. Retrieved October 25, 2004, from *www.ed.gov/nclb/methods/whatworks/whatworks.html*.

U.S. Department of Education. (2006a). Early Reading First Program. Office of Elementary and Secondary Education, Early Reading First Program. Retrieved May 10, 2008, from *www.ed.gov/programs/earlyreading*.

U.S. Department of Education. (2006b). Office of Elementary and Secondary Education, Oveview information. Retrieved May 10, 2008, from *www.ed.gov*.

U.S. Department of Education. (2008). *Reading First impact study: Interim report*. Washington DC: Author. Retrieved May 8, 2008, from *ies.ed.gov/ncee/pdf/20084016.pdf*.

Valdes, F. (1998). Under contruction: LatCrit consciousness, community and theory. *La Raza Law Journal, 10*, 3–56.

Varadharajan, A. (2000) *Reclaiming indigenous voice and vision*. Vancouver: University of British Columbia Press.

Villenas, S., Deyhle, D., & Parker, L. (1999). Critical race theory and praxis: Chicano(a)/Latino(a) and Navajo struggles for dignity, educational equity and social justice. In L. Parker, D. Deyhle, & S. Villenas (Eds.), *Race is . . . race isn't: Critical race theory and qualitative studies in education* (pp. 31–52). Boulder, CO: Westview.

Watts, J. (2006). "The outsider within": Dilemmas of qualitative feminist research within a culture of resistance. *Qualitative Research, 6*(3), 385–402.

Weis, L., & Fine, M. (2004). Introduction to compositional studies in four parts: Critical theorizing and analysis on social (in)justice. In L. Weis & M. Fine (Eds.), *Working method: Research and social justice* (pp. xv–xxiv). New York: Routledge.

Wenglinsky, H. (2002). How schools matter: The link between teacher classroom practices and student academic performance. *Education Policy Analysis Archives, 10*(12). Retrieved December 14, 2006, from *epaa.asu.edu/epaa/v10n12/*.

West, M. W., & Davis, F. E. (2005). *Research related to the Algebra Project's intervention to improve student learning in mathematics*. Technical report prepared for the State of Virginia Department of Education, Richmond, VA.

Whitmore, E., Gujit, I., Mertens, D. M., Imm, P. S., Chinman, M., & Wandersman, A. (2006). Embedding improvements, lived experience, and social justice in evaluation practice. In I. Shaw, J. Greene, & M. Mark (Eds.), *The Sage handbook of evaluation* (pp. 340–359). Thousand Oaks, CA: Sage.

Williamson, C. (2007). *Black deaf students: A model for educational success*. Washington, DC: Gallaudet University Press.

Wilson, A. (2005). The effectiveness of international development assistance from American organizations to deaf communities in Jamaica. *American Annals of the Deaf, 150*(3), 202–304.

Witkin, B. R., & Altschuld, J. W. (1995). *Planning and conducting needs assessment*. Thousand Oaks, CA: Sage.

World Health Organization. (2007). *Is it all about sex?* Copenhagen, Denmark: WHO Regional Office for Europe. Retrieved January 21, 2008, from *www.euro.who.int/document/ens/en66.pdf.*

Wright, H. K. (2003). An endarkened feminist epistemology?: Identity, difference and the politics of representation in educational research. *Qualitative Studies in Education, 16*(2), 197–214.

Yazzie, R. (2000). Indigenous peoples and postcolonial conolialism. In M. Battiste (Ed.), *Reclaiming indigenous voice and vision* (pp. 39–49). Vancouver: University of British Columbia Press.

Yin, R. (2003). *Case study research: Design and methods* (3rd ed.). Thousand Oaks, CA: Sage.

Author Index

Subject Index

About the Author

Donna M. Mertens, PhD, is Professor in the Department of Educational Foundations and Research at Gallaudet University, where she teaches advanced research methods and program evaluation to deaf and hearing students. She received the Distinguished Faculty Award from Gallaudet in 2007. The primary focus of her work is transformative mixed-methods inquiry in diverse communities that prioritizes ethical implications of research in pursuit of social justice. A past president of the American Evaluation Association (AEA), Dr. Mertens provided leadership in the development of the International Organization for Cooperation in Evaluation and the establishment of the AEA Diversity Internship Program with Duquesne University. She received AEA's highest honor for service to the organization and the field. Her recent books include *The Handbook of Social Research Ethics*; *Research and Evaluation in Education and Psychology: Integrating Diversity with Quantitative, Qualitative, and Mixed Methods*; *Research and Evaluation Methods in Special Education*; and *Parents and Their Deaf Children: The Early Years*. She is widely published in the *Journal of Mixed Methods Research*, *American Journal of Evaluation*, *American Annals of the Deaf*, and *Educational Evaluation and Policy Analysis*. Dr. Mertens conducts and consults on evaluations as well as leads professional development activities on research and evaluation in many national and international settings. Examples include the United Nations Development Fund for

Women (UNIFEM) initiative to address the Millennium Goals for women in Africa; cultural exchange programs for deaf students between Costa Rica and Gallaudet University; mixed-methods researchers at Fitzwilliam College of Health Sciences, Cambridge University; technology to improve teacher preparation; breast cancer screening project for indigenous peoples in Newfoundland; early intervention programs for deaf children of Jewish and Bedouin families in Israel; and education for deaf, blind, and mentally challenged students in Egypt.